HANDBOOK OF
PSYCHODERMATOLOGY

HANDBOOK OF PSYCHODERMATOLOGY

Second Edition

Editor-in-Chief

Abdul Latheef EN MD DVD FRCP(Glasgow) FIMSA MSc(Psychology)
Professor and Head
Department of Dermatology and Venereology
Government Medical College Kozhikode
Kerala, India

Assistant Editor

Smitha Prabhu S MD(DVL) FRCP(Edinburgh)
Additional Professor
Department of Dermatology and Venereology
Kasturba Medical College Manipal
Manipal Academy of Higher Education Manipal
Karnataka, India

Chief Advisor

Shrutakirthi D Shenoi MD
Professor and Head
Department of Dermatology
Kanachur Institute of Medical Sciences
Mangaluru, Karnataka, India

Forewords

Mohammad Jafferany	Chandani Udagedara
Vijay Zawar	Saraswoti Neupane
Om Prakash Singh	Mohammad Mahmudur Rahman

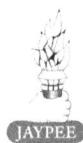

JAYPEE BROTHERS MEDICAL PUBLISHERS
The Health Sciences Publisher
New Delhi | London

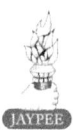 **Jaypee Brothers Medical Publishers (P) Ltd**

Headquarters
EMCA House
23/23-B, Ansari Road, Daryaganj
New Delhi 110 002, India
Landline: +91-11-23272143, +91-11-23272703
+91-11-23282021, +91-11-23245672
E-mail: jaypee@jaypeebrothers.com

Corporate Office
Jaypee Brothers Medical Publishers (P) Ltd.
4838/24, Ansari Road, Daryaganj
New Delhi 110 002, India
Phone: +91-11-43574357
Fax: +91-11-43574314
E-mail: jaypee@jaypeebrothers.com

Overseas Office
JP Medical Ltd.
83, Victoria Street, London
SW1H 0HW (UK)
Phone: +44-20 3170 8910
Fax: +44(0)20 3008 6180
E-mail: info@jpmedpub.com

Website: www.jaypeebrothers.com
Website: www.jaypeedigital.com

© 2024, Jaypee Brothers Medical Publishers

The views and opinions expressed in this book are solely those of the original contributor(s)/author(s) and do not necessarily represent those of editor(s) or publisher of the book.

All rights reserved. No part of this publication may be reproduced, stored or transmitted in any form or by any means, electronic, mechanical, photocopying, recording or otherwise, without the prior permission in writing of the publishers.

All brand names and product names used in this book are trade names, service marks, trademarks or registered trademarks of their respective owners. The publisher is not associated with any product or vendor mentioned in this book.

Medical knowledge and practice change constantly. This book is designed to provide accurate, authoritative information about the subject matter in question. However, readers are advised to check the most current information available on procedures included and check information from the manufacturer of each product to be administered, to verify the recommended dose, formula, method and duration of administration, adverse effects and contraindications. It is the responsibility of the practitioner to take all appropriate safety precautions. Neither the publisher nor the author(s)/editor(s) assume any liability for any injury and/or damage to persons or property arising from or related to use of material in this book.

This book is sold on the understanding that the publisher is not engaged in providing professional medical services. If such advice or services are required, the services of a competent medical professional should be sought.

Every effort has been made where necessary to contact holders of copyright to obtain permission to reproduce copyright material. If any have been inadvertently overlooked, the publisher will be pleased to make the necessary arrangements at the first opportunity.

Inquiries for bulk sales may be solicited at: jaypee@jaypeebrothers.com

Handbook of Psychodermatology / Abdul Latheef EN

First Edition: 2016
Second Edition: **2024**
ISBN: 978-93-5696-457-0

Contributors

Abdul Latheef EN MD DVD
FRCP(Glasgow) FIMSA MSc(Psychology)
Professor and Head
Department of Dermatology and Venereology
Government Medical College
Kozhikode
Kerala, India
drlatheef90@gmail.com

Abhineetha Hosthota MBBS MD
Professor and Head
Department of Dermatology
The Oxford Medical College Hospital and Research Center
Bengaluru, Karnataka, India
abhineethahosthota@yahoo.com

Archana AG MBBS MD DNB
Specialist Dermatologist
Department of Dermatology, Venereology and Leprosy
Skinsecrets
Kochi, Kerala, India
archanaaggn@gmail.com

Bishurul Hafi NA MD(DVL) DNB
FECSM LDPRT
Consultant Dermatologist
Revive Skin Clinic
Kozhikode, Kerala, India
bishuru@gmail.com

Eepsita Mishra MBBS MD
Senior Resident
Department of Psychiatry
Postgraduate Institute of Medical Education and Research (PGIMER)
Chandigarh, India
dr.eepsitamishra@gmail.com

Harish M Tharayil MD DPM MBA
Professor and Head
Department of Psychiatry
Government Medical College,
Kozhikode
Kerala, India
drharishmt@gmail.com

Isabella Tan MD(Trainee)
Medical Student
Department of Dermatology
Robert Wood Johnson Medical School, Rutgers University
New Brunswick, New Jersey, USA
ijt11@rwjms.rutgers.edu

Julaila Thasneem MA(Psychology) PGDRP
Developmental Psychologist
Department of Developmental Pediatrics
Christian Medical College
Vellore, Tamil Nadu, India
julailathas@gmail.com

Contributors

Madhulika Mhatre MD FRUGHS
Consultant Dermatologist
Wockhardt Hospitals
Mumbai, Maharashtra, India
dr.madhulika@hotmail.com

Manjot Marwah Sharma MD
Dermatologist and Hair Transplant Surgeon
National Hair Clinic
Hamirpur, Himachal Pradesh, India
drmanjotmarwah@hotmail.com

Mahesh MM MPhil(Clinical Psychology) PhD(Psychology)
Assistant Professor in Psychology
Research and Post Graduate Department of Psychology
Sri C Achutha Menon Government College
Thrissur, Kerala, India
drmaheshmkarun@gmail.com

Meghashree G MD
Assistant Professor
Department of Dermatology
Kanachur Institute of Medical Sciences
Mangaluru, Karnataka, India
megha91leo@gmail.com

Minu Ulpurath MBBS MD
Senior Resident
Department of Dermatology
Government Medical College Kozhikode
Kozhikode, Kerala, India
minuup2010@gmail.com

Mohammad Jafferany MD FAPA MCPS(Dermatology)
Professor of Psychodermatology, Psychiatry and Behavioral Sciences
Central Michigan University College of Medicine/CMU MedicalEducation Partners
Past President, Association for Psychocutaneous Medicine of North America
President, World Psychodermatology Day
President and Chair, Scientific and Organizing Committee32nd Annual APMNA Meeting, March 7 2024, San Diego, California, USA

Rakesh Bharti MD
Consultant, Department of Dermatology, Venereology and Leprology, Bharti Derma Care and Research Center
Amritsar, Punjab, India
rakeshbharti1@gmail.com

Ravindra Neelakanthappa Munoli MD(Psychiatry)
Additional Professor
Department of Psychiatry
Dr NR Acharya Memorial Hospital
Udupi, Karnataka, India
ravindra.nm@manipal.edu

Satnam Singh Palia MBBS FRCPSYCH DPM
Consultant Psychiatrist (Retired)
Mental Health Review Tribunal City, UK
sspalia@hotmail.com

Contributors

Savitha Soman MBBS MD(Psychiatry)
Additional Professor
Department of Psychiatry
Kasturba Medical College, Manipal
Manipal, Karnataka, India
savithasoman@yahoo.com

Shikha Shah MD DNB
Senior Resident
Department of Dermatology,
Venereology and Leprology
Postgraduate Institute of Medical
Education and Research (PGIMER)
Chandigarh, India
srs4894@gmail.com

Shrutakirthi D Shenoi MD
Professor and Head
Department of Dermatology
Kanachur Institute of Medical
Sciences
Mangaluru, Karnataka, India
dr.shrutakirthi@kanachur.edu.in

Shubh Mohan Singh MD
Professor
Department of Psychiatry
Postgraduate Institute of Medical
Education and Research (PGIMER)
Chandigarh, India
shubhmohan@gmail.com

Shweta Rai Mphil(Clinical Psychology) PhD
Additional Professor
Department of Clinical Psychology
Manipal College of Health
Professions (MCHP)
Manipal Academy of Higher
Education (MAHE)
Manipal, Karnataka, India
shwetaraisrcp@gmail.com

Smitha Prabhu S MD(DVL)
FRCP(Edinburgh)
Additional Professor
Department of Dermatology and
Venereology
Kasturba Medical College Manipal
Manipal Academy of Higher
Education
Manipal, Karnataka, India
drsmithaprabhu@yahoo.com

Sreejayan Kongasseri
MD(Psychiatry) FRANZCP
Consultant Psychiatrist
Department of Psychiatry
Northern Health, Melbourne,
Australia
Sreejayan.k@gmail.com

Sreekanth Sukumarakurup MBBS MD
Professor
Department of Dermatology
Government TD Medical College
Alappuzha
Vandanam, Kerala, India
drsreekanths@gmail.com

Sudipta Roy MPhil(Medical
and Social Psychology, NIMHANS)
PhD(MS University of Baroda)
Clinical Psychologist
Senior RCI Licensed Clinical
Psychologist
Director – Psy Lens, Surat
Supervisor - PPSUm of Psychology
Surat, Gujarat, India
psylensroy@gmail.com

Contributors

Swapna Bondade MBBS MD
Professor and Head
Department of Psychiatry
The Oxford Medical College
Hospital and Research Center
Anekal, Karnataka, India
swapna199@yahoo.co.in

Tarun Narang MD FRCP(Edinburgh)
Additional Professor
Department of Dermatology,
Venereology and Leprology
Postgraduate Institute of Medical
Education and Research (PGIMER)
Chandigarh, India
narangtarun2012@gmail.com

Uvais NA MBBS DPM
Consultant Psychiatrist
Department of Psychiatry
Crescent House
Chelari, Kerala, India
druvaisna@gmail.com

Varsha Gowda VM MBBS MD DNB
Associate Consultant
Department of Dermatology
Dr Kishan's Skin Care and
Aesthetic Centre
Bengaluru, Karnataka, India
varshagowda94@gmail.com

Venkataram Mysore MD DNB
DipRCPath(London) FRCP(Glasgow)
FISHRS
Dermatologist,
Dermatopathologist and Hair
Transplant Surgeon
Director
Venkat Charmalaya – Centre for
Advanced Dermatology and
Postgraduate Training Centre
Bengaluru, Karnataka, India
mnvenkataram@gmail.com

Foreword

Psychodermatology is an evolving field. Studies have demonstrated that about 35–40% of skin diseases have an associated psychological component which plays a major role in the causation and perpetuation of skin disease and impacts the prognosis and management. The skin and mind connection has recently been recognized and the field of psychodermatology has seen a surge of literature in the past three decades. Numerous psychodermatology associations have formed in various parts of the world. Recently, Association of Psychodermatology of India was formed, and Dr Abdul Latheef has been its former president. Dr Latheef is a dedicated teacher who is spreading the knowledge of psychodermatology in South Asia. He has dedicated his career toward teaching and training young dermatologists, psychiatrists, and psychologists. I have the honor of knowing him for several years and am very impressed with his humble personality and academic achievements. He has previously written a book *"Handbook of Psychodermatology"*, and this is the second edition of this book. This book fills the gaps in various disciplines of psychodermatology with updated chapters referring to the latest research in the field. The first two chapters cover introduction to psychodermatology and how to take history in patients with psychocutaneous disorders. The rest of the chapters cover all aspects of human life including pediatric, adolescent, and geriatric population and their psychodermatological ailments. Some chapters are dedicated to chronic diseases like the psychodermatology of Hansen's disease, HIV, and genitals. Several chapters are dedicated to different psychotherapeutic approaches in treating psychodermatological disorders. Overall, this book appears to be an excellent addition to the current psychodermatology literature and an exceptional guide to dermatologists, psychiatrists, and psychologists alike. It is an honor to write the foreword of this book by Dr Latheef and I wish him all the success in his future academic endeavors in spreading the knowledge of psychodermatology.

Mohammad Jafferany MD FAPA MCPS(Dermatology)
Professor of Psychodermatology, Psychiatry and Behavioral Sciences
Central Michigan University College of Medicine/CMU Medical Education Partners
Past President, Association for Psychocutaneous Medicine of North America
President, World Psychodermatology Day
President and Chair, Scientific and Organizing Committee
32nd Annual APMNA Meeting, March 7 2024, San Diego, California, USA

Foreword

Psychodermatology is an upcoming subspecialty in dermatology. Many commonly occurring diseases have psychological background, and consideration of such background forms an important part of the management. However, it is not an easy task to write on this subject.

Editors Dr Abdul Latheef, Dr Smitha Prabhu S and advisor Dr Shrutakirthi D Shenoi, took up a challenge to bring this excellent textbook on psychodermatology.

The content of the chapters is well laid. The language is simple and lucid yet it covers the subject comprehensively.

I am sure that this book "*Handbook of Psychodermatology*" would be well sought after by our readers.

My best wishes!

Vijay Zawar MD DNB DVD FRCP(Edinburgh)
President
Indian Association of Dermatologists,
Venereologists and Leprologists (2023)

Foreword

It is my pleasure and honor to introduce the exceptional work done by Drs Abdul Latheef EN, Shrutakirthi D Shenoi, and Smitha Prabhu S—a comprehensive handbook that delves into the interplay between the skin and the mind, now emerging as the field of psychodermatology.

The fundamental connection between the skin and the brain, both originating from the ectoderm, forms the cornerstone of the relationship explored within the pages of the *"Handbook of Psychodermatology"*. The skin, as the largest sensory organ, significantly shapes our perception of beauty, which is related to an individual's self-esteem. The societal constructs surrounding beauty, therefore unfortunately, often contribute to the development of psychiatric disorders, underscoring the importance of understanding the interplay between psychological factors and dermatological disorders. Therefore, recognizing the interconnectedness of these seemingly distinct disorders of the skin and brain is paramount, as their dynamic relationship holds important implications in the management of psychodermatological disorders.

An example of this complex relationship can be found in the case of vitiligo, a condition not strictly a disease yet perceived as one due to societal norms, causing considerable distress among affected individuals. Similarly, psychiatric disorders, such as delusional parasitosis, frequently manifest initially as skin disorders, emphasizing the imperative need for an integrated approach that transcends the boundaries of both dermatology and psychiatry.

This bidirectional relationship is further underscored by the exacerbation of skin conditions like psoriasis and eczema under stress and the role of stress management to manage these disorders. Additionally, some psychiatric drugs like lithium can exacerbate dermatological conditions like psoriasis and skin rashes, necessitating a nuanced awareness among psychiatrists and dermatologists and expanding their perspectives beyond their respective traditional boundaries.

In this context, the second edition of the *Handbook of Psychodermatology* emerges as a valuable and timely resource, bridging a crucial gap in our understanding and treatment of psychodermatological diseases. This comprehensive guide not only promises but also delivers on enhancing the understanding and management of psychodermatological patients, fostering a holistic approach that recognizes the inseparable link between the mind and the skin. I am optimistic that this edition will serve as a practical and indispensable resource for both dermatologists and psychiatrists, by advancing the collective knowledge and refining the practices in the intricate and dynamic domain of psychodermatology.

Om Prakash Singh MD(Psychiatry) FRCP(Edinburgh)
International Distinguished Fellow
American Psychiatric Association
Editor-in-Chief, Indian Journal of Psychiatry
President, Psycho-Dermatological Association of India (PDAI)

Foreword

Psychodermatology is the intersection of two realms that have long been perceived as distinct, mind and skin. As I delve into the pages of this remarkable book, I invite you on a journey of discovery where we uncover the intricate connection between our psychological well-being and the health of our largest organ—skin. Being a Consultant Dermatologist working in the Government Sector in Sri Lanka over the last 20 years and observing the profound impact of our emotions, thoughts, and mental state on the health of our skin.

Psychodermatology is a captivating discipline, which challenges the traditional boundaries between dermatology and psychology. Delving deeper, we find the hidden links between stress anxiety, depression, and the manifestation on our skin—a canvas that can mirror our emotional struggles. This book *"Handbook of Psychodermatology"* uncovers these connections, shedding light on fascinating ways our inner selves reflect in our outer appearance.

In these pages, you will embark on a quest alongside esteemed editor Dr Abdul Latheef, a leading authority in Psychodermatology. All the authors belonging to a multidisciplinary team of Dermatology, Psychiatry, and Psychology are veterans in this field. They are exploring topics of psychosomatic triggers, psychotropic medications, and the influence of mindful techniques and offer us an unparalleled understating of skin–mind connections and a holistic management approach.

I invite you all to reflect, question, and apply the insights gained from these pages.

Chandani Udagedara MD
Consultant Dermatologist
National Hospital Kandy, Sri Lanka
Past President, Sri Lanka College of Dermatologists
Vice President, South Asian Association of Psychodermatology

Foreword

Skin and the brain are closely related. *"Handbook of Psychodermatology"* describes an interaction between dermatology, psychiatry, and psychology. As dermatologists are increasingly aware of the importance of psychodermatology, the rate of diagnosis of psychodermatological disorders is also high. It is high time that we have to focus on the topic and deal with psychodermatological patients with a multidisciplinary approach.

I have had the opportunity to work closely with Professor Dr Abdul Latheef and Professor Dr Shrutakirthi D Shenoi in the South Asian Association of Psychodermatology (SAAPD). The authors have enough knowledge and experience to back up their writeup.

This book provides detailed and comprehensive information about the diagnosis and management of psychodermatological disorders. It stresses the fact that the management of such dermatological conditions is beyond psychopharmacology alone. This book further highlights updates and the addition of new chapters showcasing the book's commitment to update current knowledge.

I extend my heartiest congratulations to the authors and editors of the book for their one more successful venture. It is one more addition to the literature and a precious gift to the field of psychodermatology globally. I would like to thank the authors and the editors of the book and wish this book to reach more and more readers each day. There is a lot more to benefit from its readership.

Saraswoti Neupane MD
President
Society of Dermatologists, Venereologists and
Leprologists of Nepal (SODVELON)
Vice President
South Asian Association of Psychodermatology (SAAPD)

Foreword

Psychodermatology is a very important subject. Public and professional awareness is increasing day by day. Healthy skin is needed for healthy mind and healthy mind is needed for healthy skin. In our daily practice, we have many patients of psychodermatological illness.

Both Professor Dr Abdul Latheef EN and Professor Dr Shrutakirthi D Shenoi are very experienced and learned persons in this subject for many years. I have had the opportunity to work with them for the last few years in South Asian Association of Psychodermatology (SAAPD). They try to describe different common diseases of psychodermatology in a very simple and palatable way so that everyone can easily learn this subject. Hopefully this book *"Handbook of Psychodermatology"* will be very popular among all physicians, especially Dermatologists, Psychiatrists, and Psychologists of South Asia within a very short time.

I thank the editor, authors, and publisher and all those who are involved in this great work. This book will be a good guide for management of psychodermatological diseases for all physicians. I wish a great success for this book.

Mohammad Mahmudur Rahman
MD MBBS BCS(Health) Retired MD(Dermatology and Venerology)
Associate Professor and Head
Department of Dermatology and Venereology
East West Medical College, Dhaka, Bangladesh
Secretary General, South Asian Association of
Psychodermatology (SAAPD)
Organizing Secretary, Society of Dermatologic Surgeons
of Bangladesh (SDSB)

Preface to the Second Edition

Psychodermatology is getting remarkable recognition in recent years. Emotional or sociocultural factors of influence have dramatically changed the morbidity and pathogenic understanding of causality and therapy concepts in dermatology over the past decades. Since both skin and brain originate from the same ectoderm, skin diseases can affect the mind and vice versa. Psychodermatology covers all aspects of mind–body interactions in relation to the onset and progression of various skin disorders. This is the first book from India and probably from South Asia on this subject, written by a multidisciplinary team of psychiatrists, psychologists, and dermatologists for all the health professionals who treat patients with skin problems. The concept of Liaison Clinic is popular in Europe, America, and countries like Japan, Israel and Singapore and there are some isolated clinics in India. There are reports of some isolated clinics in India. This book *"Handbook of Psychodermatology"* offers a summarizing overview of clinical patterns in psychodermatology, psychoneuroimmunology, psychological aspect of cosmetic dermatology, sexually transmitted diseases, Hansen's disease, and issues in adolescents and geriatric population. A brief discussion on various psychological interventions such as cognitive behavior therapy, meditation, relaxation, habit reversal, hypnotherapy, group and family therapy and guided imageries are included. This book also discusses psychopharmacology, and the need for a psychodermatology liaison clinic. We have tried to keep the book comprehensive yet simple and reader friendly and included relevant information useful for a beginner and an expert. In this second edition, we have included more chapters relevant to this specialty. We hope we have succeeded in achieving this objective. I am fortunate to get very many experts as authors, and I express my sincere gratitude to all the authors for their contribution. I record with pride and happiness the splendid support given by Dr Smitha Prabhu S (Assistant Editor) and Dr Shrutakirthi D Shenoi (Chief Advisor). I express my special gratitude to Professor Mohammad Jafferany, Dr Vijay Zawar, Professor Om Prakash Singh, Professor Saraswoti Neupane, Dr Chandani Udagedara, and Dr Mohammad Mahmudur Rahman for blessing us with forewords. I express my sincere thanks to Shri Jitendar P Vij (Group Chairman),

Mr Ankit Vij (Managing Director), Ms Chetna Malhotra (Senior Director—Professional Publishing, Marketing, and Business Development), Ms Pooja Bhandari [Director–Production (Books and Journals)], and Ms Pragati Singh (Development Editor) of M/s Jaypee Brothers Publishers (P) Ltd, New Delhi, India, for their constant support and outstanding work in bringing out the book on time. I earnestly hope that the book will be appreciated by the readers and will serve as an instrument in the progress of psychodermatology. I welcome comments and feedback from the readers.

Abdul Latheef EN

Preface to the First Edition

Psychodermatology is getting increasing attention in recent years. Emotional or sociocultural factors of influence have dramatically changed the morbidity, pathogenic understanding of causality and therapy concepts in dermatology over the past decades. Since both skin and brain originate from the same ectoderm, skin diseases can affect the mind and vice versa. Psychodermatology covers all aspects of mind-body interactions in relation to the onset and progression of various skin disorders. This is the first book from India and probably from South Asia on this subject written by a multidisciplinary team of psychiatrists, psychologists and dermatologists for all the health professionals who treat patients with skin problems. The concept of liaison clinic is popular in Europe, America and countries like Israel and Singapore. There are reports of some isolated clinics in India.

The present book offers a summarizing overview of clinical patterns in psychodermatology, psychoneuroimmunology, psychological aspect of cosmetic dermatology and sexually transmitted diseases, psychological interventions including meditation, psychopharmacology and the need for a psychodermatology liaison clinic. We have tried to keep the book comprehensive yet simple and reader friendly, to include relevant information useful for a beginner and an expert. We hope we have succeeded in achieving this objective.

I am fortunate to get very many experts as authors, and I express my sincere gratitude to all the authors for their contribution. I record with pride and happiness the splendid work done by Dr Smitha Prabhu S (Assistant Editor) and Dr Shrutakirthi D Shenoi (Chief Advisor) without the sincere endeavors of whom the book would not have been possible.

I express my special gratitude to our National President, Dr Venkataram Mysore for blessing this venture with help, advice and contribution. Dr John Koo and Tina Bhutani (University of California, San Francisco), the pioneers in this field, deserve special thanks for blessing us with the foreword.

I express my sincere thanks to Shri Jitendar P Vij (Group Chairman), Mr Ankit Vij (Managing Director) and Mr Tarun Duneja (Director-Publishing) of M/s Jaypee Brothers Publishers (P) Ltd, New Delhi, India, for their constant support and outstanding work in bringing out the book on time.

I earnestly hope that the book will be appreciated by the readers and it will serve as an instrument in the progress of psychodermatology. I welcome comments and feedback from the readers.

Abdul Latheef EN

Contents

1. **Skin and Psyche: Introduction to Psychodermatology**   1
   Abdul Latheef EN
   - Stress and Psychoneuroimmunology *2*
   - Neurogenic Inflammation *4*
   - Stress and Immune Response *4*
   - Pruritus *6*
   - Stress and Barrier Function of the Skin *7*
   - Stress and Wound Healing *7*
   - Psoriasis *8*
   - Atopic Dermatitis *8*
   - Infections *8*

2. **Case-taking in Psychodermatology**   10
   Smitha Prabhu S
   - Approach to a Possible Psychodermatology Patient *11*
   - Counseling of a Psychodermatology Patient *16*

3. **Primary Psychiatric Disorders: Cutaneous Manifestations**   18
   Ravindra Neelakanthappa Munoli
   - Factitious Disorders/Self-inflicted Dermatitis *21*
   - Dermatoses as a Result of Delusional Illnesses and Hallucinations *37*
   - Somatoform Disorders *40*
   - Dermatoses as a Result of Compulsive Disorders *43*

4. **Secondary Psychiatric Disorders in Dermatology Patients**   47
   Sreejayan Kongasseri
   - Epidemiology *47*
   - Classification *49*
   - Special Populations *56*

5. **Psychophysiologic Skin Disorders**   62
   Shrutakirthi D Shenoi, Meghashree G
   - Alopecia Areata *63*
   - Atopic Eczema *63*
   - Psoriasis *64*

- Urticaria 65
- Lichen Planus 66
- Vitiligo 66
- Psychogenic Purpura 66
- Rosacea 67
- Acne 67
- Seborrheic Dermatitis 68
- Prurigo Nodularis 68
- Miscellaneous 68
- Management of Psychophysiologic Disorders 68

6. **Impact of Dermatological Diseases on Psyche of Patient, Family, and Society** 71
   Swapna Bondade, Abhineetha Hosthota
   - Navigating the Storm: The Patient's Journey 72
   - Psychological Impact of Skin Disease on Family: The Hidden Scars 75
   - Skin Diseases and the Psyche of Society 76

7. **Skin, Mind, and Beauty** 80
   Madhulika Mhatre, Venkataram Mysore
   - Understanding the Motivation 81
   - Concept of Self-perception 83

8. **Psychology of an Aesthetic Patient** 86
   Manjot Marwah Sharma, Venkataram Mysore
   - Disease Dermatology versus Desire Dermatology 88
   - Types of Patients and their Psychological Expectations 89
   - Intervention and Decision to Do the Procedure 94
   - Warning Signs for When Not to Do Procedures 95

9. **Dermatological and Aesthetic Issues in Adolescents** 98
   Tarun Narang, Shikha Shah
   - Adolescent Dermatology 98
   - Acne 99
   - Atopic Dermatitis 100
   - Hair Loss 100
   - Dyspigmentation 100
   - Body Dysmorphic Disorder 101
   - Social Media: The Double-edged Sword 101
   - Self-Induced Dermatoses 102

- Burden of the Disease and Impact on Quality of Life   *103*
- Assessment of Life Quality in Adolescents   *103*
- Management Aspects   *104*

10. Psychological and Neuropsychiatric Complications of HIV and STD   106
Rakesh Bharti, Satnam Singh Palia
- HIV/AIDS (Acquired Immunodeficiency Syndrome)   *106*
- Clinical Psychiatric Presentations   *108*
- Management of Psychiatric Disorders   *109*
- Sexually Transmitted Diseases   *111*

11. Psyche and Genitals: Conspicuous Associations in Psychodermatologic Perspective   113
Bishurul Hafi NA, Uvais NA
- Anogenital Itch   *115*
- Mucocutaneous Pain Syndromes   *117*
- Persistent Genital Arousal Disorder   *117*
- Body Dysmorphic Disorder and Genitals   *118*
- Small Penis Syndrome   *119*
- Venereophobia   *120*
- Genital Dermatillomania   *121*
- Psychological Effects of Genital Mutilation   *121*
- Disorders of Sex Development   *122*
- Postorgasmic Illness Syndrome   *122*
- Semen Contact Allergy   *123*
- Koro Syndrome   *123*
- Dhat Syndrome   *124*

12. Psychiatric Morbidities in Hansen's Disease   128
Minu Ulpurath, Abdul Latheef EN
- Types of Stigma   *128*
- Causes for Stigma   *129*
- Effects of Stigma on Patients   *129*
- Approach to Psycho Social Aspects of Leprosy   *132*

13. Psychodermatological Issues in Geriatric Population   136
Archana AG, Abdul Latheef EN
- Changes in Aging Skin   *138*
- Dermatological Diseases with Psychiatric Morbidity in Elderly   *138*
- Psychological Morbidity   *145*

14. **Sleep in Dermatology** — 150
    Savitha Soman
    - Physiology of Sleep *151*
    - Interface Between Skin and Sleep *152*
    - Dermatological Disorders and Sleep Problems *152*
    - Other Sleep Disorders Related to Skin Problems *156*
    - Assessment of Sleep *157*
    - Management *158*

15. **Suicide Prevention in Patients with Dermatological Conditions** — 163
    Shubh Mohan Singh, Eepsita Mishra
    - Suicide and Suicidality in Dermatoses *165*
    - Understanding the Psychological Impact of Dermatological Conditions in Relation to Suicide *165*
    - Recognizing Suicide Warning Signs *170*
    - Collaborative Care Approach *170*
    - Psychological Interventions *171*
    - Pharmacological Considerations *171*
    - Patient Education and Empowerment *172*
    - Creating a Supportive Environment *173*
    - Crisis Intervention and Referral Procedures *173*
    - Public Health Initiatives and Policy Recommendations *174*

16. **Assessment Tools and Questionnaires in Psychodermatology** — 178
    Sreejayan Kongasseri
    - Diagnostic Scales *179*
    - Screening Tools *179*
    - Substance Use *181*
    - Quality of Life *182*
    - Stigma *182*
    - Disability *183*
    - Suicidal Risk *183*
    - Children *184*
    - Disease-specific Scales *184*

17. **Psychodermatology Counseling: A Holistic Approach to Skin and Mind** — 186
    Sudipta Roy
    - Introduction to Psychodermatology: Understanding the Skin–Mind Connection *186*

- Assessment and Evaluation in Psychodermatology Counseling 194
- Therapeutic Approaches in Psycho-dermatology Counseling 196
- Building Resilience and Coping Skills 198
- Addressing Body Image and Self-esteem 199
- Family and Social Support in Psychodermatology 200
- Ethical Considerations in Psychodermatology Counseling 201
- Case Studies and Practical Applications 201
- Future Directions in Psycho-dermatology Counseling 202

18. **Psychological Intervention in Psychodermatological Conditions: Part 1** 205
    Shweta Rai
    - Habit Reversal 206
    - Relaxation Procedures 207
    - Cognitive Behavior Therapy 213
    - Supportive Therapy 217

19. **Psychological Interventions in Psychodermatological Conditions: Part 2** 219
    Abdul Latheef EN, Julaila Thasneem
    - Psychoeducation 219
    - Hypnotherapy 221
    - Behavior Therapy 227
    - Group Therapy 229
    - Family Therapy 229
    - Neurolinguistic Programming 230

20. **Meditation: An Experience beyond Words** 232
    Sreekanth Sukumarakurup
    - Meditation as Medication: Exploring the Medical Benefits of Meditation 234
    - Classification 234
    - Premeditation Steps 238
    - Meditation Steps 239

21. **Mindfulness-based Therapies for Dermatological Disorders** 244
    Mahesh MM
    - Mindfulness-based Therapies: An Overview 245
    - The Process of Mindfulness in Skin Disorders 246
    - Rationale for Mindfulness-based Therapies in Skin Disorders 247

Contents

22. Drug Treatment of Psychodermatological Conditions — 256
Harish M Tharayil
- Working Classification   258
- Choosing a Drug: Some Tips   259
- Antipsychotics   261
- Depression   266

23. Dermatological Adverse Effects of Psychotropic Medications — 272
Savitha Soman
- Cutaneous Adverse Effects with Specific Drug Classes   273
- Cross Reactions   275
- Risk Factors   276
- Morphology of Cutaneous Lesions   277
- Diagnosis   279
- Treatment   282

24. Psychodermatology Liaison Clinic — 286
Shrutakirthi D Shenoi, Varsha Gowda VM
- Scope   287
- Liaison Clinics   288
- Sample of a Case Record in a Liaison Clinic   288
- Advantages of Psychodermatology Approach   290
- Difficulties Encountered at Liaison Clinic   290

25. Research in Psychodermatology: Unveiling the Mind–Skin Connection — 291
Isabella Tan, Mohammad Jafferany
- Scope of Psychodermatology Research   292

Index — 299

CHAPTER 1

Skin and Psyche: Introduction to Psychodermatology

Abdul Latheef EN

> **Key Messages**
> - Skin and brain, both originate from the same ectoderm, skin diseases can affect psyche and vice versa.
> - Skin is a part of NICE (neuro-immuno-cutaneous-endocrine) system; stress can induce or exacerbate many dermatological conditions.
> - Psychiatric comorbidity in dermatological outpatients ranges from 30 to 40%, and in inpatients, it is up to 60%.
> - Anxiety, depression, adjustment disorders, and social withdrawal are common problems.

"Man is made by his beliefs—as he believes so he is."
—***Bhagavad Gita***

"There is a part in our body, if it is healthy the whole body is healthy, if it is sick the whole body is sick, that is mind."
—**Prophet Muhammad**

INTRODUCTION

The age old adage 'face is the mirror of mind' is applicable not only to the face but to the whole skin of our body. This dictum has acquired tremendous importance in recent decades. The mind and body are considered as a single unit instead of mind versus body dualism, and this stresses the need for holistic approach of disease management. Formerly, the biomedical concept of disease was very prevalent, which compared the human body to a machine and the doctor was like a technician doing the repair work of human machine, where the mind was completely neglected. But in this recent concept, the mind has very important role in health, disease causation, and healing.

Every dermatologist knows that chronic skin diseases, especially on visible areas, may lead to considerable emotional and psychosocial stress in the affected individuals, more so if the lesion is disfiguring or tends to heal with scars. In the same way, emotional or psychological disorders may trigger skin diseases also.

The relationship between skin and psyche is getting increasing attention and several theories postulate psychophysiological mechanisms underlying various dermatological disorders. Emotional or sociocultural factors of influence have dramatically changed the morbidity, pathogenic understanding of causality, and therapy concepts in dermatology over the past decades. Since both skin and brain originated from the same ectoderm, skin diseases can affect mind and vice versa. Psychosomatic dermatology addresses skin diseases in which psychogenic causes, consequences, or concomitant circumstances have an essential and therapeutically important influence. In the narrower sense, it covers every aspect of intra- and interpersonal problems triggered by skin diseases and the psychosomatic mechanisms of eliciting or coping with dermatoses.

The skin is a complex system made up of blood vessels, nerves, glands, and muscle elements, many of which are controlled by the autonomic nervous system and can be influenced by psychological stimuli. They have the capacity to cause autonomic arousal and are capable of affecting the skin and the development of various skin disorders. In dermatology practice, various studies have shown that psychiatric morbidity in outpatients ranges from 30 to 40%, and in inpatients it is up to 60%. Anxiety, depression, adjustment disorders, and social withdrawal are common problems.

STRESS AND PSYCHONEUROIMMUNOLOGY

Skin is a part of NICE (neuro-immuno-cutaneous-endocrine) system and stress can induce or exacerbate many of the pathogenic mechanisms in a variety of dermatological conditions. Various researches in this field for last 30 years have established the close relationship between central nervous system (CNS) and the immune system. Stressors activate two major neural pathways—hypothalamo-pituitary-adrenal (HPA) axis and sympathetic nervous system. The hypothalamus secretes corticotropin-releasing hormone (CRH), arginine and vasopressin. CRH release activates the HPA axis, leading to release of adrenocorticotropic hormone (ACTH) from the pituitary gland. ACTH induces downstream release of glucocorticoids from the adrenal cortex. Activation of the noradrenergic pathways by CRH results in secretion of norepinephrine and epinephrine from the adrenal medulla and norepinephrine by the peripheral sympathetic nervous system. CRH and noradrenergic neurons in the CNS innervate and stimulate each other producing complementary effect. The activation of these two neurochemical pathways and release of hormones and transmitters have profound downstream effects on immune function. As a result, the body produces innumerable hormones, cytokines, and other neurohumoral chemical mediators, which trigger and maintain the skin disease without much response to therapy. Neurons use different groups of chemical signals for transferring information. They release neurotransmitters, neuropeptides, and gases such as nitric oxide and even cannabinoids. Neurons often produce one or more neuropeptides and a conventional neurotransmitter [glutamate gamma amino butyric acid (GABA), glutamate, or dopamine]. They regulate neuronal communication by exerting effect on specific cell-surface receptors of other neurons which in turn produce a number of changes in human behavior. They can also produce a biological impact on local blood flow, gene expression, glial cell morphology, and synaptogenesis. Positive life conditions, solid social support network, happy personal relationships, etc., can increase natural killer (NK) cell activity, lymphocyte function, the immune system response to the hepatitis B vaccine and immunity (mitogen tests). Good humor, laughter, and happiness increase the lymphocyte count, lymphocyte activity, and serum IgA level. Relaxation techniques and hypnosis have been found to improve NK cell activity and cell effectiveness lowering stress hormone levels in blood and decreasing herpes virus activity. Aerobic physical exercise stimulates production of white blood cells, NK cells, and T cells, and endorphins. Similarly, peer support and good group can increase the lymphocytes and NK cell numbers and activity. Stressful events may play a significant role in allergies and autoimmune diseases such as systemic lupus erythematosus, rheumatoid arthritis, systemic sclerosis, mixed connective tissue disease, and Sjögren's syndrome. Feelings of helplessness and negative emotions can trigger the growth or spread of malignancy. Neuropeptides, neurotransmitters, catecholamines and neurotrophins play an important role in regulating the immune response.

NEUROGENIC INFLAMMATION

Neurogenic cutaneous inflammatory response is triggered by the stress-induced products of cutaneous sensory nerve endings. The skin is innervated primarily by sensory C-fibers. Their free nerve endings contain neuropeptides, such as substance P (SP), calcitonin gene-related peptide (CGRP), and pituitary adenylate-cyclase-activating polypeptides (PACAP). These bind to receptors on cutaneous blood vessels, inducing vasodilatation, increased vessel permeability, chemotaxis, exocytosis, and activation of neutrophils. These peptides, in conjunction with keratinocyte-derived CRH and nerve growth factor (NGF) act on mast cells resulting in the degranulation of these cells, secretion of tumor necrosis factor alpha (TNF-α), histamine, and tryptamine leading to cutaneous inflammation. It is also observed that stress will increase the production and release of proinflammatory cytokines and nitric oxide from macrophages and this leads to selective redistribution of immune cells from one organ to another (e.g., reduction in number and percentage of cells in the peripheral blood and concomitant increase of immune cells in the skin).

Stressors also activate intracellular transcription factors that play a central role in mediating the physiological effects of proinflammatory cytokines. Altogether, stress has a significant role in the initiation and maintenance of cutaneous inflammatory response.

STRESS AND IMMUNE RESPONSE

Acute or Mild Stress

Studies conducted in laboratory animals have shown that brief and mild stressors enhance acquired immunity. In a series of experiments in rats, it has been shown that a brief stressor (2 hours of physical restraint or shaking) applied before antigen challenge significantly enhances delayed-type hypersensitivity (DTH). Similarly, rodents exposed to acute or mild stressors or both before antigen presentation have been reported to enhance humoral immunity by producing more antibodies than control groups. But if the intensity or duration of stress is increased, opposite effect is observed even if the same stressor type is used. It is observed that the enhancing effect of immunity is due to the stress-related release of corticosteroids and epinephrine, however, chronic stress or chronic administration of corticosteroids suppresses the immunity. Human studies with parachute jumping and first-time public speaking as stressors have shown many enumerative changes in the immune cells. These changes include increase in total white blood cells count, CD8 T cell, NK cells, NK cell activity, and CD4/CD8 ratio. But it also decreases the number of total B and T cells. It also favors the production of T helper type 1 (Th1) cytokine Interferon-gamma (IFN-γ). In humans, it is also observed that acute stress rapidly evolves into chronic stress in terms of immune system effect.

Chronic or Severe Stress

Chronic or severe stressors in animals and humans are associated with alterations in immune system that leads to development of diseases. Studies conducted in individuals appearing for examinations and those caring a demented spouse have shown that both cellular and humoral immunity are affected adversely. The ability to suppress the activity of latent viruses decreases and it also interferes with antibody production after vaccination.

The enumerative changes include increase in circulating white blood cells, Th2 cytokines IL-4, IL-10, but decrease in CD4 (helper), CD8 (cytotoxic) cells, ratio of CD4/CD8 cells, B cells, T cells, and NK cells. Chronic stressors also suppress delayed-type hypersensitivity (DTH), NK cell activity, memory T-cell response, Th1-cytokines IFN-γ, and IL-2 production.

In short, chronic or severe stress leads to activation of the HPA axis that results in the secretion of catecholamines and glucocorticosteroids. They have a profound effect on immunity, inducing a Th2 shift by upregulating the production of Th2-cytokines, interleukin (IL)-4, IL-10, and IL-13, and by suppressing Th1-cytokine IL-12 production and macrophages. In this manner, chronic stress inhibits cell-mediated immunity, favoring antibody-mediated and allergic responses. This combined effect on the Th1–Th2 balance may explain why the activity of some diseases such as autoimmune diseases, including pemphigus or conditions with Th2 predominance, like atopic eczema appears to deteriorate during periods of stress **(Flowchart 1)**.

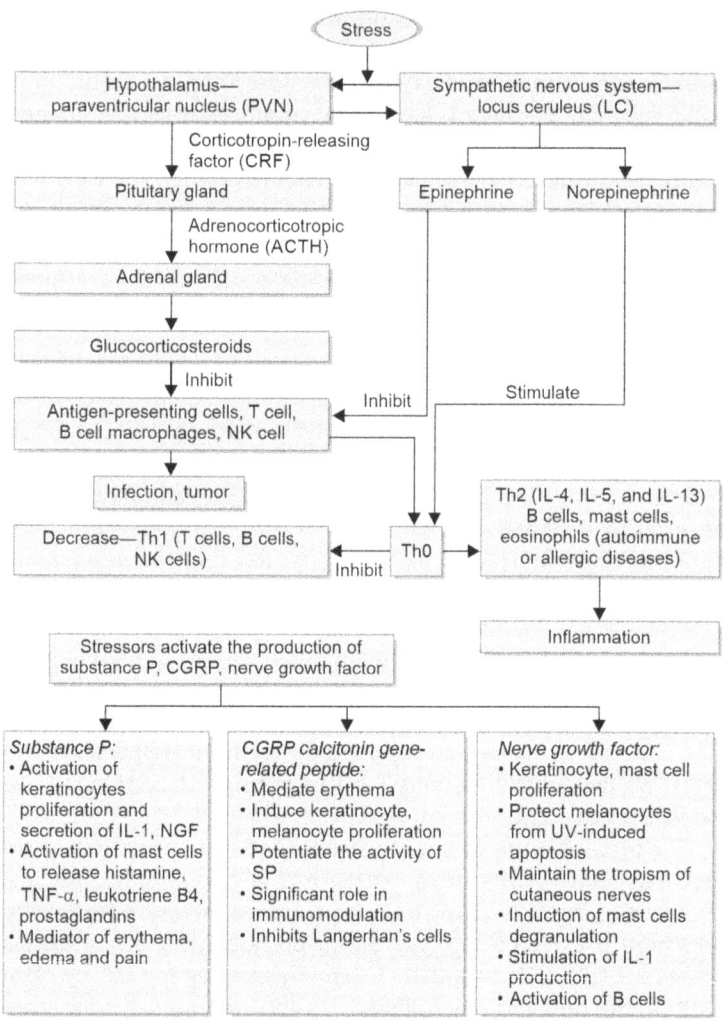

Flowchart 1: Effect of stress on skin.
(CGRP: calcitonin gene-related peptide; IL: interleukin; NGF: nerve growth factor; NK: natural killer; SP: substance P; Th: T helper; TNF: tumor necrosis factor)

PRURITUS

Pruritus or itching is an unpleasant sensation, similar to pain, that can be generalized or localized. It is a complex emotional and sensory experience produced by primary psychiatric or psychophysiological disorders. Diseases of the nervous system can cause neurological itching as with neuropathies, or anxiety, sexual problems, psychic mania, psychiatric conditions, etc. Functional brain imaging studies have observed the regions of brain associated with itching and found that many areas are activated by itch stimuli. The possible roles of these areas in itch perception along with differences in the cerebral mechanisms of healthy subjects and chronic itch patients have been discussed. The central itch modulation system, cerebral mechanisms of pleasurable sensation evoked by scratching, and the mechanism of contagious itch have also been investigated. Several nervous system activities might be responsible for itching. Cholinergic nerve fibers produce acetylcholine and vasoactive intestinal peptide (VIP), which stimulate the eosinophils to produce histamine and activate the peripheral itch receptors situated in the epidermis. The histamine activates the H2 and H3 brain receptors and stimulates the CNS neurons to release opioid peptides that also stimulate the peripheral itch receptors. In addition, type-C sensory nerve fibers are also stimulated producing neuropeptides, SP, neurokinin A, and NGF that further stimulates the itch receptors. Itch receptors can also be indirectly activated by prostaglandins and IL-2.

STRESS AND BARRIER FUNCTION OF THE SKIN

The barrier function of the skin gets impaired during period of stress. Stress liberates histamine and vasoactive neuropeptides and causes hemodynamic changes such as variation in skin temperature, blood flow, and sweat response which in turn contribute to increased transepidermal water loss. Altered skin-barrier function creates increased susceptibility to cutaneous inoculation with environmental agents (e.g., allergens such as dust mites, dander, bacteria, and viruses) that are potential precipitants of atopic flares.

STRESS AND WOUND HEALING

It is observed that wounds healed significantly slower in healthy students during periods of examinations compared with non-stressful times. Delayed healing is seen in couples with poor marital relationships. Thus, the process of wound healing is affected by stressful life conditions and can be improved through psychological intervention and/or changes in lifestyle. The mechanisms which occur in the nervous system, both central and peripheral, that alter innate and cellular immunity in the skin in response to wound healing require further studies.

PSORIASIS

Emotional stressors have been reported to precede the onset and flares of psoriasis. It is observed that psoriatic patients who suffered traumatic sensory denervation had resolution of lesions in the areas innervated by the sectioned nerves and the disease reappeared when nerve fibers regenerated. Psoriatic plaques display increased nerve fiber density and altered content of neuropeptides such as SP, CGRP, vasoactive intestinal peptide, and NGF. High expression of NGF mediates T cell and keratinocyte proliferation, mast cell migration, degranulation, and memory T-cell chemotaxis, which are hallmarks of psoriasis. It is also noted that stress reduction interventions have successful result in psoriasis management.

ATOPIC DERMATITIS

Patients with atopic dermatitis (AD) have severe impairment in their quality of life, resulting in significant emotional distress that leads to exacerbation of the disease. AD patients have upregulation of glucocorticoid receptors on peripheral leukocytes and there is a cytokine shift from Th1 to Th2 immune response. Stress-induced local and systemic secretion of epinephrine and norepinephrine also accelerate the Th2 differentiation by production of IL-13 and IL-4. There is also a redistribution of lymphocytes and eosinophils in atopic skin. Psychotherapeutic procedures for stress reduction such as insight-oriented psychotherapy, cognitive behavior therapy, psychoeducation, hypnosis, and biofeedback have been reported to be effective in improving the skin manifestations of AD patients.

INFECTIONS

Various studies have demonstrated that stressors have deleterious effects on the evolution of bacterial and viral infections of the skin. It is observed that stress can lead to the activation of herpes simplex virus remaining dormant in the dorsal nerve root ganglion.

CONCLUSION

Stress and mental tension are the inseparable part of modern life producing innumerable health hazards to the humanity. All human organs are linked with mental health, especially the skin. Stressors are acting as a trigger in the onset or chronic progression of many psychophysiological conditions such as psoriasis, AD, urticaria, lichen planus, alopecia areata, vitiligo, prurigo nodularis, autoimmune diseases like systemic lupus erythematosus, scleroderma, pemphigus, and infections like recurrent herpes simplex infection, reactions in Hansen's disease, etc. Hence, stress management is very essential along with standard dermatological management for an early and better clinical response.

FURTHER READINGS

1. Ader R, Feilten DL, Cohen N. Psychoneuroimmunology, 3rd edition. New York: Academic Press; 2001.
2. Charles L, Raison MD, Pearce DB, Miller AH. Immune system and central nervous system. In: Sadock BJ, Sadock VA (Eds). Kaplan and Sadock's Comprehensive Textbook of Psychiatry, 9th edition. New York: Lippincott Williams and Wilkins; 2009.
3. Juan F, Honeyman JF. Psychoneuroimmunology and the skin. Acta Derm Venereol. 2016;(Suppl 217):38-46.
4. Hassan I, Haji ML. Understanding itch: an update on mediators and mechanisms of pruritus. Indian J Dermatol Venereol Leprol. 2014;80:106-14.
5. Misery L, Alexandre S, Dutray S, Chastaing M, Consoli SG, Audra H, et al. Functional itch disorder or psychogenic pruritus: suggested diagnosis criteria from the French psychodermatology group. Acta Derm Venereol. 2007;87: 341-4.
6. Dhabhar FS, McEwen BS. Enhancing versus suppressive effects of stress hormones on skin immune function. Proc Natl Acad Sci USA. 1999;96:1059.
7. Harth W, Gieler U, Kusnir D, Tausk FA (Eds). Clinical Management in Psychodermatology. Germany: Springer Publication; 2009.
8. Jaremka LM. Synergistic relationships among stress, depression, and troubled relationships: Insights from Psychoneuroimmunology. Depress Anxiety. 2013;30(4):288-96.

CHAPTER 2

Case-taking in Psychodermatology

Smitha Prabhu S

> **Key Messages**
> - Both skin and brain originate from ectoderm. Diseases of one can affect the other. Unless we treat both the conditions simultaneously, therapeutic response will be less. So a detailed history-taking is essential to look out for the skin-mind connection.
> - History-taking is an art to be acquired through repeated practice based on the best available knowledge.

INTRODUCTION

Patient–doctor interaction is more complex than just treatment of disease. Patients have varied expectations from doctor, including being a confidante, guide, or even a friend at times, rather than just a healer of their diseases. They often expect miracles, even in chronic and extensive disease.

It is a well-known fact that up to 40% of dermatology patients have underlying psychological or psychiatric issues, either primary or secondary, to varying extents. Recognizing such patients is of utmost importance, as medical treatment of the dermatological disease alone may not suffice many a time. The underlying psychological/psychiatric distress is sometimes well hidden by the patient and comes into light only with a thorough and empathetic history taking.

Case-taking is an art to be honed by repeated practice. Nevertheless, there are a few facts to keep in mind while taking history, and examining the patient, in any field of medicine, be it dermatology, psychiatry, or psychodermatology.

CHAPTER 2: Case-taking in Psychodermatology

Psychodermatology, an interface between dermatology and psychiatry dealing with both the psyche and skin of the patient, is currently one of the upcoming specialties in psychiatry as well as dermatology with much potential for further development. A psychodermatological consultation is more time consuming than the conventional dermatological consult, as the patient requires more time to build confidence and to come out with the psychological problems. A dermatologist requires good relationship skills, empathy, and a basic understanding of psychodermatology to be an efficient psychodermatologist.

The interrelationship between mind, disease, environment, as well as genetic predisposition and interpersonal relations play a great part in disease progress and response to treatment.

A dermatologist should acquire basic skills in counseling, and may have to refer patient to a psychotherapist or psychiatrist if detailed psychotherapy or psychopharmacotherapy is indicated.

APPROACH TO A POSSIBLE PSYCHODERMATOLOGY PATIENT

A possible psychodermatology patient is one who has primary psychiatric problem who comes with dermatoses, or one who has secondary psychiatric problems due to chronic, persistent, or disfiguring diseases or some minor or major stressors, which act as a trigger in common dermatological conditions such as psoriasis, atopy (psychophysiological conditions). Dermatological drugs can also cause psychological or psychiatric conditions **(Table 1 and Box 1)**.

Table 1: Classification of psychodermatological disorders.

Psychophysiological disorders	Skin diseases exacerbated by stress: Acne, psoriasis, atopic dermatitis, and urticarial
Primary psychiatric disorders	Dysmorphophobia, delusion of parasitosis, and trichotillomania
Secondary psychiatric disorders	Psychosocial impact of skin disease such as anxiety and depression
Comorbidity with psychiatric disorders	Impact of skin disease on a primary psychiatric problem

> **BOX 1: New proposed classification of psychodermatological disorders.**
>
> *Group A: Primary psychodermatological disease—examples*:
> - Alopecia areata
> - Atopic dermatitis
> - Chronic spontaneous urticaria
> - Psoriasis
> - Vitiligo
>
> *Group B: Primary psychodermatological illness—examples:*
> - Body dysmorphic disorder
> - Delusional infestation
> - Dysesthesias (e.g., burning mouth syndrome, vulvodynia)
> - Psychogenic pruritus
> - Self-inflicted skin lesions
>
> *Group C: Secondary psychodermatological disorder:*
> - Secondary dermatologic disease related to psychiatric medications—examples:
>   - Acne: Lithium
>   - Alopecia: Carbamazepine, fluoxetine, lithium, and valproic acid
>   - Photosensitivity: Antipsychotics and tricyclic antidepressants
>   - Skin pigmentation: Clozapine
>   - Stevens–Johnson syndrome and toxic epidermal necrolysis: Carbamazepine and lamotrigine
> - Secondary psychiatric illness related to dermatologic medications—examples:
>   - Depersonalization: Minocycline
>   - Mood disorders: Isotretinoin, methotrexate, and systemic steroids
>   - Psychoses: Dapsone and hydroxychloroquine
>   - Sedation and drowsiness: Antihistamines
>
> *Source*: Adapted from Ferreira BR, Jafferany M. Classification of psychodermatological disorders. J Cosmet Dermatol. 2021;20(6):1622-4.

Pointers toward psychodermatology patient examination:
- Always conduct patient consultation in a private area, with least external disturbance.
  I have noticed in my practice that patients open up only if confidentiality and privacy is assured, especially when relating to delicate issues such as spousal relations, sexual problems, and interpersonal strifes.

- Greet the patients with warmth, give them a seat and make them comfortable.
- A patient is always slightly apprehensive of the doctor and what a medical visit implies. Unless we seem nonconfrontational and nonthreatening, they never disclose full facts of either disease, or attendant psychosocial issues.
- Initially, a general history-taking in presence of the bystander can be done to get preliminary information regarding dermatology condition and psychological well-being. After that, the bystander may be requested to be outside the consultation room and will be called as and when needed (in front of others, patient usually will not disclose highly personal confidential matters).

Then start more detailed history-taking:
- In the beginning of a consultation, never ask potentially embarrassing questions such as—"Are you stressed out?"; "Is your disease related to any psychological problem?". The immediate response will be a denial in most cases. Many dermatology patients will not accept a psychological cause for their ailments. Indirect questions such as—"How is your sleep and appetite? Do you experience any lack of energy or lack of interest in common pleasurable activities?", etc., help in opening up patients' to the doctor's line of questioning. Direct or leading questions followed by detailed history-taking are then possible.
- Keep asserting that many skin diseases have direct relationship with mind, so that patients do not feel embarrassed or confused while being asked about their intimate details. Some examples of direct questions are:"How is this disease affecting you?; Has this disease caused any problem in your day-to-day life in any manner–work, relationships, friendships, studies, concentration, etc.?". Direct questions should be asked only when there is some rapport or positive eye contact with the patient.
- Keenly observe the body language of the patient: How the patient talks, behaves, and also for nonverbal clues such as eye contact, gloomy face, tears, change in pitch and tonality of voice, tremors, etc., from patient or relatives. Look for any strife between patient and relative while asking questions and also observe for any hidden signs of anxiety, agitation, and depression.
- Many a times, a careful observation unearths matters which would otherwise remain hidden. A nervous tic, or frequent lip lick, or

even blinking away tears can be easily missed. Many bystanders interfere and try to dominate during history-taking, especially in case of children, parents, and spouses. Observing the interpersonal play can give a clue as toward the troubles faced by the patient at the family and social front.
- Ensure confidentiality, if deemed necessary, by sending out bystanders, students, nurses, etc., from the room.

Many patients are shy and withhold information in front of their relatives or friends, especially so in case of very personal and sexual problems. The sexual and psychological stigma or isolation can sometimes be elicited only under strict privacy. We have to emphasize our nonjudgmental attitude before asking highly private questions.
- Enquire about the condition, duration, response to previous treatment, if any, and possible cause or any other factor deemed important by the patient.

Longer duration, frequent relapses, and less than expected response to treatment can be equated to more psychological stress. Try to verify if the patient is conscientiously taking the treatment prescribed in the last visit. Indirect questions such as have you finished the prescribed medicine, if so, how many days ago? How many tubes of cream you used in the past? When do you make time to apply the cream, etc., help a long way in assuring whether the patient has been compliant.
- Enquire about occupation/studies/imminent exams or placement stress.

People involved in occupation which necessitates dealing with many people are often psychologically more affected by socially disabling diseases such as psoriasis, vitiligo, and severe acne. It is observed that many students are under very high educational stress. Refractory prurigo nodularis is common in such group as they tend to scratch at or pick at their lesions as a stress reduction method. Some students may not be initially aware of this but later on they will be on the lookout for this behavior.
- Enquire about sleep, appetite, and hobbies, which may give an indirect indication toward the mental health of the patient.

Reduced or excessive sleep, insomnia, unexplained weight gain or loss, irritable bowel syndrome, etc., can point toward psychological morbidity.

CHAPTER 2: Case-taking in Psychodermatology   15

- Enquire about absenteeism, the working atmosphere, and any adjustments the patient has to make in view of the disease. Any disease which warrants frequent absenteeism can cause havoc with job opportunities and promotions, thus, imposing more psychological burden.
- Ask leading questions, only if the patient seems comfortable, as to interpersonal relationship with spouse, children, close family members, friends:
   ○ Any incident where the patient had to suffer humiliation about the disease
   ○ Any incidence of ostracism due to the disease
   ○ Any feeling of guilt, frustration, and helplessness, and episodes of panic
   ○ As to feeling of unworthiness, persistent sadness interfering with day-to-day activities and suicidal ideation.
- While taking history, try to differentiate between frank delusions, psychosis, or dermatoses secondary to psychoses, which primarily require psychiatric therapy. A tendency toward hypochondriac behavior also should be looked out for.
- If history feels incomplete, or if the patient holds back in the first visit, try to elicit more in subsequent visits, but being careful not to intimidate the patient or make them give up on the consultation.
- Family history is important as many dermatological as well as psychological conditions as these conditions have a genetic background.
- While examining, look for hidden signs of psychiatric distress—nail biting, skin biting, hesitation cuts, patchy hair loss, and neglectful hygiene.
- Ask leading questions to diagnose or exclude common psychiatric comorbidities in dermatology like depression, anxiety, adjustment disorder, obsessive compulsive disorder, etc. (clinical details discussed in the respective chapters). A very detailed history taking as done in psychiatry is usually not needed in psychodermatology.
- After a diagnosis is arrived at, if the patient fits into any of the below diagnoses, he or she requires a psychiatric/psychological help:
   ○ A primary psychiatric disorder
   ○ Secondary psychiatric comorbidity?
   ○ Underlying stressors that trigger or exacerbate the existing dermatological condition

In a primary care setting, where there is no psychodermatology liaison clinic or a psychiatrist at hand, and if the dermatologist has the basic knowledge in counseling and pharmacotherapy, they may attempt to manage the patient on their own.

The following situations make it is advisable to seek a psychiatric/psychological consultation:
- Primary psychiatric disorder (dysmorphophobia, delusional disorder, and trichotillomania)
- Major secondary psychiatric comorbidity (major depression with suicidal ideation, severe social withdrawal)
- Tendency for substance abuse
- Lack of insight
- Lack of response to treatment.

Patient may not cooperate with, or even be hostile to abrupt orders as to get a psychiatric consultation done. Such a situation should be tactfully handled. Patients with delusions and factitious disorders are very difficult to manage and extreme tact and gentle handling is required to prevent the patient from being angry or abusive.

Having a psychodermatology liaison clinic or a psychiatrist within the dermatology clinic helps to a great extent in such cases.

A psychodermatology practitioner should have a special ability to prescribe common psychotropic and antidepressant medications with a good knowledge of their effects and side-effects, good relationship skills, and the ability to recognize the need for a psychologist or psychodermatologist at the earliest.

COUNSELING OF A PSYCHODERMATOLOGY PATIENT

Patients do not easily accept that they need a psychological or psychiatric intervention, because, according to them, they suffer purely from a skin disease, and not a mental disease. Hence, it is very essential that the patient should be explained in simple terms why their skin disorder is linked to their psyche. A simple diagram drawn on a piece of paper while simultaneously explaining this goes a long way in helping the patient understand the skin mind body connection. The interrelationship between mind and skin should be stressed upon, i.e., brain and skin has a common origin, and anything that affects the skin can affect the brain and hence, your mind, and vice versa, is a simple way to put forth a complex idea to the patient. They should be made to realize that approaching a psychiatrist or psychologist is nothing to be ashamed of and they will not be stamped as a "mental or mad patient." The need to regularly take dermatological as well as psychiatric medications prescribed should be stressed upon. The need for regular consultations also should be explained. The symptoms of the disease should be integrated with the psychological signs as well as fears and dysfunction of the patient, and explained in simple terms. We should let them know that we are there to help them, any time and conquering over the disease is a teamwork.

CONCLUSION

A good psychodermatologist needs to be open with good communication skills, knowledge about psychopharmacology medications, and the ability to recognize as to when a patient requires psychiatrist's help. Self-awareness and empathy are as important as technical skill and medical knowledge.

FURTHER READINGS

1. Ferreira BR, Jafferany M. Classification of psychodermatological disorders. J Cosmet Dermatol. 2021;20(6):1622-4.
2. Gordon-Elliott JS, Muskin PR. Managing the patient with psychiatric issues in dermatologic practice. Clin Dermatol. 2013;31:3-10.
3. Lawrence-Smith G. Psychodermatology. Psychiatry. 2009;8:223-7.
4. Poot F, Sampogna F, Onnis L. Basic knowledge in psychodermatology. J Eur Acad Dermatol Venereol. 2007;227-34.
5. Gibson R, Williams P, Hancock J. An introduction to the assessment and management of psychodermatological disorders. BJ Psych Advances. 2021;27(5):305-12.

CHAPTER 3

Primary Psychiatric Disorders: Cutaneous Manifestations

Ravindra Neelakanthappa Munoli

> **Key Messages**
> - Primary psychiatric disorders can lead to self-inflicted secondary dermatological diseases.
> - Common conditions are anxiety, depression, delusions, obsessive compulsive disorder, etc.
> - Their management is essential before dermatological management for a successful result of the skin problem.

INTRODUCTION

Psychodermatology or psychocutaneous medicine has evolved as branch over decades, and many definitions have been used to explain the term. The revised definition of psychodermatology or psychocutaneous medicine is "a branch of medicine which addresses dermatoses or physiological changes in skin, in which psychosocial factors play role in etiopathogenesis, progression, exacerbation, treatment or prognosis; further it addresses all dermatoses, in which psychological disorders can be seen as comorbidities, either as primary conditions or as secondary conditions due to dermatoses or as treatment (with dermatological treatment or with psychotropics) emergent conditions and all of these will require comprehensive psychocutaneous approach of assessment and intervention".

Just like the definition, the classification of psychodermatological disorders also has evolved over time. Various classifications are mentioned in **Box 1**. In International Classification of Disease-11 (ICD-11) the section of "sensory and psychological disorders affecting the skin" covers psychodermatological disorders. The unit has been classified as in **Box 1**.

CHAPTER 3: Primary Psychiatric Disorders: Cutaneous Manifestations

BOX 1: Classification of psychodermatological disorders.

I. *Classification by Koo et al. (2003)*:
  - Psychophysiological disorders
  - Primary psychiatric disorders
  - Secondary psychiatric disorders
  - Cutaneous sensory disorders

II. *Classification by Bewley et al. (2014)*:
  - Primary dermatologic disorders caused by or associated with psychiatric comorbidity
  - Primary psychiatric disorders which present with skin diseases or changes

III. *Classification by Reichenberg et al. (2018)*:
  - Primary dermatologic conditions causing secondary psychiatric conditions
  - Primary dermatologic conditions exacerbated by stress or psychiatric conditions
  - Primary psychiatric conditions that manifest as skin concerns

IV. *Classification by Ferreira et al. (2020)*:
  - Psychophysiological dermatoses
  - Primary psychopathology focused on the skin
  - Cutaneous sensory disorders
  - Dermatoses or disfiguring skin conditions leading to psychosocial comorbidity

V. *Classification by Ferreira and Jafferany (2021)*:

  Group A: Primary psychodermatological disease—in this group, the primary dermatoses have psychological stress, a psychological mechanism, and/or psychopathology as main elements either for inducing or for worsening. For example, alopecia areata, atopic dermatitis, chronic spontaneous urticarial, psoriasis, vitiligo

  Group B: Primary psychodermatological illness—in this group of dermatoses there are skin symptoms, with or without secondary self-induced skin lesions (such as excoriations), without a primary dermatosis. For example, body dysmorphic disorder, delusional infestation, psychogenic pruritus, self-inflicted skin lesions, dysesthesias like burning mouth syndrome, vulvodynia

  Group C: Secondary psychodermatological disorder—in this group, psychiatric complications of medications prescribed in dermatology and dermatological consequences of psychotropics are included:
  - Secondary dermatologic disease related to psychiatric medications
  - Secondary psychiatric illness related to dermatologic medications. For example:
    ○ Depersonalization: Minocycline
    ○ Mood disorders: Isotretinoin; methotrexate; systemic steroids

Continued

Continued

- ○ Psychoses: Dapsone; hydroxychloroquine
- ○ Sedation and drowsiness: Antihistamines skin disease, skin symptoms, or mental illness—linked with exogenous factors—drug reactions connecting dermatology and psychiatry

VI. *International Classification of Diseases-11 (ICD-11)*:
  Sensory and psychological disorders affecting the skin:
  - Disturbances of cutaneous sensation:
    - ○ EC90 Pruritus
    - ○ EC91 Prurigo
    - ○ EC92 Mucocutaneous or cutaneous pain syndromes
    - ○ EA83.0 Lichen simplex
    - ○ EC9Y Other specified disturbances of cutaneous sensation
  - Psychological or psychiatric conditions affecting the skin
  - Self-inflicted skin disorders:
    - ○ ED00 Artefactual skin disorder
    - ○ ED01 Simulated skin disease
    - ○ ED02 Painful bruising syndrome
  - 6B25 Body-focused repetitive behavior disorders:
    - ○ 6B25.0 Trichotillomania
    - ○ 6B25.1 Excoriation disorder
    - ○ 6B25.Y Other specified body-focused repetitive behavior disorders
    - ○ 6B25.Z Body-focused repetitive behavior disorders, unspecified
  - ED0Y Other specified self-inflicted skin disorders
  - 6B22 Olfactory reference disorder:
    - ○ 6B22.0 Olfactory reference disorder with fair to good insight
    - ○ 6B22.1 Olfactory reference disorder with poor to absent insight
    - ○ 6B22.Z Olfactory reference disorder, unspecified
  - 6B21 Body dysmorphic disorder:
    - ○ 6B21.0 Body dysmorphic disorder with fair to good insight
    - ○ 6B21.1 Body dysmorphic disorder with poor to absent insight
    - ○ 6B21.Z Body dysmorphic disorder, unspecified
  - ED2Y Other specified psychological or psychiatric conditions affecting the skin
  - Neurological conditions affecting the skin

In all the classifications, the abnormality in primary psychodermatological disorders has been abnormality of psyche or mind which in turn can lead to dermatological diseases. On evaluation, such patients will have underlying psychological problems like anxiety,

Table 1: List of primary psychiatric disorders.	
Factitious disorders/ self-inflicted dermatitis	• *Dermatitis artefacta syndrome*: As dissociated (not-conscious) self-injury behavior • *Dermatitis paraartefacta syndrome*: Disorders of impulse control, often as manipulation of an existing specific dermatosis (often semiconscious, admit self-injury) • *Malingering*: Consciously simulated injuries and diseases to obtain material gain • *Special forms*, such as the Gardner–Diamond syndrome, Münchausen syndrome, and Münchausen-by-proxy syndrome
Dermatoses as a result of delusional illnesses and hallucinations	• Delusional parasitosis • Body odor delusion (bromhidrosis) • Hypochondriacal delusions • Body dysmorphic delusions
Somatoform disorders	• Somatization disorders • Hypochondriacal disorders • Somatoform autonomic disorders (functional disorders) • Persistent somatoform pain disorders (cutaneous dysesthesias) • Other undifferentiated somatoform disorders (cutaneous sensory disorders)
Dermatoses as a result of compulsive disorders	• Washing eczema • Primary lichen simplex chronicus

depression, delusions, obsessive–compulsive disorder (OCD), etc., which need to be addressed first before the dermatological management for a successful therapeutic response of the skin problem. Some of these lesions may be self-inflicted.

For the ease of understanding, the comprehensive list of primary psychiatric disorders with cutaneous manifestations is mentioned in **Table 1**.

FACTITIOUS DISORDERS/SELF-INFLICTED DERMATITIS

According to ICD-11, factitious disorders are characterized by "feigning, falsifying, or intentionally inducing or aggravating medical, psychological, or behavioral signs and symptoms or injury in oneself or in another person associated with identified deception". A pre-existing disorder or disease may be present, but the individual intentionally aggravates existing symptoms or falsifies or induces additional symptoms. Individuals with factitious disorders seek treatment or otherwise present themselves or another person as ill, injured, or impaired based on the feigned, falsified, or self-induced signs, symptoms, or injuries. The deceptive behavior is not solely motivated by obvious external rewards or incentives (e.g., obtaining disability payments or evading criminal prosecution). This is in contrast to malingering, in which clear external rewards or incentives motivate the behavior.

In context of psychodermatology, this section includes the disorders in which the lesions are created/mimicked by the person. It indicates mutilation of self (without suicidal intent) or reference person leading to damage to a particular organ with relevant symptomatology. The prevalence of factitious disorders ranges from 0.05 to 0.4% in the general population. Except for malingering, this is seen mostly in women (5–8:1) and onset will be during puberty or early adulthood.

These disorders can be classified into the following:
- *Dermatitis artefacta syndrome*: In this, the person's self-injurious behavior is dissociated from the consciousness as such
- *Dermatitis paraartefacta syndrome*: It represents impulse control disorder (not able to control the urge to manipulate), often present as a manipulation of an existing specific dermatosis (often semiconscious, admit self-injury)
- *Malingering:* Consciously simulated injuries and diseases to obtain material gain
- *Special forms*, such as the Gardner–Diamond syndrome, Münchausen syndrome, and Münchausen-by-proxy syndrome

Dermatitis Artefacta Syndrome

Dermatitis artefacta syndrome is caused by the deliberate harm by a fully aware or dissociated patient on skin, hair, nails, or the mucosa to attract attention, satisfy a psychological need, or evade responsibility. The patients usually hide the responsibility for their actions from their doctors. By default, it should be part of differential diagnosis of all recurrent, chronic, and unexplainable dermatoses.

Clinical Features

Epidemiology
Prevalence in pediatric population is 1 case in 23,000 persons. There is female preponderance (female–male ratio reported to vary from 20:1 to 4:1). The condition is poorly recognized and under-reported and usually occurs between late adolescence (11–14 years) and early adulthood. It is important to remember that no age group is exempted from being diagnosed with this condition. No racial or ethnic predisposition has been noted.

History
The patient may be in good health and may have history of (h/o) chronic dermatoses, personal/family h/o psychiatric disorder, personal h/o chronic medical illness or pain symptoms, presence of psychosocial stressors, h/o multiple consultations, and usage of multiple medications in the past with poor response. Various psychosocial conflicts, emotional immaturity, unconscious motivations, and disturbed interpersonal relations have been implicated as the etiological factors.

Evolution of Symptoms
Often, history will be unclear about onset and progression of symptoms/lesions. Phenomenon of "*la bella Indifference*" is often seen; that is patients will explain about their symptoms but appear emotionally uninvolved, as if it is happening to someone else. Reactions of pain, frustration, anger, etc., which are expected to result from lesions, are not seen.

Suspicion should arise where clinical presentation is with atypical (1) localization, (2) morphology, (3) histology, and (4) unclear therapeutic responses. "Atypical is the typical feature." In addition, an attempt should be made to gather details about the role of foreign bodies, toxins, infections, or infectious materials. Types and sites of lesions are mentioned in **Table 2**.

Psychological Basis
It may manifest as a self-injurious behavior which is dissociated from the consciousness, often considered as an expression/activation of the childhood traumas indicating a nonverbal expression. The behavior usually occurs in dissociative states; that is, the patient will be unable to remember or remember partially and unable to comprehend the event emotionally.

Table 2: Dermatitis artefacta.

Morphology of lesions (polymorphic and bizarre)	Sites	Differential diagnosis
Superficial erosion (50%)	Face (45%)	Emotionally unstable personality disorders—borderline
• Hyperpigmented macule or purpura (30–42%) • Excoriation (17%)	Distal upper extremity (i.e., hand and forearm; 24%)	• Schizophrenias, schizotypal and delusional disorders • Hypochondriacal delusion, parasitosis, monosymptomatic psychosis
Deep necrosis, ulceration (17%)	Lower extremities (31%)	Affective disorders with psychotic symptoms, juvenile autism
• Irritant dermatoses (17%) • Papules (17%) • Crusts (8%) • Scars pinpoint, star shaped, atypically shaped (8%) • Onychodystrophy • Other keratoses, tattoo like	• Trunk (24%) • Upper arm (7%) • Scalp (7%)	• Substance use—acute intoxications, substance withdrawals • Brain—psychiatric manifestations with organic basis, syndrome, dementias • Epilepsies—temporal lobe epilepsy, seizure • Religious/cultural phenomenon, sexual act • Intention to die • *Comorbid with other diseases/syndromes*: Neurosyphilis, chronic encephalitis, Cornelia de Lange, Lesch–Nyhan syndrome, Rett syndrome

Pathophysiology

It is thought to be due to interplay of biological (genetic factors to be precise), psychological, and social factors, and these interact with a person's past history of psychiatry illness or presence of family history of mental health aberrations. Mild forms are seen following interpersonal conflicts, substance abuse, and also as a comorbid condition in depression, anxiety, and OCDs.

Management

The skin lesions should be dealt with appropriately, but the underlying psychiatric disorder should be treated promptly. Unless the psychiatric problem is tackled, the chance of recurrence is very high. Complementary adjuvant therapies may include cognitive behavior therapy, biofeedback, relaxation techniques, and hypnosis.

Drugs include selective serotonin reuptake inhibitors (SSRIs), tricyclic antidepressants (TCAs), typical (e.g., pimozide), and atypical antipsychotics (e.g., risperidone, olanzapine). Topical antimicrobials; oral antibiotics (for infected skin lesions).

Prognosis

Mild cases, secondary to identifiable psychosocial stressors, usually have a good outcome. However, if these are associated with chronic dermatologic or medical issues, prognosis is poor. Continuous or repeated episodes of self-mutilation may result in disfiguring scars on exposed areas of the body. Dermatitis artefacta is a long-term disorder, and patients need regular follow-up with a dermatologist and a psychiatrist because relapses are common.

Case Vignette

A 34-year-old lady presented with unexplained ulcers over face and neck of 1-year duration. History revealed that she was separated from husband following his infidelity and frequent quarrels. After this, she started staying alone; while at home, she would remain preoccupied with her relationship with husband and would cry, and during these times she would go on scratching her forehead and neck unknowingly. Examination revealed excoriations, ulcerations, crusts, and raw wounds. Adequate wound management was done. After ruling out other disorders, she was diagnosed as dermatitis artefacta and was started on antidepressant, escitalopram. Behavior therapy was started with coping skill training and issue of separation, and its consequences were explained. Subsequently, over a period of 6 months, the wounds healed and there were no recurrences.

Dermatitis Paraartefacta Syndrome

In this condition, the core feature is a patient's loss of control in context of skin's structural manipulation. Here, the primary lesion would be minimal which in turn gets traumatized excessively and this is the characteristic feature of this condition also. Subsequently, it leads to pronounced skin damage and the findings will be clinically serious. When traced, impulse control disorder emerges as the most common underlying mental health condition. The common patterns of dermatitis paraartefacta are mentioned in **Table 3**.

Table 3: Patterns of dermatitis paraartefacta syndrome.	
Skin and mucosa	• Skin-picking syndrome (epidermatillomania, neurotic excoriations) • Acne excoriée • Pseudo-knuckle pads • Morsicatio buccarum • Cheilitis factitia
Integument	• Onychophagia, onychotillomania, onychotemnomania • Trichotillomania, trichotemnomania, trichoteiromania

Skin-picking Syndrome (Epidermatillomania, Dermatillomania, Neurotic Excoriations)

Often seen in impulse-control disorders, skin-picking syndrome is a form of DPS, in which the patient will inflict injury to skin or mucosa which in turn will serve in reducing underlying emotional tension. The manipulation may be on an insect bite reaction/acne/folliculitis/eczema or a normal skin. This is characterized by recurrent picking of one's own skin leading to skin lesions, accompanied by unsuccessful attempts to decrease or stop the behavior. This condition is more commonly seen in women. The average age for the onset of this condition varies between 3rd and 5th decade.

Evolution

Initially, there will be feeling of tension which gradually and progressively builds up. This need not be always associated with itching. Subsequently, there will be skin picking leading to excoriation of the skin. After this act, the patient feels satisfied or relieved. This proceeds in a vicious cycle. These acts can be of any variety including pulling of skin structures, picking of skin, poking into the skin, prodding, tearing of skin, and squeezing of the skin. It can be episodic, irregular, or constant. Patient pick at areas until they can pull the material out of the skin, also referred to as *"pulling a thread from the skin."* The numbers of lesions are usually in the range of few to hundreds. These lesions will be seen in almost all stages of the development. One of the extreme variants of this condition is "prurigo nodularis".

Sites

Multiple body sites can be involved, but the most common sites usually seen are the face, hands, and arms. These are mentioned in **Table 4**.

CHAPTER 3: Primary Psychiatric Disorders: Cutaneous Manifestations

Table 4: Skin-picking syndrome.

Morphology of lesions (polymorphic)	Sites (accessible areas)	Differential diagnosis
Excoriations, erosions, crusting atrophic and hyperpigmented scars secondary to self-inflicted trauma	• Arms and legs • Face (acne excoriée)	• Prurigo nodularis • Lichen simplex chronicus • Insect bite reaction

Individuals may pick at healthy skin, at minor skin irregularities, at lesions such as pimples or calluses, or at scabs from previous picking. Most individuals pick with their fingernails, although a substantial minority use tweezers, knives, or other objects. Camouflaging and concealing the evidence of skin picking is commonly seen in such patients. Gathering information from multiple sources and a detailed physical examination will be essential **(Table 4)**.

Disorder Symptomatology

People with excoriation disorder tend to spend a lot of time, sometimes few hours per day, on their behavior. By the time it comes to clinical attention, several months or years would have passed. Certain rituals around the skin are seen such as examining it, manipulating it, or picking/eating it.

Psychological Basis

These behaviors have a psychological basis which may vary from anxiety, stress, worries, and depression. Here, the tension gets built up which is reduced with the behavior and this results in pleasure. This pleasure will reinforce the particular behavior. Not all individuals will be happy after the behavior and many will feel ashamed or express their inability to control on the behaviors. Insight among these individuals will vary with excoriation disorder reporting varying degrees of awareness of their skin-picking behavior. This is part of impulse-control disorders, and exacerbation is preceded by some psychosocial stress in nearly 30–90% of patients. It can also be understood as an urge or compulsion to manipulate the skin structure. Depression can be seen as a comorbidity in this.

Management

In mild cases: Psychoeducation or supportive psychosomatic primary care.

In moderate-to-severe cases: Behavioral therapies like supportive psychotherapy, cognitive behavior therapy, and habit reversal and relaxation techniques are particularly indicated and successful.

Drugs: Benzodiazepines or SSRIs are used.

Prognosis

The prognosis is generally better because of the patient's insight.

Acne Excoriée

Acne will be a concern for many and at times an individual tends to manipulate the acne which is a form of skin-picking syndrome. The manipulation will be in the form of rubbing the acne repeatedly, pressing the acne repeatedly, and frequent squeezing of the acne and to do this an individual may use a sharp object or commonly fingernail. Psychologically, individuals will report of build-up of an urge/anxiety which they find it difficult to resist; at times, it will be an impulsive act also. This behavior leads to skin lesions in the form of simple erosions to ulcerations also. Subsequently, scarring is seen with discoloration of the site. It is commonly seen in women gender, and the usual mean age of occurrence is around 30 years. The lesions will vary in size (millimeters to several centimeters) and shape (linear/angular to circular/oval) and are grouped along sites of the body that are easily accessible and usually exposed. Ultimately, the repeated picking results in erosions, ulcerations, and long-term scarring with hyper- or hypopigmentation. Psychiatric comorbidities in this condition are of both neurotic spectrum, like anxiety, body dysmorphic disorder, OCD, depression, social anxiety disorder, and of psychotic spectrum disorder like delusional disorder in addition to comorbid personality disorders. The usual acne areas like cheek area in front of ears, forehead area, area near the hairline, or chin areas are involved. Evaluation and management are similar to those of DPS. Due to face involvement, the patient may feel embarrassed, guilty, and stigmatized. So, disease-coping strategies need to be addressed first. N-acetylcysteine in the dose range of 600–1,200 mg/day has shown to be beneficial. The condition tends to fluctuate in association with stress and life events. Despite remission, some may continue the habit of picking the area. Recurrence of even milder acne may trigger the condition again.

> ### Case Vignette
>
> A 32-year-old lady was seen following referral for evaluation of anxiety features. She had presented with complaints of acne and arm skin lesions. History revealed that since 2 years, she had increased responsibility at workplace following promotion. She found it difficult to handle both personal and professional life. She was noticed to get angry easily on family members and shout at colleagues. She felt that her acnes are increasing, so she would try to burst them, squeeze them, and pull them out; it is only after this that she would feel better. Sometimes, there would be bleeding at the site. Also, she would go on picking skin and would remove dermal tissue and throw it telling it was dirt. Further evaluation revealed that she had anankastic and low frustration tolerance traits in personality. She would get anxious if work was not done on time. She was diagnosed with anxiety disorder and skin-picking syndrome and was started on escitalopram (SSRI) and clonazepam. Relaxation techniques were taught; subsequently, coping skills and ways to handle pressure situations were addressed.

Pseudo-knuckle Pads

Usually seen in mental retardation, pseudo-knuckle pads are padlike, rough, hypertrophic, slightly scaly skin lesions. These lesions are usually results of trauma in the form of repeated rubbing of the knuckles or persistent massaging of knuckle area or recurrent chewing of the area around the knuckle or repeated/persistently sucking of the skin around knuckle joints. Management includes understanding the underlying concept or mechanism of act and promoting suppression of act and supportive skin-care measures. Since it is commonly seen in individuals with subnormal intelligence, using behavioral techniques as therapy mode will be of help and in other individuals, when associated with stress, stress-reduction strategies can be explored and healthy coping mechanisms have to be taught.

Morsicatio Buccarum

In this condition, patients will have continuous, unconscious sucking and chewing on the oral mucosa. The lesions in this condition are in buccal mucosa and gums near tooth base. The lesions are like white patches which will be sharply demarcated and are benign in nature. Again, compulsive disorders may be the underlying condition. It is found more often among denture wearers without other psychiatric symptoms.

Cheilitis Factitia (Lip-licker's Dermatitis)

Usually seen in children, here the person will be having compulsive licking behavior affecting discrete, symmetric, sharply delineated areas beyond the outline of the lips, frequently associated with traumatizing lip chewing. The outcome of these behaviors is irritant contact dermatitis. This in turn leads to skin changes which will be eczematous in nature and in turn these will predispose to a secondary impetiginization of the specific area. The behavior of lip-licking can be psychologically explained on the basis of impaired impulse control. Management includes understanding the basis/mechanism for lip-licking. A comprehensive psychoeducation about the causes, manifestations to both patients and their caregivers/parents/guardians, and specific techniques to control the underlying urge can be explained to patients.

Onychophagia, Onychotillomania, Onychotemnomania

Usually these are behaviors that are normally seen in population and not disease entities as such. These become troublesome when the behavior leads to problems in structure or function of nail appendages.

Onychophagia (Nail Biting or Nail Chewing)

A person bites, chews, and swallows nail fragments. These behaviors may result in infections (fungal, bacterial) or inflammation of the nail appendages, bleeding can be seen, and the repeated trauma may lead to certain malformations of the involved area commonly visible as significant shortening of the distal nail plate. Usually, it is seen in nearly 45% adolescents, so not everyone with this condition will have an underlying psychological problem. In few cases, unresolved conflicts or tension may exist.

Onychotillomania

These are a form of self-induced nail diseases. The underlying behaviors for this will include paronychium trauma. There will be a recurrent insult to the nail/cuticle in the form of picking, manipulation, or removal of cuticle. As a consequence, nail dystrophy or onychodystrophy can be seen or at times paronychias also.

Onychotemnomania

In this condition, there will be trauma to nail fold or nail bed because of a person's act of cutting nails much shorter than what is expected.

Trichotillomania, Trichotemnomania, Trichoteiromania
Trichotillomania

Trichotillomania literally means a compulsive urge to pull out one's hair. ICD-11 defines it as a disorder characterized by "recurrent pulling of one's own hair leading to significant hair loss, accompanied by unsuccessful attempts to decrease or stop the behavior". The hair-pulling is usually preceded by mounting tension and is followed by a sense of relief or gratification. This diagnosis should not be made if there is a preexisting inflammation of the skin or if the hair-pulling is in response to a delusion or a hallucination.

Epidemiology: The exact incidence is unclear. It is diagnosed in all age groups; the onset is more common during preadolescence and young adulthood. This is more common in children as compared to adults (in proportion of 7:1). Female predominance increases with age. "Automatic" hair pulling occurs in approximately three-quarters of adult patients with trichotillomania.

Clinical features: Commonly scalp hair, rarely from eyebrows, eyelashes, pubic hair, and torso hair, with hair loss being minimal to extensive are its clinical features. Clinical examination will reveal a typical presentation which will have three-phase zones:

Zone 1: Long hair (normal hair, unaffected hair, no pathology will be visible).

Zone 2: Missing hair (recent hair loss/alopecia as a result of hair pulling).

Zone 3: Hair in the phase of regrowth which will be short and will not be regular unlike the normal hair (irregular hair growth area because of growing hairs in alopecia area which in turn get affected by repeated hair pulling).

There is a term called "Rapunzel syndrome" in which the individual suffering from trichotillomania will eat/swallow (trichophagia) the plucked hairs repeatedly and the swallowed hairs get accumulated in the stomach forming a hair ball with a tail at times (known as tricobezoar), and these need surgical interventions.

The episodes of hair pulling can occur periodically for brief periods which will be in different times of the day. At times, these episodes can be seen for prolonged periods also, sometimes for hours. The individuals will not come to clinical attention at the beginning as it will not be glaringly obvious in the beginning and the patient does not consider it as an issue. By the time they reach clinical services, few months or years would already have passed.

Diagnosis: This condition is diagnosed mainly based on the clinical examination. When confirmation is needed or when the presentation is not clear, scalp biopsy is considered. Scalp biopsy shows a normal, noninflamed dermis in which there will be empty anagen hair follicles and normally growing hair. Specific hair morphology which are seen: Hair shafts are bizarrely fractured, there will be pigment casts, distorted and curled hair bulb (trichomalacia), and there can be perifollicular hematoma. Trichogram will show a reduced telogen rate.

Psychological basis: Typically, it is an impulse-control disorder and as a feature of this disorder, prior to hair pulling there is a gradual escalation and building up of anxiety/tension. This is followed by an urge to pull or pluck the hair. After plucking the hair, the individual feels relieved and the tension/anxiety subsides. There will be a sense of satisfaction; an individual experiences a sort of pleasure or feels relaxed after the act. It will be difficult to find any psychopathology as such in childhood trichotillomania patients. In children, it may be usually a habitual disorder or may be associated with thumb sucking and/or nail biting. In adults, the comorbid conditions are depression, anxiety disorder, and OCD.

Management
Children: Elicit any stressor. Parental education about the disorder is essential; then behavior-modification strategies are to be followed—usually habit reversal techniques are used.

Adolescents and young adults: Habit reversal techniques.

Habit reversal therapy: The basic assumption in this form of therapy is that the behavior is more like a habit which gets triggered in situations or is usually preceded by something. Individuals are taught to identify these triggers/situations in which they have an urge to pull/pluck their hair. Subsequently, they will be taught about how to substitute this behavior of hair plucking with some other behavior.

Components: The therapy has many components and the integral part of it is relaxation training. Other components include the following:
- *Awareness training/self-monitoring*: In the initial couple of sessions, the person's goal is to recognize the triggers/situations

which lead to hair pulling or to find the premonitory features prior to the hair pulling.
- *Competence behavior*: Subsequently, an individual is supposed to substitute the behavior of hair pulling/picking with other behaviors which can be more conducive and adaptive which can include fist clenching to cease the urge or redirecting one's hand movements toward ears or squeezing a rubber ball.
- *Generalization of behavior*: Once behavior is substituted, the individual needs to practice the newly learnt skill in varying situations to ingrain it in the usual routine life.
- *Stimulus control*: Another essential aspect is to make changes in the environment based on the identification of the triggers. This will help in reducing the emergence of any opportunities for the individual to go for any hair pull/pluck or pick. Simple modifications can include asking individuals to be in the vicinity or keep the room door open at workplace/home as the act is usually done when alone and the presence of people around will prevent this, wearing a cap or scarf to cover the scalp, wearing gloves when alone, or try to strap the fingers used for plucking hairs.
- *Cognitive restructuring*: In this, the individual's thought process is evaluated and any distorted belief is made aware of. Subsequently, the distorted belief is discussed and replaced with a more adaptive understanding which in turn translates into a healthy behavior.
- *Acceptance and commitment therapy (ACT)*: Here, the person is taught to recognize and accept one's own thoughts and urges but to avoid acting on those urges.
- *Pharmacotherapy*: Several medications have been tried and have shown significant results in hair-pulling disorder and skin-pricking disorder. The following medications can be used:
  - *N-acetyl cysteine (NAC)*: It can be tried in the adequate dose range of 1,200–2,400 mg/day for an adequate duration of 3 months.
  - *Selective serotonin reuptake inhibitors (SSRIs)*: For trichotillomania and other disorders in OCD spectrum including impulse control disorders, SSRIs are the usual first line of choice of drugs. Another drug which has been found to be effective is clomipramine.
  - *Second-generation antipsychotics (SGAs)/atypical antipsychotics*: Antipsychotics are usually the second line of option or at times are added as add-on drugs in these. Among SGAs, olanzapine is the preferred drug because of effectiveness.

However, other antipsychotics aripiprazole, risperidone, and typical antipsychotic haloperidol have also been of benefit in few studies.
- *Naltrexone*: It is an opioid antagonist which is usually preferred in the treatment of addiction disorders to reduce the craving or urge of substance seeking. This principle is the basis of using this drug in trichotillomania where the individual's urge to pull/pluck hair needs to be reduced.
- *Liaison approach*: These conditions can have best outcomes when managed in liaison with psychiatry and clinical psychology departments. Usually, the diagnosis is made after excluding the mimicking conditions. Invariably comorbid mental health ailments exist which must be addressed by a psychiatrist. Addressing comorbid conditions will also help in preventing relapses.

Prognosis: Childhood/adolescent cases usually have a good prognosis but the onset at later life will not have good prognosis.

Case Vignette

A 16-year-old adolescent girl was brought by father with the complaint that his daughter is having hair loss since 6 months. History revealed that it started 6 months ago, during her 10th standard main examination. She reported that she was anxious during that period so unknowingly, while studying, she would pluck scalp hairs and put them in book which she was reading. She would go on doing this daily. After her exams got over, she continued this hair plucking; while watching TV she would just pluck scalp hairs, sometimes eyebrows and throw them or sometime would eat them. There was no specific reason for this, but she would feel anxious if she did not do it; after plucking hair, she would feel relieved and would continue this act. On examination, she had scalp hairs of different lengths, hairs were broken, and some patchy hair loss was also noticed. She was admitted and was diagnosed with trichotillomania and started on fluoxetine for relief of anxiety and compulsive behavior. Habit reversal techniques and relaxation exercises are taught. She was followed up regularly and she stopped hair plucking.

Trichotemnomania
It is a rare entity, in which the hair is intentionally cut off.

Trichoteiromania (Greek teiro, "I scratch")
In this condition, there is pseudoalopecia. This is the result of recurrent scratching and rubbing of the scalp.

The differences between these are mentioned in **Table 5**.

Malingering

Malingering is defined as "intentional and conscious creation and elaboration of physical or psychiatric symptoms, in order to obtain tangible benefit". A variety of injuries are seen: Mechanical injuries from pressing, rubbing, biting, cutting, stabbing, or burning; self-inflicted infections with wound-healing impairments, abscesses, mutilations, acid burns, or other toxic damages to the skin.

Since is the injuries intentional and conscious, they are hardly amenable to interventions as there is no patient motivation. So, after rapport building and confirmation, confrontation is the best way to proceed in such patients with caution to avoid any act of self-harm.

Table 5: Trichotillomania, trichotemnomania, trichoteiromania.

	Trichotillomania	Trichotemno-mania	Trichoteiromania
Pattern of trauma	Pulling/picking out the hair	Severing/cutting off the hair	Scratching which leads to hair break
Examination findings	*Three phases*: Normal hair, patch of hair loss, hair in regrowing phase	There will be hair stubble which appears as shaved and pseudoalopecia	Hair with normal thickness but broken in few areas; white hair stubble with ragged ends
Investigation: Trichogram	Reduction in the telogen rate	No abnormality	Reduction in proportion of telogen; root appears dystrophic

Special Forms

Gardner–Diamond Syndrome (Autoerythrocyte Sensitization or Painful Ecchymoses Syndrome or Psychogenic Purpura or Painful Bruising Syndrome)

Gardner–Diamond syndrome (autoerythrocyte sensitization or painful ecchymoses syndrome or psychogenic purpura or painful bruising syndrome) is a rare condition, and this is seen mostly in young females but it can occur in males and children/adolescents also.

Clinical Features

In this condition, there are blue patches which are painful and they appear periodically. In addition, the individual will have multiple somatic complaints and psychiatric symptoms. The usual affected sites are extremities, but legs are more commonly affected. There will be a burning pain after the initial itching sensation; then ecchymoses and erythematous plaques will appear. All these will heal within 1–2 weeks without any scarring as this happens periodically. However, there will be symptoms related to lesions in the internal organs, like pain in abdomen, hematuria, headache, paresthesias, menorrhagia, and vomiting, diarrhea.

Münchausen Syndrome

Münchausen syndrome is characterized by the triad of hospital wandering, pathological lying, and self-injury. It denotes malingering/simulation of acute diseases with a demonstrative dramatic description of complaints and false information. Dermatological manifestations are less reported.

Münchausen-by-proxy Syndrome

In this syndrome, primary caretakers injure own children. This is being done to get in touch with the health professionals. Usually, the mother inflicts injuries and seeks medical intervention. Bleeding, seizures, clouding of consciousness up to and including respiratory arrest, diarrhea, vomiting, fever, and skin changes with scratching, acid burns, or occlusions may be seen.

# DERMATOSES AS A RESULT OF DELUSIONAL ILLNESSES AND HALLUCINATIONS

Delusion of Parasitosis/Ekbom's Syndrome

In this, the patient has delusion that his body is infested with parasites. It is a rare disease, and the exact prevalence rate is unknown.

Clinical Profile

Usually, it is seen in middle aged/elderly socially isolated females. They complain of itching, tingling, pain, or formication, coupled with the subjective certainty that the symptoms are being caused by insects, mites, worms, or other parasites. They justify this by reporting of perceptions (tactile hallucinations) that insects were crawling in body, burrowing, and biting at multiple places; in addition, they report of visualizing (visual hallucinations) them. Manipulations of the skin in an attempt to remove the assumed parasites are common acts which lead to excoriations, erosions, cuts, and burns. They may apply various lotions, antimicrobial ointments, and chemicals, and sometimes burn the area also. They will remove the assumed pathogen (which usually will be foreign matter, skin structures, fibers) and bring them to the clinician in small boxes.

Differential Diagnosis

Psychiatric disorders–psychotic disorders: Schizophrenia, mania with psychotic symptoms, severe depression with psychotic symptoms, formication, during cocaine withdrawal (cocaine bugs), or withdrawal from alcohol or amphetamine. Physical illnesses like neurosyphilis, stroke, and multiple sclerosis.

Management

Antipsychotic medication can be started and pimozide has shown to be the most effective antipsychotic in these. Due to a better response and favorable side effects, second-generation antipsychotics like olanzapine, risperidone, and amisulpride are preferred. Due to certain cardiac side effects, pimozide is less preferred.

> **Case Vignette**
>
> A 56-year-old diabetic male was referred from plastic surgery department for evaluation of self-harm attempt as he had burned his scalp. History revealed that he was working as a forest officer; while he went for rounds couple of years ago, he felt some insects had entered his body. Subsequently, he started reporting of insects crawling underneath his skin and moving around all over. He would try to pick them up and would remove some skin/scalp tissue. As it continued, he started rubbing tobacco over body to kill insects, unsatisfied with response; he thought insects will die if exposed to heat. So, he would hold his head over flame for 1/2–1 hour. While doing so, he ended up burning his scalp. On examination, there were excoriations, ulcerations, and dark pigmentation of skin of the whole body. He was diagnosed with delusional parasitosis and started on treatment with pimozide and was psychoeducated about illness. Over a period of follow-ups, his symptoms have decreased.

Bromhidrosis

Bromhidrosis is characterized by subjective unpleasant odor resulting from physiological sweat. Another variant is chromhidrosis, in which there is secretion of subjectively colored sweat. This is also known as olfactory reference disorder and in the recent classification of ICD 11, this is a distinct category. The patient would try to check his smell repeatedly. He would apply perfumes to mask the smell. In addition, the person seeks reassurance from others that there is no smell. First, an attempt has to be made to educate the patient about the ailment and the person has to be conveyed that there will be physiological normal variations. Low-dose antipsychotics will be of help in individuals who lack insight.

> **Case Vignette**
>
> A 36-year-old clerk working in the government sector presented with complaints of sweat smelling foul. History revealed that he was working in office and sharing hall along with others. Since 6 months, he started noticing that whenever people pass him, they would rub nose. Then he started feeling that his sweat was smelling foul. He would inhale and feel foul smell. He would enquire with colleagues, friends, and family members, who all denied any smell. But he was not convinced and would

get foul smell. He would use deo sprays repeatedly and would take bath thrice daily. Despite this, he felt that his sweat continued to smell foul. He was diagnosed with bromhidrosis. As his conviction was almost at delusional level, he was started on low-dose antipsychotic—pimozide—and explained about illness. There was partial improvement in the next couple of months.

Hypochondriacal Delusions

Hypochondriacal delusion is characterized by persistent, delusional belief/preoccupation with the fear or conviction of suffering from a serious physical disease. The delusions vary with a patient's social/educational/cultural and economic background. In the past, patients were more concerned about syphilis; currently, patients present with delusion of having contracted acquired immunodeficiency syndrome (AIDS). Usually, delusions will be of life-threatening disease or cancer. Before arriving at diagnosis, schizophrenia and anxiety disorders have to be ruled out. In delusional cutaneous hypochondriasis, second-generation antipsychotics are usually the first line of drugs. In patients where the diagnosis is unclear and appears like somatoform disorder, SSRIs can be used. All these have to be supplemented with psychotherapy for better outcomes.

Case Vignette

A 42-year-old barber was referred from medicine for evaluation of anxiety. He presented with complaints of having typhoid since 2 years. History revealed that he was diagnosed with typhoid 3 years ago, during which he had abdominal pain, felt tired, and felt his face had become dark. After treatment, he recovered well. However, 2 years ago he started noticing that his face was becoming dark, so he concluded that he was suffering from typhoid again. He started feeling weak, would remain preoccupied with illness, and stopped working. Then he went for investigations, which came as negative. He felt that it was faulty and went to a metro city and got evaluated; there also it was negative. Not satisfied with the report, he would go on getting investigated to the extent of visiting five laboratories per day. Also, he would feel that his face was becoming darker day-by-day. After evaluation, he was admitted and diagnosed with hypochondriacal disorder and started on escitalopram (SSRI), and cognitive behavioral therapy was initiated. Distraction techniques and relaxation techniques were also taught.

Body Dysmorphic Delusions

Body dysmorphic delusion consists of an "excessive preoccupation with an uncorrectable, imagined deficiency or disfigurement in the outward appearance, which is at delusional level". The preoccupation leads to dysfunction in multiple domains like social, occupational, family, personal, and other domains, and this makes them seek corrective procedures in the imagined disfigurement. Schizophrenia should be excluded. It is usually comorbid with OCD, depression, social anxiety disorder, and anxious avoidant personality disorder. Prevalence of this varied from 0.75 to 12% in different studies. It is usually seen in females in their 30s. Women's complaints are confined mainly to face, breast, hair, nose, and stomach, while men's concern is confined to hair, nose, ear, genitals, and body build. Suicidal ideation and suicide attempts are common (up to 30%).

Management

In case of poor insight, it is difficult to intervene. Since the perceived abnormality is dermatological, an individual will find it difficult to accept psychiatric intervention. If insight is good, they can be easily psychoeducated and will accept pharmacological interventions.

SOMATOFORM DISORDERS

In these patients, unexplained somatic complaints will be there. In context of dermatology, the symptoms can be unexplainable itching, dysesthesias, or nonobjectifiable hair loss.

Somatization Disorder

In this condition, there are multiple somatic complaints and these will be clinically significant complaints every time the individual visits the clinician. These will occur repeatedly and the individual will seek medical intervention. Multiorgan (gastrointestinal, sexual, neurological) symptoms are seen with pain being a common symptom. In dermatology, *ecosyndrome* is proxy of somatization disorders. Here, the individual will have multiple complaints and these will be attributed to plenty of intolerances. In this, the individual has a conviction that environmental toxins have made him/her sick.

CHAPTER 3: Primary Psychiatric Disorders: Cutaneous Manifestations

In the "total allergy syndrome," numerous "allergies" are held responsible for the complaints ("allergic to everything"). The individual will explain about presumed etiology as exposure to toxins in the environment, without any proof.

These disorders are summarized in **Table 6**.

Table 6: Overview of somatoform disorders in dermatology.

Somatoform disorder		Dermatoses
Somatization disorder	Environment syndrome	Ecosyndrome, multiple chemical sensitivity syndrome, sick-building syndrome
	Special forms	Food allergies, sperm allergy, detergent allergy, light allergy electrosmog, amalgam-related complaint syndrome
Hypochondriacal disorder	Hypochondriacal disorder in the actual sense	• Infections (fungal, parasitic, viral, bacterial) • Neoplasia
	Body dysmorphic disorder	• Whole body involvement: Dorian Gray syndrome • *Regional involvement*: Genitals, breast, head
	Special form	Botulinophilia
Somatoform autonomic function disorder	• Hyperhidrosis • Erythrophobia • Goose bumps	
Persistent somatoform pain disorder	Cutaneous dysesthesias	• Glossodynia—orofacial pain syndrome • Trichodynia • Anodynia, phallodynia, vulvodynia

Other somatoform disorders	Sensory complaints	• *Itching*:
		  ○ Localized somatoform itching
		  ○ Generalized somatoform itching (pruritus sine materia)
		• Paresthesias
		• Burning
		• Stabbing

Psychogenic Pruritus

Here, the patient has intractable or persistent itch, not ascribed to any physical or dermatological illness. The diagnostic criteria for this are listed in **Box 2**. The subtypes are described in **Table 7**.

Clinical Features

Itching/scratching episodes have abrupt onset and abrupt termination. These usually occur when the individual is not focusing on anything and at night or while relaxing.

Most Common Sites

Sites which are easily accessible to fingers are commonly involved like genitals, arms, and legs.

BOX 2: Diagnostic criteria for psychogenic pruritus.

Three compulsory criteria are as follows:
1. Localized or generalized pruritus sine material
2. Chronic pruritus (>6 weeks)
3. Absence of a somatic cause

Three additional criteria from the following seven:
1. A chronological relationship of pruritus with one or several life events that could have psychological repercussions
2. Variations of intensity associated with stress
3. Nocturnal variation
4. Predominance during rest or inaction
5. Associated psychological disorders
6. Pruritus that is improved by psychogenic drugs
7. Pruritus that is improved by psychotherapy

Table 7: Subtypes of psychogenic pruritus.

Compulsive type	Impulsive type	Mixed type
Skin excoriation is done as a response to obsession or anxiety	Skin excoriation is done for pleasure, arousal, or for decreasing tension	Both features are present
Individual is fully aware while doing it	At time, individual does it automatically	–
Tries to resist at times	No resistance is seen as such	–

There will be a history of a stress preceding to the onset of this condition. Further, comorbid anxiety and/or depression is commonly seen. It is diagnosed when other cutaneous and systemic conditions have been ruled out after detailed evaluation and investigations.

Management
Usually, psychotherapy helps. In addition, SSRIs are useful.

> **Case Vignette**
>
> A 46-year-old lady working as labor in a construction firm came with complaints of generalized itching since 6 years. History revealed that she felt that her workplace is clogged with dust and other chemicals, which leads to itching all over body. Further, she reported that, while working, she would not have any itch; however, after her dinner, when she lies down for sleep, she starts getting itch, especially in inguinal region/groin and back. She would feel relieved after scratching. Even on days when she did not go for work, she would have itching. While at home, watching TV, or relaxing, she would start getting itch. Further, she expressed that there are financial restraints and husband abuses alcohol. She was diagnosed with psychogenic pruritus and started on sertraline (SSRI), and supportive psychotherapy was initiated; also, habit reversal techniques were used as behavioral measures.

DERMATOSES AS A RESULT OF COMPULSIVE DISORDERS

Compulsive thoughts/obsessions are repeated/recurrent, persistent thoughts/impulses/ideations which will be irrational and intrusive and evoke significant anxiety. Compulsive acts are the behaviors as a response to the obsessions. Compulsive disorders may also be present as comorbidity with certain dermatoses. They are mentioned in **Box 3**.

Washing Eczema

Here, the patient has an obsession of contamination with germ, dirt, and infections. This leads to anxiety and distress; to relieve this anxiety, the patient repeatedly washes hands, feet, face, etc. The washing practice may be very frequent to the extent of 50–200 times or duration of washing may be more like 5–10 minutes for hand washing, 1 hour for bathing, etc. Also, washing method and using soap to wash will be

> **BOX 3: Categorization of compulsive disorders.**
>
> *Certain compulsive disorders*:
> - Washing eczema
> - Primary lichen simplex chronicus
>
> *Frequent compulsive disorders*:
> - Trichotillomania
> - Body dysmorphic disorder
> - Cutaneous hypochondrias
> - Special multifactorial dermatoses (anal eczema, seborrheic eczema)

in excess. All these lead to eczematous changes, mycotic infections, and nail dystrophies.

Management includes pharmacotherapy with SSRIs, TCAs, and low-dose antipsychotics clubbed with cognitive behavioral therapy focusing on exposure to dirt and preventing response of washing.

Primary Lichen Simplex Chronicus

Primary lichen simplex chronicus is a chronic pruritic lichenoid plaque. In this condition, there is thickening of the skin areas. This is usually provoked and maintained by repeated rubbing or scratching. An emotional disorder is primarily seen along with this; occasionally, it is associated with atopic eczema.

Sites Involved

It is commonly seen in posterior neck, extensor aspect of the extremities, axillae, and genital area.

Psychiatric Symptoms

Obsession of itch and compulsion of scratching are seen.

Differential Diagnosis

It is a group of prurigo diseases (prurigo simplex acuta, prurigo simplex subacuta, and prurigo simplex chronica), paraartefactas.

Management

Pharmacotherapy with SSRIs, TCAs, and low-dose antipsychotics clubbed with cognitive behavioral therapy focusing on preventing scratching/rubbing are recommended.

CONCLUSION

Primary psychiatric disorders are widely prevalent in the population with dermatological disorders. Recent research in this area has lead to conceptual understanding and classification of these disorders, which are divided into subgroups for the ease of understanding, evaluation and interventions. Many of these will require a comprehensive evaluation from dermatological and psychological aspects. Psychopharmacotherapy and psychotherapy have evidence in managing these conditions and these should be prioritized in managing these conditions.

FURTHER READINGS

1. Baranska-Rybak W, Cubala WJ, Kozicka D, Sokołowska-Wojdyło M, Nowicki R, Roszkiewicz J. Dermatitis artefacta: Along way from the first clinical symptoms to diagnosis. Psychiatr Danub. 2011;23(1):73-5.
2. Bewley A, Magid M, Reichenberg JS, et al. Introduction. In: Bewley A, Taylor RE, Reichenberg JS, Magid M (Eds). Practical Psychodermatology. Chichester: Wiley Blackwell; 2014. pp. 3-10.
3. Chamberlain SR, Menzies L, Sahakian BJ, Fineberg NA. Lifting the veil on trichotillomania. Am J Psychiatry. 2007;164(4):568-74.
4. Demaret A. Nail-biting, hair-plucking, and grooming. Ann Med Psychol (Paris). 1973;2:235-42.
5. Ehsani AH, Toosi S, Shahshahani MM, Arabi M, Noormohammadpour P. Psychocutaneous disorders: an epidemiologic study. J Eur Acad Dermatol Venereol. 2009;23(8):945-7.
6. Ferreira BR, Jafferany M. Classification of psychodermatological disorders. J Cosmet Dermatol. 2021;20:1-3.
7. Ferreira BR, Jafferany M, Patel A (Eds). Classification and terminology of psychodermatologic disorders. In: The Essentials of Psychodermatology. Cham: Springer International Publishing; 2020. pp. 37-46.
8. ICD-11 for Mortality and Morbidity Statistics. (2023). [online] Available from https://icd.who.int/browse11/l-m/en [Last accessed January, 2024].

9. Koo JYM, Lee CS (Eds). General approach to evaluating psychodermatological disorders. In: Psychocutaneous Medicine: Basic and Clinical Dermatology. New York: Marcel Dekker; 2003. pp. 1-12.
10. Millard L. Dermatitis artefacta in the 1990s. Br J Dermatol. 1996;135:27.
11. Munoli RN. Psychodermatology: An overview of history, concept, classification, and current status. Ind J Priv Psychiatry. 2020;14:85-91.
12. Phillips KA, Menard W. Suicidality in body dysmorphic disorder: A prospective study. Am J Psychiatry. 2006;163:1280-2.
13. Radmanesh M, Shafei S. Underlying psychopathologies of psychogenic pruritic disorders. Dermatol Psychosom. 2001;2:130-3.
14. Reichenberg JS, Kroumpouzos G, Magid M. Approach to a psychodermatology patient. G Ital Dermatol Venereol. 2018;153:494-6.
15. Veale D. Body dysmorphic disorder. Postgrad Med J. 2004;80:67-75.
16. Wong JW, Nguyen TV, Koo JY. Primary psychiatric conditions: dermatitis artefacta, trichotillomania and neurotic excoriations. Indian J Dermatol. 2013;58(1):44-8.

CHAPTER 4

Secondary Psychiatric Disorders in Dermatology Patients

Sreejayan Kongasseri

> **Key Messages**
> - Patients with dermatological illness suffer high rates of psychiatric comorbidity, particularly those with chronic dermatoses.
> - The secondary psychological disturbance could be syndromal psychiatric disorders or psychological reactions to the skin conditions.
> - The effective treatment of these disorders is facilitated by a close liaison between dermatologist, psychiatrist, and psychologist.

INTRODUCTION

This category of disorders includes patients who have psychological symptoms secondary to the skin disorder, which is usually chronic and disfiguring, taxing on the patient's coping skills and affecting their self-confidence, interpersonal relationships, and quality of life. The course of such dermatoses is characterized by exacerbations and remissions, and the patients' initial enthusiasm to new treatments wanes off leading to a stage where they have to learn to live with the condition. How successfully they are to be able to do this depends on their psychological resources and resilience.

EPIDEMIOLOGY

Compared to general population, psychosomatic disorders are more prevalent among dermatological patients. The rates are twice among inpatients than among outpatients. The prevalence of psychiatric disorders among dermatological patients is slightly higher than that of neurological, oncology, and cardiac patients combined. In a multicenter European study conducted to assess the psychological burden of skin diseases, which included 3,635 patients and 1,359 controls, clinical depression was present in 10.1% patients (controls 4.3%), clinical anxiety in 17.2% (controls 11.1%), and suicidal ideation was reported by 12.7% of all patients (controls 8.3%). Only patients with psoriasis had significant association with suicidal ideation. Patients with psoriasis, atopic dermatitis, hand eczema, and leg ulcers had the highest association with anxiety and depression. **Table 1** summarizes the prevalence rates of psychiatric disorders in various dermatological populations.

Table 1: Studies on prevalence of psychiatric disorders in various dermatological conditions.

Study	Dermatological disorder	Prevalence
Dalgard et al. 2015	All skin diseases	• Depression 10.1% (controls 4.3%) OR 2.40 (1.67–3.47) • Anxiety 17.2% (controls 11.1%) OR 2.18 (1.68–2.82) • Suicidal ideation 12.7% of all patients (controls 8.3%) OR 1.94 (1.33–2.82)
Shenoi et al. 2013	All patients in a psycho-dermatology clinic	• Depression (17%) • Adjustment disorder (5%) • Anxiety disorders (2.5%)
Altunay et al. 2020	Acne	Psychiatric morbidity (21%)
Samuels et al. 2020	Acne vulgaris	Meta-analysis significant association with depression ($r = 0.22$) and anxiety ($r = 0.25$)
Colon et al. 1991	Alopecia areata	Psychiatric morbidity (76%)
Sellami et al. 2014	Alopecia areata	• Depression (38%) • Anxiety (62%)
Mattoo et al. 2002	Vitiligo	Psychiatric morbidity (25%)
Matoo et al. 2001	Vitiligo	• Adjustment disorder (56%) • Depression (31%)
Matoo et al. 2001	Psoriasis	• Adjustment disorder (62%) • Depression (33%)

Continued

Continued

Study	Dermatological disorder	Prevalence
Olivier et al. 2010	Psoriasis	• Hazard ratio • Depression (1.39) • Anxiety (1.31) • Suicidality (1.44)
Mathur et al. 2023	• Chronic plaque • Psoriasis	• Depression 49.3% • Anxiety 28.6% • Suicidal ideation 7.8% • Alcohol use disorder 16.4%
Arbabi et al. 2011	Pemphigus	Psychiatric morbidity (74%)
Slattery et al. 2011	Atopic dermatitis (adolescents)	• Depression (9%) • Anxiety (26%) • Social anxiety (14%)
Cvetkovski et al. 2006	Hand eczema	Depression (9%)
Onderdijk. 2013	Hidradenitis suppurativa	Depression (9%) not different from controls
Sawant et al. 2015	Lichen planus	Depression (25%)
Brenaut et al, 2019	Prurigo	• Depression 37% • Anxiety 29% • Suicidal ideations 19%

CLASSIFICATION

The psychiatric disorder in a patient with a dermatological condition could be due to various reasons: As a comorbid condition, as an emotional reaction to the chronic dermatological condition or as an adverse effect of treatment for the dermatological condition:

- *Secondary psychiatric disorder as a comorbidity*: There could be common predisposing factors for dermatoses and psychiatric disorder. Cytokines and inflammatory factors, which are elevated in conditions like psoriasis, can also predispose to depression; however, alopecia areata, which does not have abnormal cytokine levels, is also associated with depression. Brain-derived neurotrophic factor (BDNF) has been seen to be reduced in vitiligo and depression. Medical conditions like diabetes, hypothyroidism, and systemic lupus erythematosus can cause dermatoses and organic psychiatric disorders (secondary to medical cause).

- *Secondary psychiatric disorder as a reaction to dermatoses*: In addition to its physiological functions, skin is also an organ of importance in social interaction. The initial social assessment of a person by another is solely based on skin and facial features. Under the influence of media, the modern society's preoccupation with body image is ever increasing. Chronic skin diseases are often disfiguring and cause embarrassment and discrimination. A person's perception of body image, self-esteem, and confidence is lowered and leads to a strained relationship with the partner and sexual dysfunction. Others may consider the condition as contagious and actively avoid the patient. This leads to discrimination, stigmatization, and social isolation. The stigma is not just external (from the society) but also internal (from the patient). Many patients cope with this and may not develop psychological morbidity. Those with maladaptive coping develop depression, anxiety disorders (including social anxiety), adjustment disorders, substance abuse, and suicidal ideations. How well one is able to cope depends on their childhood experiences and personality traits. Excessive importance to physical attractiveness, sensitivity to criticism, poor self-esteem, inability to maintain relationships, high neuroticism, and use of maladaptive defences are some factors that predict poor coping. Patients with psoriasis have been reported to have higher scores for alexithymia (deficiency in understanding, processing and describing emotions) which was associated with both anxiety and depression scores. Psychological morbidity is higher among patients with chronic, resistant, and exposed site dermatoses. Teenagers with acne were perceived by others as shy, nerdy, stressed, lonely, boring, unkempt, unhealthy, introverted, and rebellious. They reported lower self-confidence or shyness, difficulty finding dates, problems making friends, challenges with school, and trouble getting a job. Associated psychiatric condition results in further worsening of their quality of life, poor compliance to treatment, and poor doctor–patient relationship. Fear of certain medications like corticosteroids, methotrexate, and cyclosporine may have a negative impact on treatment adherence. The dermatological malignancies could be associated with excessive anxiety about recurrence after treatment and body image disturbance after surgery.
- *Secondary psychiatric disorders as treatment-emergent psychiatric conditions*: The drugs used for treatment of dermatoses can cause

psychiatric symptoms, especially in the elderly and those with pre-existing psychiatric disorders. Such adverse effects lead to emotional suffering, increase in disability, length of stay in the hospital, mortality (including suicide), noncompliance, lack of recovery from the primary condition, harm to others and self, and increased utilization of healthcare services.

Table 2 shows some of the psychological adverse effects of dermatological medications. Management includes reducing dose or substituting with another medication. In severe cases, psychotropics may be required to treat the condition. Patients who are on medications that are known to cause psychological adverse effects should be screened frequently.

Many patients may not have a syndromal psychiatric diagnosis; nevertheless, their mental health could be significantly affected

Table 2: Psychological adverse effects of dermatological medications.

Medications	Psychological adverse effects
Antiretrovirals (Efavirenz, Zidovudine, Abacavir, Nevirapine, Combivir)	Depression, suicidal thoughts, auditory hallucinations, psychosis
Cephalosporins	Euphoria, delirium, delusions, depersonalization, illusions. Renal disease is a risk factor
Corticosteroids	Psychosis, delirium, mania, depression: 1–3% incidence, may be dose-related, can also occur during withdrawal
Estrogens	Panic attacks, depression
Fluoroquinolone antibiotics	Acute psychosis, confusion, agitation, depression, hallucinations, paranoia, Tourette-like syndrome, mania
H1 antihistamines	Hallucinations, confusion, agitation, delirium: With first-generation drugs. Rarely, with second-generation agents
H2 antihistamines	Delirium, confusion, psychosis, mania, aggression, depression, nightmares: Especially in the elderly and seriously ill
Nonsteroidal anti-inflammatory drug	Depression, paranoia, psychosis, confusion, anxiety: More common with indomethacin

Continued

Continued

Medications	Psychological adverse effects
Procaine derivatives (procainamide procaine penicillin G)	Fear of imminent death, hallucinations, illusions, delusions, agitation, mania, depersonalization, psychosis
Acyclovir	Hallucinations, fearfulness, confusion, insomnia, hyperacusis, paranoia, depression: At high doses and renal failure
Amphotericin B	Delirium
Dapsone	Insomnia, agitation, hallucinations, mania, depression: May occur even with low doses
Isoniazid	Psychosis, hallucinations, mania
Isotretinoin	Depression, suicidality
Thalidomide	Reversible dementia

Source: The Medical Letter, Volume 50, Issue 1301/1302, December 15/29, 2008.

due to the psychological reaction to the dermatoses. The secondary psychological disturbances can be broadly divided as given in the following text.

Psychosocial Reactions

Disfigurement

Disfigurement is a condition which causes a visible difference on the skin and lowers its aesthetic value. It could be congenital (e.g., hemangiomas) or acquired (e.g., trauma, vitiligo) leading to negative social experiences resulting in excessive preoccupation with appearance and excessive scanning for others' reactions and many times misinterpreting them. The visibility of the disfigurement and how different the lesion is from others determine its significance. Culture (whether there is emphasis on physical appearance), coping styles, social interaction skills, family environment, and social support mediate the distress. The developmental stage of the subject's life also plays an important role in experiencing distress. A disfigurement in child could affect the parent's attitude and affect the bonding between them. In adolescence, it could lead to poor peer acceptance, bullying, and difficulties in interaction with the opposite gender. In adulthood, it can be a barrier to desired employment and partner intimacy. For most people, by old age, the significance of physical attributes comes down and it is easier to adjust to the disfigurement. Surgical procedures can help normalize appearance. Educating the patient, providing a realistic evaluation of their situation, supportive therapy, cognitive behavioral therapy, and social skills training are useful nonpharmacological management strategies. Changing faces is a self-help group that has been successful in reducing distress by their interventions. A possibility of associated body dysmorphophobia or depression should be considered if the distress is more than what would be expected for the lesion.

Stigmatization

According to Goffman, stigma is an attribute that extensively discredits an individual, reducing them "from a whole and usual person to a tainted, discounted one." Stigma consists of five components: (i) identifying and labelling human differences, (ii) stereotyping, (iii) separating "them" from "us", (iv) experience of discrimination, and (v) loss of their status and inability to exercise power. Stigma may be internalized (from the individual toward self) or externalized (from the society). Conditions like psoriasis and vitiligo are associated with stigma. Stigmatization endangers personal identity, social life, and economic opportunities.

Internalized stigma is managed by supportive therapy and psychoeducation. Externalized stigma is managed by changing the attitudes of the society toward dermatological illness through health education and media campaigning.

Impaired Quality of Life

The terms "quality of life" and, more specifically, "health-related quality of life" refer to the physical, psychological, and social domains of health, seen as distinct areas that are influenced by a person's experiences, beliefs, expectations, and perceptions. Chronic dermatoses cause poorer quality of life. The quality of life is further impacted by the secondary psychiatric disorders. Improvements in quality of life can be brought about by a comprehensive management plan that includes medical, psychological, and social inputs.

Suicide

Suicidal expressions range from being weary of one's life (taedium vitae), a wish that one is better off dead (death wishes), suicidal ideation, suicidal plans, suicidal attempts, and completed suicide, and this often progresses in a continuum, making it necessary to detect the initial presentations to prevent mortality. Chronic illness is a risk factor for suicide. In studies, psoriasis, acne, and atopic dermatitis have been associated with suicidal thoughts. The percentage of patients with suicidal ideas was found to be highest for psoriasis (2.5–21.2%) followed by atopic dermatitis (2–18%) and acne (8%). Patients with eczema and urticaria were not at a higher risk of developing suicidal ideations. Presence of depression increases the risk of suicide. Clinicians should regularly inquire for suicidal ideations in their assessments and if screened positive, the patient should be referred to a mental health professional who would complete a risk assessment and management. Treatment plan will involve medications for comorbid psychiatric disorders and psychotherapy. Negotiating a "no suicide contract"—a written promise that the patient would not end their life for a specific short period of time—and providing them with contacts to call can be an effective safety plan in a dermatology clinic.

Psychiatric Disorders

Depression

Depression is characterized by sad mood, marked loss of pleasure in activities, poor concentration, low self-esteem or inappropriate guilt, hopelessness, suicidal thoughts, disturbed sleep or excessive sleep, changes in appetite, agitation or slowness, and fatigue. A diagnosis of depression can be made if 5 out of these 10 symptoms occur most of the day for 2 weeks [International Classification of Diseases 11th revision (ICD-11)]. Persistent depressive disorder (dysthymia) is mild but a long-term (chronic) form of depression lasting at least for 2 years, usually with stressors in the background. Patients with depression may complain of pains or may report symptoms (e.g., pruritus) more than that is expected from their clinical severity. Mild depression can be managed by cognitive behavioral therapy or interpersonal therapy. Moderate-to-severe depression requires a combination of medication and psychotherapy for effective treatment. Selective serotonin reuptake inhibitors (SSRIs; escitalopram, fluoxetine, sertraline, vortioxetine), serotonin norepinephrine reuptake inhibitors (SNRIs; mirtazapine, venlafaxine, desvenlafaxine, duloxetine), and tricyclic antidepressants are evidence-based treatment for depression. Drugs like mirtazapine and tricyclics have antihistaminergic action that may help with pruritus. Agomelatine is a newer antidepressant that works on the melatonin receptors and does not have the side effects of SSRIs and SNRIs. Bupropion acts by inhibiting the dopamine and norepinephrine uptake.

Anxiety Disorders

Anxiety disorders are characterized by anxiety associated with autonomic arousal. Chronic anxiety can lead to cognitive symptoms (like poor concentration) and physical symptoms (pains). Anxiety can be comorbid with depression. Panic disorders are episodes of intense anxiety occurring out of the blue lasting for a few minutes to hours. Though patients may have good interepisodic recovery initially with time, anxiety persists in between the episodes. Generalized anxiety disorder is characterized by free floating anxiety with excessive and disproportionate anxiety about several aspects of life, such as work, social relationships, or financial matters. Phobias present as persistent anxiety on being exposed to a situation or an object which the patient commits to great lengths in avoiding. Anxiety is typically disproportional to the actual danger posed and is recognized as irrational. Patients with disfiguring conditions may develop social phobia. Dermatologists also come across patients with needle phobias and blood phobias during a procedure.

Treatment consists of SSRIs or SNRIs with cognitive behavioral therapy. An episode of acute anxiety may be managed with benzodiazepines. However, patients have a high risk of developing dependence, and long-term prescription of benzodiazepines is discouraged.

Adjustment Disorders

Adjustment disorders are emotional disorders with depressive or anxiety symptoms that are precipitated by a negative life event and cause significant personal and socio-occupational dysfunction. The onset of a dermatological condition could precipitate adjustment disorder.

Psychosis

Psychosis is usually an adverse reaction to medications, mostly corticosteroids. The prominent symptoms are hallucinations (perceptions without stimuli) and delusions (beliefs that are not true). The patient presents as paranoid, and thinking may be affected. Their judgment may be impaired which may lead to non-cooperation with treatment, aggression and difficulties for caregiver. Management includes ensuring safety and liaison with a psychiatrist. The patient may need to be managed in a psychiatric inpatient unit for containment. The implicated medication is stopped and an alternative considered. If the ongoing treatment is necessary, dose reduction may be the option. Due to acuity of their presentation, antipsychotics will be required for symptomatic management. Second-generation antipsychotics (e.g., risperidone, quetiapine, olanzapine, aripiprazole) are the first-line treatment for psychosis.

Delirium

Delirium occurs due to impairment in brain functioning owing to various risk factors. It presents as confusion, disorientation, memory disturbances, sleep disturbances, hallucinations, fearfulness, delusions, and agitation. Delirium can be caused by a wide array of causes. Metabolic abnormalities, infections, and medications will be particularly important in a dermatology patient. Old age, polypharmacy, cognitive impairment, sensory impairment, and substance use are risk factors to developing delirium.

Low-dose antipsychotics and environmental manipulation are strategies used in management. Medications like benzodiazepines and anticholinergic agents can worsen delirium.

Substance Abuse

Substances are used to cope with stress or as self-medication for anxiety or depression. Alcohol and tobacco are the commonly used substances. Use of substances can complicate the dermatological condition and their treatment. Management includes pharmacological and nonpharmacological strategies.

SPECIAL POPULATIONS

Psychological difficulties in children do not present with typical symptoms as described among adults. A child with emotional problems may present with poor socialization, school refusal, academic decline, conduct problems, oppositional behavior, enuresis, or even regression of milestones in severe disturbances. Skin disorders and associated psychological disorders can cause impairment in emotional and cognitive development and predispose to psychiatric disorders and poor adjustment in adulthood. Treatment is provided through the child-mother-doctor triad.

Geriatric population with emotional difficulties can present with physical complaints, and an underlying psychological component can be easily missed. Often, psychological problems are considered to be part of old age and the treatment is delayed. Since it is often believed that elderly are less concerned about their body image, the impact of disfigurement due to dermatological conditions may be underestimated. Agism on the part of treating dermatologist, caretakers, and sometimes the patients themselves may lead to the elderly receiving suboptimal care and incomplete resolution of the symptoms due to less aggressive management than that would have been given to a younger person.

CONCLUSION

Psychiatric disorders are often associated with a dermatological condition. It can be difficult to determine if it is a comorbidity or a reaction to the dermatoses. Nevertheless, they cause significant impairment for the patient, worsen their quality of life, and complicate treatment. Depression is the most common presentation. Suicide is a significant cause of death among young population. Symptoms of psychiatric disorders can be masked by physical presentations, and it takes an alert clinician to identify them. Asking questions on mental health routinely in a dermatology clinic is an effective way to screen for these disorders. The treatment is a combination of pharmacology and psychotherapy. The treatment is best offered in liaison with mental health professionals in a dermatology clinic. Successful treatment of psychological disorder ensures better recovery and patient satisfaction.

Case Vignette 1

A 24-year-old lady presented to the psychodermatology clinic with lesions over the leg which were diagnosed as chronic dermatitis. She had a normal childhood development and did not have any significant medical or psychiatric illness previously. Five years back, her parents had died in a road accident. She was now staying with her uncle's family and her brothers were staying with another aunt. There was minimal interaction between them and the brothers were not ready to take her responsibility. During this period, she was suffering from unresolved grief due to her parents' death. Four months back, she had developed skin lesions. She was treated by many dermatologists with unsatisfactory outcomes before she consulted our clinic. Her aunt believed that the condition could be contagious and she needs to take extra precautions so that others would not get it. The aunt was also often critical of her and not happy that she was not helping in the household work. The aunt often blamed her for being a financial burden due to the skin condition on which they had spent a lot of money. Over the last 3 months, she reported of worsening of sadness, not being able to work as before due to tiredness and loss of interest in activities that she used to enjoy before. She often thought that she had become a burden on others. She would cry often when alone and would think of ending life to get out of the misery. She had even thought of ways to end her life. However, she did not go ahead with the plans because she was worried about the bad name she would bring to her uncle's family. Her sleep routine and appetite were disturbed. She reported to have become slow in all the activities. She was diagnosed to have severe depression and unresolved grief. She was prescribed escitalopram and a no-suicide contract was made. She was also taken up for supportive psychotherapy to help her cope with her grief and the stress due to her dermatological condition. This case highlights the role of psychosocial reactions to dermatoses leading to depression in a vulnerable individual.

Case Vignette 2

A 65-year-old man presented with 35 years' history of psoriasis to our psychodermatology clinic. The clinical course was characterized by frequent remissions and exacerbations. For the last 2 years, he had never reached complete remission. He had a normal childhood and did not have any significant past history. Eight years back, his wife had passed away and he was living with his sister. He did not have any children. He was working as an unskilled laborer but due to his illness was not able to go for work regularly. Most of his earning was spent on his medications. He had to sell his house few years back to clear the debts. Though his sister was supportive, her children would often be critical toward him. He reported of being sad most of the time for the last 10 years. In a day, his mood would cheer up when he would meet his friends and when he was with his sister. He also had difficulty in sleeping. He would sleep only for 4–5 hours per day and would feel unrefreshed on the next day morning. He often thought that he would have been better off dead. Eight years back, when his wife died his mood had worsened and he started drinking alcohol excessively for 3 months. After that his alcohol consumption had come down and now he drinks once or twice a month. He had also observed that his skin lesions would worsen when his emotional problems increased. He was diagnosed as dysthymia and was prescribed duloxetine. He was also taken up for supportive psychotherapy.

Case Vignette 3

A 25-year-old college student presented to our psychodermatology clinic with depigmentation around mouth for the last 1 year. She had a normal childhood development. She was above average in studies and had taken part in many dance and singing programs. She placed importance to looking good and considered herself one among the good-looking women in the college. She reported that after the lesions appeared, she has been excessively worried about them. She felt that they have caused a significant damage to her body image perception. She would think that the people are looking at her and may be making fun of her. Her self-esteem had become low. She lost her confidence and would feel anxious when she presented in front of her class or when she had to appear on stage. Sometimes, her anxiety would be so high that she would have palpitations, sweating, tremors, and dizziness. This affected her performance which in turn made her more anxious. She would always think that she was being scrutinized by others. She stopped meeting people or going out with them. Her interaction with the opposite gender also came down. She was diagnosed to have social anxiety and was treated with escitalopram. She was also taken up for cognitive behavior therapy for her social anxiety.

Case Vignette 4

A 23-year-old man presented to our psychodermatology clinic with lesions over the face for the last 6 months. He was diagnosed to have Darier's disease. He had a normal development and was attending college for postgraduation. He had limited benefits from treatment. He was reported to be an extrovert and was above average in studies. The lesions on his face were disfiguring. He reported of difficulties in attending college and facing peers. On some occasions, when he had attended classes due to parent's coercion, he reported of people looking at him in a "weird" way and many of them asking him about his condition repeatedly. Some of his friends were avoiding him. He refused to go to college anymore and was homebound. He would not meet his friends or talk to them if they called him over the phone. He started feeling lonely and would be sad most of the time. His mood would lift up only when he watched his favorite movies. People coming home would fill him with dread and would start feeling anxious. His sleep was disturbed due to constant worrying. He was upset about losing a year in college as he had not taken exams. The thoughts of having to attend classes with his juniors next year made him anxious. He would often think that he is better off dead; however, he was hopeful that his condition would be cured. A diagnosis of adjustment disorder was made and he was prescribed sertraline. He was also taken up for supportive therapy by the clinical psychologist.

FURTHER READINGS

1. Altunay IK, Özkur E, Dalgard FJ, Gieler U, Aragones LT, Lien L, et al. Psychosocial aspects of adult acne: data from 13 European countries. Acta dermato-venereologica. 2020;100(4):adv00051.
2. Arbabi M, Ghodsi Z, Mahdanian A, Noormohammadi N, Shalileh K, Darvish F, et al. Mental health in patients with pemphigus: an issue to worth consideration. Indian journal of dermatology. 2011;56(5):541.
3. Brenaut E, Halvorsen JA, Dalgard FJ, Lien L, Balieva F, Sampogna F, et al. The self-assessed psychological comorbidities of prurigo in European patients: a multicentre study in 13 countries. J Eur Acad Dermatol Venereol. 2019;33(1):157-62.
4. Chung WL, Ng SS, Koh MJ, Peh LH, Liu TT. A review of patients managed at a combined psychodermatology clinic: a Singapore experience. Singap Med J. 2012;53(12):789-93.
5. Colón EA, Popkin MK, Callies AL, Dessert NJ, Hordinsky MK. Lifetime prevalence of psychiatric disorders in patients with alopecia areata. Compr Psychiatry. 1991;32(3):245-51.
6. Cvetkovski RS, Zachariae R, Jensen H, Olsen J, Johansen JD, Agner T. Quality of life and depression in a population of occupational hand eczema patients. Contact dermatitis. 2006;54(2):106-11.
7. Dalgard FJ, Gieler U, Tomas-Aragones L, Lien I, Poot F, Jemec GBE, et al. The psychological burden of Skin Diseases: A Cross-Sectional Multicenter Study among Dermatological Out-Patients in 13 European Countries. J Invest Dermatol. 2015;135(4):984-91.
8. Gupta MA, Gupta AK. Depression and suicidal ideation in dermatology patients with acne, alopecia areata, atopic dermatitis and psoriasis. Br J Dermatol. 1998;139:846-50.
9. Harth W, Gieler U, Kusnir D, Tausk FA. Prevalence of somatic and emotional disorders. In: Clinical management in psychodermatology. 1st ed. Berlin Heidelberg: Springer-Verlag; 2009. p. 7.
10. Harth W, Gieler U, Kusnir D, Tausk FA. Secondary emotional disorders and comorbidities. In: Clinical management in dermatology. 1st ed. Berlin Heidelberg: Springer-Verlag; 2009. p. 123.

11. Mathur A, Neema S, Sahu R, Radhakrishnan S. Anxiety, depression and harmful use of alcohol in severe chronic plaque psoriasis: A cross-sectional study. Med J Armed Forces India. 2023;79(4):464-9.
12. Mattoo SK, Handa S, Kaur I, Gupta N, Malhotra R. Psychiatric morbidity in vitiligo and psoriasis: a comparative study from India. J Dermatol. 2001;28(8): 424-32.
13. Mattoo SK, Handa S, Kaur I, Gupta N, Malhotra R. Psychiatric morbidity in vitiligo: prevalence and correlates in India. J Eur Acad Dermatol Venereol. 2002;16(6):573-8.
14. Olivier C, Robert PD, Daihung DO, et al. The risk of depression, anxiety, and suicidality in patients with psoriasis: a population-based cohort study. Arch Dermatol. 2010;146(8):891-5.
15. Onderdijk AJ, Van der Zee HH, Esmann S, Lophaven S, Dufour DN, Jemec GBE, et al. Depression in patients with hidradenitis suppurativa. J Eur Acad Dermatol Venereol. 2013;27(4):473-8.
16. Picardi A, Lega I, Tarolla E. Suicide risk in skin disorders. Clin Dermatol. 2013;31(1):47-56.
17. Samuels DV, Rosenthal R, Lin R, Chaudhari S, Natsuaki MN. Acne vulgaris and risk of depression and anxiety: A meta-analytic review. J Am Acad Dermatol. 2020;83(2):532-41.
18. Sawant NS, Vanjari NA, Khopkar U, Adulkar S. A study of depression and quality of life in patients of lichen planus. Scientific World Journal. 2015:2015:817481.
19. Sellami R, Masmoudi J, Ouali U, Mnif L, Amouri M, Turki H, et al. The relationship between alopecia areata and alexithymia, anxiety and depression: a case-control study. Indian J Dermatol. 2014;59(4):421.
20. Shenoi SD, Prabhu S, Nirmal B, Petrolwala S. Our experience in a psycho-dermatology liaison clinic at Manipal, India. Indian J Dermatol. 2013;58(1):53.
21. Slattery MJ, Essex MJ, Paletz EM, Vanness ER, Infante M, Rogers GM, et al. Depression, anxiety, and dermatologic quality of life in adolescents with atopic dermatitis. J Allergy Clin Immunol. 2011;128(3): 668-71.

CHAPTER 5

Psychophysiologic Skin Disorders

Shrutakirthi D Shenoi, Meghashree G

> **Key Messages**
> - Skin and mind are inter-related.
> - Stress can precipitate or aggravate skin disease (stress responders).
> - Keys to treatment—stress management and specific dermatologic treatment.

INTRODUCTION

Skin and psyche (mind) are inter-related. The relation between stress and certain skin disorders is well-established. Stressors are events or factors that disturb one's mental balance. Reaction to stress depends on the genetic makeup of the individual and how one perceives the event. The perception depends on external factors such as life events, natural environment and individual factors such as attitude, temperament and previous experiences.

Stress activates hypothalamo-hypophyseal-adrenal axis and sympathetic nervous system to liberate glucocorticoids and catecholamines, respectively. Both inhibit Th1 response (suppress cell-mediated immunity) and promote Th2 response. This activates mast cells, eosinophils and B-cells causing inflammation.

In addition, the skin is not only a target for mediators, but also an active participant through local hypothalamic–pituitary–adrenal (HPA) axis, peripheral nerves and skin cells including mast cells, immune cells and keratinocytes. Stress disturbs epidermal permeability barrier. It also liberates histamine and vasoactive neuropeptides; and causes variation in skin temperature, blood flow, and sweat response, which contribute to itch-scratch cycle.

Psychophysiologic skin disorders are those conditions that are either precipitated or aggravated by stress (in stress responders) and include alopecia areata, atopic eczema, psoriasis, and urticaria. All these conditions are not uniformly affected by stress. There are persons who are nonstress responders, where mental stress does not play any role. The role of stress in lichen planus, vitiligo, psychogenic purpura, rosacea, acne and seborrheic dermatitis is unclear.

ALOPECIA AREATA

Alopecia areata is a T-cell-mediated autoimmune disease characterized by localized patches of hair loss on the scalp, sometimes involving other areas such as beard, moustache, and eyebrows. The hairs regrow after varying periods of time. Progressive cases of alopecia totalis and universalis have an unfavorable prognosis.

Various precipitating factors such as febrile illnesses, drugs, and trauma have been reported. Stressors can also act as potential triggers for alopecia areata. Stressful life events such as personal, family, and job-related problems have been reported in the preceding 3 months of the onset of the disease. In children, stressful events are mostly related to school (beginning of school, examinations, problems with school-mates/teachers, too much of homework) and home (family fights, birth of sibling). Corticotropin-releasing hormone (CRH), the key stress hormone, is present in the hair follicle. Stress affects local CRH expression and HPA activity causing hair loss.

ATOPIC ECZEMA

Atopic eczema is a common endogenous dermatitis characterized by pruritus, recurrent eczema, and an atopic diathesis. It starts in the 2nd or 3rd month of age and continues into adulthood. Various factors such as genetics, infections, weather, food, tobacco, and aero-allergens such as house dust mite and stress have been implicated. Several studies have shown association of stress with onset of flares and worsening of atopic dermatitis. In children, stress and family environment are predictors of symptom severity.

Prenatal distress, maternal stress during pregnancy, postpartum depression, and perceived stress in the mother are associated with increased risk of atopic dermatitis in the child.

A study suggested that high maternal sensitivity significantly protects against atopic dermatitis whereas poor maternal-infant relationship quality in the form of low sensitivity, high unresponsiveness, and high controlling behavior during interaction with the infant resulted in increased risk of atopic dermatitis. Another study which included 66 infants with atopic eczema showed that when the mother performed infantile massage, it resulted in lower eczema area and severity index (EASI) and infantile dermatitis quality of life (QOL) scores and less number of relapses. The tactile contact between mother and infant during massage reduced stress-related hormones and led to relief in the symptoms of eczema.

In atopic dermatitis, a blunted HPA axis responsiveness with a concurrent overactivity of the sympathetic adrenomedullary system may increase susceptibility to inflammation causing stress-related worsening of eczema. The reduced endogenous cortisol production under stress would impair anti-inflammatory effect of this hormone. Patients with atopic dermatitis, thus, have a hyperacute response to stress with T-cell and mast cell activation, HPA dysregulation, neurogenic inflammatory mediator expression, and release and disruption of normal epidermal barrier function.

In atopic eczema, there is typically itch–scratch cycle. Stressors cause itching, and scratching initially relieves it. With time, constant scratching causes structural inflammatory changes causing more itching and more scratching leading to a vicious cycle. Patients find it difficult to refrain from scratching. Atopic dermatitis is typically referred to as "the itch that rashes." Psychotherapeutic interventions such as stress management and relaxation training can reduce itching and scratching causing improvement.

PSORIASIS

The etiology of psoriasis is multifactorial involving genetic and environmental factors. Among the latter, stress has an important role in the onset and exacerbation of psoriasis. In normal individuals, stress activates HPA axis and sympathetic adrenal-medullary (SAM) axis. But in psoriasis, stress reduces HPA response and upregulates the SAM response. Hence, stress reduces cortisol levels, increases the levels of epinephrine and norepinephrine, both of which stimulate the release of mast cells, affect skin barrier function, and upregulate proinflammatory cytokines.

The proportion of patients who are stress responders ranges from 37 to 78%. Majority of patients feel that stress is a more important aggravating factor than others such as foods and weather. The incubation period between stress and exacerbation varies from 2 days to 1 month. Differences have been found in patients whose psoriasis has flared following stress (stress responders) compared to those who did not flare with stress. Stress responders had more flares during 6 months prior to admission, had more disease-related daily stress, and relied more on the opinions of others.

Stress responders tend to self-report greater disease severity compared to nonstress responders even though their PASI is identical. They also have been reported to have more lesions in the visible areas than nonvisible areas. Apart from increasing the severity of psoriasis, stress also affects outcome of treatment. Patients with high levels of worry tend to clear 2–3 times slower those with low worry. A small study has shown that patients with psoriasis who underwent photochemotherapy, who listened to mindfulness meditation tapes, improved faster than those who did not listen.

Early-onset psoriasis (onset before the age of 40 years) is triggered more readily by stress than late-onset psoriasis, attributable to the fact that younger psoriatics have greater difficulties in assertion and expression of anger, which adversely affects their ability to cope with stress. An interesting fact is stress-induced psoriatics have a better long-term prognosis, especially if they have high levels of insight. Thus, identification of such patients early in their disease and incorporating psychological interventions along with standard skin care may improve the course of the disease.

URTICARIA

Urticaria is characterized by localized or generalized wheals with or without angioedema. In nearly 70% of cases, an underlying cause cannot be determined. Psychological factors play a role in about 50% of patients. Several studies have reported that urticaria patients frequently have had stressful life events before the onset of the disease. The effect of stress is mediated by CRH, which is known to cause degranulation of mast cells. This hormone is elevated during stress and in depression.

A variant of urticaria known as adrenergic urticaria is induced by intense emotions and exercise associated with high levels of catecholamines in the blood. Intradermal injection of adrenaline reproduces the wheal. Propranolol, a beta adrenergic antagonist, is the treatment of choice.

LICHEN PLANUS

Although lichen planus is a T-cell-mediated inflammatory dermatoses, various triggers have precipitated the condition such as stress, drugs, and infections. Stressful events in the family such as death of someone close, personal problems such as examinations may have some role in the onset and extension of lichen planus. Psychosocial stressors have also been implicated in oral lichen planus.

VITILIGO

Vitiligo is a common depigmentary condition affecting the melanocytes. Various theories such as autoimmune, neural, and reactive oxygen species theory have been put forth, in addition to genetic predisposition. It has been found in studies that vitiligo patients experience more number of stressful events than controls, suggesting that psychological distress may contribute to the onset of disease.

PSYCHOGENIC PURPURA

Psychogenic purpura, also called as Gardner–Diamond syndrome or autoerythrocyte sensitization syndrome is a spontaneous recurrent painful ecchymosis, most commonly in women, that is always preceded by severe stress and emotional trauma. Psychiatric comorbidity such as depression may be present. Although a psychological basis is postulated for the occurrence, the precise mechanism is not understood. Some patients demonstrate a positive intradermal test wherein autologous RBCs or 0.5 mL blood is injected intradermally. There is immediate erythema with itching followed by the typical purpuric lesion within 48 hours.

ROSACEA

Rosacea is a chronic skin condition characterized by facial erythema with telangiectasia, papules, and pustules occurring predominantly over the central parts of face such as forehead, nose and cheeks. It primarily affects women between 30 and 50 years of age. The exact cause of rosacea is unknown but various triggers have been implicated such as emotional stress, extremes of temperature, sunlight, hot beverages, spicy foods, and alcohol. Studies have shown increased sympathetic nerve activity in the facial skin in response to trigger events. Neurovascular interactions with release of proinflammatory and vasodilatory neuropeptide mediators are key to the pathogenesis of certain types of rosacea.

ACNE

Acne vulgaris is a common disease of the pilosebaceous apparatus with polymorphic lesions affecting the face, chest back, and upper arms. The classical lesions include open and closed comedones, erythematous papules, nodules, cysts, and scars. Triggering factors for acne include high glycemic diet, hormones, cosmetic use and smoking.

Emotional stress can have a significant impact on acne. It has been found that examination stress can worsen acne. Stress leads to increased secretion of adrenal androgens causing sebaceous hyperplasia and comedones. Stress also releases neuropeptides from peripheral nerves causing proliferation and differentiation of sebaceous gland with increased sebum secretion. Sleep deprivation causing stress can cause acne in adult females.

In acne excoriee, during stressful periods, patients pick at their acne causing hyperpigmented crusted lesions. Usually, there is associated psychiatric comorbidity such as depression, anxiety, dysmorphophobia, or obsessive-compulsive disease.

SEBORRHEIC DERMATITIS

Seborrheic dermatitis is a chronic inflammatory condition characterized by erythematous scaly patches over the scalp, face, chest and back, sometimes affecting the groins, gluteal cleft, and genitals. Dandruff is the mildest variety occurring over the scalp. The exact cause is not known. The yeast *Malassezia* is implicated in causing the inflammation. Other precipitating factors include humidity, season, trauma, and emotional stress.

PRURIGO NODULARIS

Prurigo nodularis is an itchy condition characterized by hyperpigmented excoriated and hyperkeratotic papules and nodules over the forearms and legs. It may be associated with atopy, stress, renal disease or HIV. Associated anxiety and depression are seen in many patients.

MISCELLANEOUS

Household stress has been a contributory factor for poor wound healing. Pemphigus vulgaris, herpes labialis, and generalized pruritus have also been related to stress.

Coronavirus disease 2019 (COVID-19) pandemic-related psychosocial stress was linked with exacerbations of pre-existing skin conditions such as psoriasis, eczema, telogen effluvium, atopic dermatitis, urticaria, herpes zoster, and vitiligo.

MANAGEMENT OF PSYCHOPHYSIOLOGIC DISORDERS

Treatment of a psychophysiological condition involves a two-pronged approach. Firstly, the role of stress in the initiation and exacerbation of the condition has to be ascertained and managed. Secondly and most important is the treatment of the dermatological disease. Ideally, these patients should be managed in a psychodermatology liaison clinic alongside clinical psychologists and psychiatrists.
- Stepwise plan for psychophysiologic disorders
- Standard dermatological management

- Psychological intervention (depending on the situation we can use singly or in combination):
  - Psychosomatic primary care
  - Psychoeducation
  - Cognitive behavior therapy
  - Relaxation therapy
  - Mindful stress reduction
  - Hypnosis
  - Guided imageries
  - Habit reversal
  - Supportive therapy
  - Disease coping skill training
  - Group therapy
  - Family therapy
- Psychopharmacotherapy (depending on the psychiatric comorbidity)

Liaising is not always possible. A dermatologist can play the role of a psychodermatologist too. Chronic dermatoses, some acute, e.g., acute urticaria should be viewed as potential psychophysiologic cases. If any stressor has precipitated the disease, the effect on the patient has to be assessed. Acute stressor, e.g., loss of a loved one may not only precipitate the skin disease but also cause secondary depression. Chronic stressors such as work pressures, relationship problems, and financial difficulties perpetuate skin and psychiatric problems in susceptible people.

CONCLUSION

In stressful situations, patients should be encouraged to practice nonpharmacological interventions such as engaging in hobbies, listening to music, practicing yoga, going for walks, and other relaxation techniques. Hypnosis and cognitive behavior therapy are some of the advanced psychological treatments. Psychiatric comorbidities should be treated with appropriate psychotropic drugs.

Every person should be educated about the disease regarding its course, aggravating factors. The importance of adhering to the treatment and regular follow-up should be impressed upon the patient.

FURTHER READINGS

1. Tausk FA, Nousari H. Stress and the skin. Arch Dermatol. 2001;137(1):78-82.
2. Ito T. Recent advances in the pathogenesis of autoimmune hair loss disease alopecia areata. Clin Dev Immunol. 2013:348546.
3. Suárez AL, Feramisco JD, Koo J, Steinhoff M. Psychoneuroimmunology of psychological stress and atopic dermatitis: pathophysiologic and therapeutic updates. Acta Derm Venereol. 2012;92:7-15.
4. Heller MM, Lee ES, Koo JY. Stress as an influencing factor in psoriasis. Skin Therapy Letter. 2011;16:1-4.
5. Manaloche L, Seceleanu-Petrescue D, Benea V. Lichen planus and stressful events. J Eur Acad Dermatol Venereol. 2008;22:437-41.
6. Papadopoulos L, Bor R, Legg CL, Hawk JL. Impact of life events on the onset of vitiligo in adults. Preliminary evidence for a psychological dimension in aetiology. Clin Exp Dermatol. 1998;23:243-8.
7. Jafferany M, Bhattacharya G. Psychogenic purpura—Gardner–Diamond syndrome. 2015;17. doi: 10.4088/PCC.14br01697. eCollection 2015.
8. Chiu ABS, Chon SY, Kimball AB. The response of skin disease to stress. Changes in the severity of acne vulgaris as affected by exam stress. Arch Dermatol. 2003;139:897-900.
9. Manolache L, Petrescu-Seceleanu D. Stress involvement as trigger factor in different skin conditions. World J Dermatol. 2013;2:16-26.
10. Kimyai-Asadi A, Usman A. The role of psychological stress in skin disease. J Cut Med Surg. 2001;5:140-5.
11. Chan CWH, Law BMH, Liu YH, Ambrocio ARB, Au N, Jiang M, Chow KM. The Association between Maternal Stress and Childhood Eczema: A Systematic Review. Int J Environ Res Public Health. 2018;25:395.
12. Graubard R, Perez-Sanchez A, Katta R. Stress and Skin: An Overview of Mind Body Therapies as a Treatment Strategy in Dermatology. Dermatol Pract Concept. 2021;11.
13. Rousset L, Halioua B. Stress and psoriasis. Int J Dermatol. 2018;57:1165-72.
14. Pendlebury GA, Oro P, Haynes W, Merideth D, Bartling S, Bongiorno MA. The Impact of COVID-19 Pandemic on Dermatological Conditions: A Novel, Comprehensive Review. Dermatopathology (Basel). 2022;29:212-43.
15. Lin L, Yu L, Zhang S, Liu J, Xiong Y. The positive effect of mother-performed infant massage on infantile eczema and maternal mental state: A randomized controlled trial. Front Public Health. 2023;11:10.

CHAPTER 6

Impact of Dermatological Diseases on Psyche of Patient, Family, and Society

Swapna Bondade, Abhineetha Hosthota

> **Key Messages**
> - Dermatological diseases are not merely superficial conditions; they can have profound psychological consequences for patients, families, and society. The close link between skin and brain can lead to a complex interplay between physical symptoms and emotional distress.
> - The visible manifestations of skin conditions often lead to social stigma, discrimination, and isolation, affecting self-esteem, body image, and overall mental well-being.
> - The emotional burden of living with a loved one suffering from a dermatological disease can significantly impact family dynamics, relationships, and mental health within the family unit.
> - Dermatological diseases can lead to discrimination and prejudice in various social settings, including workplaces, schools, and public spaces. This can have significant consequences for employment, education, and overall quality of life.
> - Recognizing the psychological and social dimensions of skin diseases is crucial for providing effective and holistic care. This requires a multidisciplinary approach that addresses not only the physical symptoms but also the emotional and social needs of patients and their families.
> - Education and awareness campaigns can play a vital role in dispelling myths and misconceptions surrounding skin diseases. By fostering empathy and understanding, we can create a more inclusive society where individuals with skin conditions can thrive.

INTRODUCTION

The skin, often hailed as the "organ of expression," stands sentinel between our inner selves and the relentless external forces of the world—an intricate interface that marks our first point of contact with the world. As the largest organ of the body, its responses to both physiological and psychological stimuli illuminate a profound relationship between the skin and the myriad factors shaping our internal and external realms.

Skin conditions, often perceived as solely physical ailments, carry a weighty and multifaceted psychological burden that ripples beyond the individual, impacting families, communities, and society. This burden, invisible yet deeply impactful, requires us to shift our gaze beyond the surface and delve into the intricate tapestry woven between skin and psyche.

Coping with these skin conditions becomes a multifaceted journey, dictated by an individual's personality, the support of their familial bonds, and the intricate web of their social networks. The skin, in its uniqueness, presents a dual nature—both a canvas for the visible manifestations of distress and a cryptic realm harboring hidden struggles.

NAVIGATING THE STORM: THE PATIENT'S JOURNEY

For individuals living with skin conditions, the psychological burden can be a daily storm to weather. Let us explore some of the key challenges they face.

Negative Body Image and its Fallout: The Shattered Mirror

Body image, the subjective perception of one's own physical appearance, can be profoundly impacted by skin diseases. While often conceptualized as an internal struggle in psychiatric disorders like dysmorphophobia and bulimia nervosa, in the context of dermatological conditions, it becomes a tangible reality etched onto the skin. Visible and disfiguring skin conditions like alopecia, vitiligo, and psoriasis disrupt the very basis of body image, leading to a cascade of negative consequences.

Changes in skin surface and color can trigger a distorted body image, breeding feelings of shame, inadequacy, and social disconnection. This is particularly pronounced when lesions affect sensitive areas like genitalia, fueling anxieties about rejection and intimacy. The resulting emotional vulnerability and insecurity erode self-confidence, impacting communication and social interaction. Individuals with chronic skin conditions are at an increased risk for developing social phobia, anxiety, depression, and even suicidal ideation.

Research underlines the bidirectional relationship between negative body image and skin diseases. Studies have shown that a negative body image can exacerbate existing skin conditions, creating a vicious cycle of psychological distress and physical manifestation. This highlights the need for a holistic approach that addresses both the physical and the psychological aspects of skin diseases.

Coping Mechanisms: A Double-edged Sword

Adapting to chronic skin conditions can be an arduous mental battle. Patients often develop maladaptive coping mechanisms like avoidance, secrecy, or self-blame, further hindering their quality of life. Social gatherings become battlegrounds, public spaces transform into minefields, and intimacy becomes a distant dream. The constant struggle to manage the physical symptoms and the fear of judgment can take a toll on mental well-being, creating a vicious cycle that is difficult to break free from.

The fear of stigma and negative societal reactions can lead to social withdrawal and isolation. Patients may avoid public spaces or social gatherings, opting for the confines of their homes, where the judgmental gaze of others feels less intrusive. This self-imposed exile can have far-reaching consequences, impacting career prospects, personal relationships, and overall well-being. The world shrinks, opportunities dwindle, and the feeling of being an outsider becomes pervasive.

Quality of Life

The impact of skin diseases on health-related quality of life (HRQoL) is undeniable, far exceeding just physical symptoms. Studies consistently report negative impacts on HRQoL across various conditions like psoriasis, acne, lupus erythematosus, alopecia, urticaria, and vitiligo. Notably, factors like age, disease duration, severity, and even socioeconomic status significantly influence HRQoL in specific conditions. Despite being among the most common global diseases, the impact of skin conditions remains underestimated. This underestimation can be attributed to the often-invisible nature of the emotional and social burdens these conditions carry.

Dermatological diseases like vitiligo and psoriasis can lead to social withdrawal, impaired relationships, sexual dysfunction, stigmatization, anxiety, and difficulty finding work, ultimately contributing to a significantly reduced HRQoL.

Comorbid Mental Health Issues: The Shadowed Companion

Skin diseases often walk together with various psychiatric comorbidities, including depression, anxiety, phobias, and obsessive-compulsive disorders. These comorbidities can significantly complicate the management of both the skin condition and the mental health issues, creating a tangled web of challenges that require a multifaceted approach. Imagine battling the physical discomfort of a skin condition while simultaneously navigating the emotional turmoil of depression or the debilitating grip of anxiety. This is the reality for many individuals, making the journey toward healing even more arduous.

Anxiety and depression: The constant emotional turmoil associated with negative body image, stigma, and social isolation can trigger anxiety and depression. Individuals may experience excessive worry, hopelessness, and even suicidal ideation.

Obsessive-compulsive behaviors: Individuals may develop compulsive behaviors like excessive skin picking, scratching, or applying topical medications, fueled by anxiety and a desire to control the condition.

Chronic stress and fatigue: The ongoing physical and emotional demands of managing a skin disease can lead to chronic stress and fatigue, further impacting mental well-being and daily functioning.

PSYCHOLOGICAL IMPACT OF SKIN DISEASE ON FAMILY: THE HIDDEN SCARS

The visible nature of many skin conditions often fuels societal stigma, leading to feelings of shame, isolation, and discrimination. Family members, too, can bear the brunt of this stigma, experiencing anxiety about their own perceptions and navigating social interactions with heightened sensitivity. This stigma can significantly affect relationships, creating a sense of exclusion and hindering open communication within families.

Family members, often thrust into the role of caregivers, face their own set of challenges. The constant stress of supporting a loved one with a skin condition can lead to feelings of overwhelm, frustration, and exhaustion. Maladaptive coping mechanisms, such as chronic fatigue, low mood, burnout, and even depression and anxiety, are not uncommon among caregivers.

Child and Parents: A Shared Burden

When a child suffers from visible or severe skin disorders, the psychological burden often falls first on their parents. Congenital or acquired conditions like ichthyosis, epidermolysis bullosa, and autoimmune diseases present unique challenges for families. Parents grapple with accepting and adjusting to their child's illness, struggling to express empathy while navigating their own anxieties and fears. Studies reveal that 36–42% of parents in this situation experience anxiety disorders, and 26–36% struggle with depression. The emotional turmoil is further amplified by societal stigma and misinformation, leading some parents to reject or blame their child, adding to the child's already fragile sense of self. Inferiority, low self-esteem, body image distortion, and social withdrawal are tragically common consequences for these children.

However, amidst the darkness, a beacon of hope emerges. Recognizing the child's need for unwavering love and support alongside proper medical treatment is paramount. Parents must remember that their child is not defined by their skin, and their unconditional love can significantly impact the child's coping mechanisms and resilience.

Spouses/Partners: Navigating Intimacy and Acceptance

Intimacy thrives on a delicate balance of physical and emotional connection. Skin conditions can disrupt this equilibrium, particularly within marriages and partnerships. When one partner battles a skin disease, the other's support becomes a lifeline. Yet, lacking or inadequate support can exacerbate disease-related stress, breeding interpersonal conflicts and eroding the foundation of the relationship. Marital harmony, sexual intimacy, and emotional attachment become casualties in this struggle. Fear of proximity, negative perception of the affected partner, and even sexual criticism can become the new reality.

The emotional fallout is often devastating. Persistent depression, known as dysthymia, can engulf the partner who feels their sense of belonging shattered. To counteract this, acceptance of the condition and active coping with its complexities are crucial. Unconditional love, unwavering support, and an empathetic stance toward both the patient and the impact on the relationship are essential for navigating this turbulent tide.

Redefining Social Norms: Embracing Difference

The fear of societal stigma often leads to social withdrawal within families affected by skin disease. Denial becomes a coping mechanism, with open discussions about the condition or the affected individual becoming taboo. Family functions are avoided, and patients themselves develop anxiety and embarrassment about public interactions, often facing the sting of ignorant and insensitive comments.

This altered social behavior significantly impacts the dynamics within the family, creating distance and isolation. Acceptance of the disease by family members, without compromising their emotional bond with the patient, is key to building resilience and fostering open communication. Support from friends and extended family also forms a crucial safety net, providing strength and emotional nourishment to both the patient and their immediate circle.

SKIN DISEASES AND THE PSYCHE OF SOCIETY

Skin diseases, while often perceived as solely physical afflictions, can have a profound impact on the collective psyche of society. This intricate interplay between skin conditions and social attitudes can be understood through several key lenses.

Stigma and Discrimination

Many skin diseases, particularly those with visible manifestations, can be associated with societal stigma and discrimination. Misconceptions and negative stereotypes surrounding certain conditions, like leprosy or psoriasis, can lead to social isolation, exclusion, and even prejudice. This can significantly impact the mental and emotional well-being of individuals living with these conditions, perpetuating a cycle of stigma and hardship.

Beauty Standards and Body Image

Cultural norms and media portrayals often define specific skin tones and appearances as desirable, creating pressure to conform to unrealistic beauty standards. Individuals with skin conditions that deviate from these norms may experience negative self-image, low self-esteem, and anxiety about their appearance. This can have broader societal implications, reinforcing discriminatory attitudes and hindering inclusivity.

Lack of Awareness and Education

Limited knowledge and understanding about skin diseases can contribute to stigma and discrimination. Misinformation and myths surrounding certain conditions can fuel fear and prejudice, leading to negative societal reactions. Educational initiatives and awareness campaigns can play a crucial role in dispelling myths, promoting empathy, and fostering understanding.

Cultural Context of Skin Disorders

The complex landscape of psychosomatic skin diseases in India is deeply intertwined with various cultural factors. Religious and spiritual beliefs, dietary habits, clothing styles, sun exposure, and socioeconomic status significantly influence disease presentation and management. One notable aspect is the association of lighter skin tones with beauty and social value, potentially leading to emotional difficulties for individuals with darker skin.

Traditional practices, while holding significant emotional and spiritual significance, require careful exploration in relation to skin health. While visiting temples, performing offerings, and immersing oneself in holy rivers may offer comfort and solace, the use of unproven remedies like urine, cow dung, or potentially harmful chemicals in rituals can aggravate certain skin conditions. Similarly, dietary patterns within households, including commonly consumed foods like brinjals, black gram, eggs, and chicken, can act as potential allergens for some individuals.

Stigma surrounding specific skin diseases, notably psoriasis and leprosy, poses a significant challenge. Societal exclusion and ostracization associated with these conditions can worsen disability and impede access to proper care. Research suggests that even vitiligo can negatively impact marriage prospects and interpersonal relationships.

CONCLUSION

In conclusion, the impact of skin diseases extends far beyond the surface, leaving deep scars on the psyche of patients, families, and society at large. Navigating the emotional turmoil of negative body image, fear, and stigma requires a holistic approach that recognizes the interconnectedness of physical and mental well-being. By empowering individuals through therapy and support groups, equipping families with resources and coping mechanisms, and fostering empathy and understanding within society, we can start to heal the invisible scars and create a world where everyone feels confident, valued, and embraced, regardless of the mark etched upon their skin. Remember, skin may be the canvas, but our true beauty lies in the resilience and compassion we cultivate in the face of adversity.

FURTHER READINGS

1. Mysore V. Invisible dermatoses. Indian J Dermatol Venereol Leprol. 2010;76:239-48.
2. Harth W, Gieler U, Tausk FA. Clinical Management of Psychodermatology. Berlin: Springer-Verlag; 2008.
3. Shuster S, Fisher GH, Harris E, Binnell D. The effect of skin disease on self image (proceedings). Br J Dermatol. 1978;99:18-9.
4. Jafferany M. Psychodermatology: A guide to understanding common psychocutaneous disorders. Prim Care Companion J Clin Psychiatry. 2007;9:203-13.

5. Colón EA, Popkin MK, Callies AL, Dessert NJ, Hordinsky MK. Lifetime prevalence of psychiatric disorders in patients with alopecia areata. Compr Psychiatry. 1991;32:245-51.
6. Korabel H, Grabski B, Dudek D, Jaworek A, Gierowski JK, Kiejna A, et al. Stress coping mechanisms in patients with chronic dermatoses. Archives of Psychiatry and Psychotherapy. 2013;3:33-40.
7. Harth W, Gieler U, Kusnir D, Tausk FA. Suicide in dermatology [Internet]. In: Clinical Management in Psychodermatology. Berlin: Springer; 2009. pp. 187-8. [online] Available from http://link.springer. com/10.1007/978-3-540-34719-4_12 [Last accessed January, 2024].
8. Chren M-M, Weinstock MA. Conceptual issues in measuring the burden of skin diseases. J Invest Dermatol Symp Proc. 2004;9(2):97-100.
9. Jones-Caballero M, Chren MM, Soler B, Pedrosa E, Peñas PF. Quality of life in mild to moderate acne: relationship to clinical severity and factors influencing change with treatment. 2007;21(2):219-26.
10. El-Khalifi A, Abulnaja A, Alajmi A. The impact of dermatological diseases on the health-related quality of life: A comprehensive review. Int J Dermatol. 2023;62(1):3-17.
11. Raikhy S, Gautam S, Kanodia S. Pattern and prevalence of psychiatric disorders among patients attending dermatology OPD. Asian J Psychiatr. 2017;29:85-8.
12. Wilhelm S, Steeves MM. Psychotic versus obsessive-compulsive symptoms in patients with psychogenic excoriation. Int J Dermatol. 2009;48(2):160-4.
13. Gupta MA, Krishnamurthy V. The concept of "greater patient" in dermatology and its psychosocial implications. Indian J Dermatol. 2011;56(1):8.
14. Manzoni AP, Weber MB, Nagatomi AR, Pereira RL, Townsend RZ, Cestari TF, et al. Assessing depression and anxiety in the caregivers of pediatric patients with chronic skin disorders. An Bras Dermatol. 2013;88:894-9.
15. Thoman-Touet SK. (1992). A qualitative study of the effect of chronic illness on marital quality. Retrospective Theses and Dissertations. [online] Available from https://lib.dr.iastate.edu/rtd/10156 [Last accessed January, 2024].
16. Eram U. Myths and Stigma Associated with Skin Diseases: A Review Article. Global J Eng Sci Res Manage. 2017;4(1):39-42.
17. Chaturvedi SK, Singh G, Gupta N. Stigma experience in skin disorders: An Indian perspective. Dermatol Clin. 2005;23:635-42.
18. Shenoi SD, Prabhu S. Role of cultural factors in the biopsychosocial model of psychosomatic skin diseases: An Indian perspective. Clin Dermatol. 2013;31:62-5.

CHAPTER 7

Skin, Mind, and Beauty

Madhulika Mhatre, Venkataram Mysore

> **Key Messages**
> - There is a close interaction between skin and the mind.
> - Perception of beauty is individual and psychological.
> - These undergo change with times with social media playing a big role.
> - Understanding the psyche is of vital importance for proper cosmetic management.

INTRODUCTION

"I cannot say often enough how much I consider beauty a powerful and advantageous quality. Socrates called it 'A short tyranny,' and Plato, 'The privilege of nature.' We have no quality that surpasses it in credit. It holds the first place in human relations; it presents itself before the rest, seduces and prepossesses our judgment with great authority and a wondrous impression."

—**Montaigne, Essays**

In 1884, Jonathan Hutchinson delivered a series of lectures emphasizing that our ancestors, despite knowing less about pathology than we do now, appreciated the significance of temperament and diathesis. While advancements in knowledge have led us to focus primarily on diseases, it is essential not to overlook the study of individual differences, which may play a crucial role in modifying disease processes. This holds true even today. The skin's ability to reflect emotions and provide insight into a person's temperament is often underestimated.

Throughout the years, research in social science has consistently established the relationship between appearance, social stereotypes, and expectations. Attractiveness significantly impacts psychological development and social relationships. This desire to enhance one's appearance has created a separate subset of patients seeking help from dermatologists, plastic surgeons, and beauty parlors. However, defining beauty, an abstract concept rooted in individual perceptions, remains a challenge. Physical beauty's importance in self-perception and social interactions emerges early in life and can influence behavioral and mental health outcomes. While innate preferences for symmetry and adaptive features influence attractiveness, social experiences, including media exposure, also shape our perceptions of beauty.

Cosmetic surgery, focused on maintaining, restoring, or enhancing physical appearance, has become more prevalent and accessible in Western society. It is essential to explore the internal and external factors motivating individuals to undergo cosmetic procedures, such as the availability of cosmetic surgeons, media influence, evolutionary interests, and personal factors.

The mind-body problem revolves around explaining the relationship between mental states and physical states within the human body, considering the mind's nonphysical nature and the body's physical existence.

Dermatologists and clinicians have long recognized the neurophysiological connections between skin appearance, perception of beauty, and overall health. Common phrases like "beauty is in the eye of the beholder" and "beauty is only skin deep" underscore the ephemeral nature of attractiveness. For instance, philosopher David Hume famously argued that beauty exists solely in the mind of the beholder, with each mind perceiving a different form of beauty. This reinforces the intricate interplay between perception, aesthetics, and individual experiences.

UNDERSTANDING THE MOTIVATION

An aesthetic patient requires a distinct and careful approach. Establishing a strong patient-doctor relationship is crucial. This involves attentively listening to their concerns, understanding the underlying motivation behind their desire for the procedure, and taking their issues seriously. Motivation in such cases can stem from either internal or external factors. External motivation might be driven by the desire to please a spouse, improve marital prospects, or secure better job opportunities. On the other hand, internal motivation arises from the aspiration to look and feel good for oneself. It is essential to recognize that dissatisfaction with appearance may lead to anxiety and could be a contributing factor to psychiatric illness. Identifying such patients is crucial, and counseling should be recommended before proceeding with cosmetic correction to address their psychopathology effectively.

It is important to note that aesthetic procedures are not intended to promote health or cure illnesses. While some research suggests that cosmetic surgery may positively impact body image, its efficacy in improving individuals' psychological health remains a subject of debate. The fact that some patients undergo multiple procedures, despite having undergone previous corrections, raises questions about the ultimate satisfaction achieved through cosmetic surgery. Understanding the patient's motivation (internal or external) becomes vital in identifying potential body dissatisfaction disorder clues.

Social pressures to look attractive and desirable can also be significant motivating factors. In such cases, even though the motivation is external, undertaking the required cosmetic procedure can uplift the patient's confidence and self-image. For example:

- A wife who experienced low self-confidence after childbirth and suspected her husband's interest in other women might seek cosmetic procedures to regain her self-esteem. In such situations, a dermatologist may need to play the roles of a physician, psychiatrist, and therapist, involving the spouse in discussions to support the patient's emotional well-being.
- The influence of social situations and peer pressure is evident in cases like a college student who refuses to attend college due to pimples. Social and print media perpetuate the notion that looking good equates to popularity, intelligence, and more friends. Fear of social rejection drives many teenagers to seek basic skin treatments and advanced aesthetic procedures.
- Emotional factors can play a role as well, as seen in the case of a 72-year-old man who sought hair removal on his ears after his wife's passing. He had fallen in love with a widow, also experiencing loneliness, and desired a change in his appearance for this new relationship.

- In another instance, a young man underwent hair transplantation to challenge his bald father, who he believed to be responsible for his own baldness.

These examples illustrate the diverse and intricate motivations driving individuals to seek aesthetic procedures, emphasizing the importance of understanding each patient's unique perspective and needs.

CONCEPT OF SELF-PERCEPTION

Self-perception encompasses our beliefs, attitudes, and images about ourselves, both positive and negative. For many, it is closely tied to body image. When an individual fixates on inaccurate and flawed body images, their perception becomes distorted, adversely impacting their self-esteem. In today's media-driven world, we are constantly bombarded with images of "beautiful people," setting unrealistic standards for the average person to attain. This constant comparison can lead individuals to focus on imagined flaws, resulting in distorted body perceptions and lowered self-esteem. Such negative body image can even lead to body dysmorphic disorder (BDD), a condition characterized by an obsession with perceived imperfections.

Common signs of BDD include repetitive checking of perceived defects, avoiding mirrors or photographs, excessive grooming, and resorting to cosmetics or clothing to conceal the supposed flaws. The power of self-talk, the subconscious voice within, plays a crucial role in shaping our perceptions, beliefs, and behaviors. Positive self-talk can be uplifting and encouraging, while negative self-talk can drain self-confidence and foster feelings of depression and self-doubt. Recognizing this process allows individuals to replace negative messages with positive affirmations, promoting a healthier mindset and improving overall well-being.

Fairness and perception of beauty: In the Indian psyche, there exists a deep-rooted craze for fairness, extending not only to the face but also to other body parts like arms, thighs, legs, and even groins. This obsession with fair skin has led to the advertisement of groin fairness creams and the indiscriminate use of hydroquinone, resulting in an increase in cases of pseudo-ochronosis. Unfortunately, even 3-year-old children are brought in with requests to become fair, and topical steroids are misused in pursuit of fairer skin. It is essential to address these harmful practices and promote a more inclusive perception of beauty.

Beauty and hair: Hair loss seems to cause a disproportionate amount of psychological stress. People's obsession with hair is on the rise, often exceeding the impact of actual hair loss. For instance, a young woman, a divorcee seeking to remarry, blamed her hair loss for her inability to find a partner, seeking hair transplantation when she had telogen effluvium due to stress. In another case, a 40-year-old man described hair loss as a "curse." Additionally, certain misconceptions about hair treatments can lead to misguided decisions, such as a woman self-administering apple stem cell injections for her anemia instead of seeking appropriate medical treatment. Hair transplantation has been dubbed "psychiatric surgery" at times, as it can significantly impact a person's appearance and self-perception.

Beauty and aging: With an aging population and increasing longevity, there is a growing desire to reverse the signs of aging. The market has been flooded with a plethora of treatments, ranging from fillers to botulinum toxin type-A (BTX-A) and lasers, offering ways to combat the effects of aging. In this quest to defy aging, some individuals turn to poorly evidenced treatments like the vampire lift and mesotherapy, seeking quick fixes without adequate consideration of potential risks. It is essential to emphasize the importance of evidence-based practices and encourage a balanced approach to aging gracefully.

CONCLUSION

While society may define beauty in certain ways, it is vital to remember that true beauty lies beyond physical appearance. Beauty is a complex interplay of perceptions, thoughts, and actions. Embracing oneself and appreciating individual uniqueness are key to nurturing self-confidence and authentic beauty, irrespective of external standards or cosmetic procedures. It is through understanding and accepting our inner selves that we can truly celebrate the beauty within each one of us.

FURTHER READINGS

1. Goldfield A, Chrisler JC. Body stereotyping and stigmatization of obese persons by first graders. Percept Mot Skills. 1995;81:909-10.
2. Hawley PH, Johnson SE, Mize JA, McNamara KA. Physical attractiveness in preschoolers: Relationships with power, status, aggression, and social skills. J School Psychol. 2007;45:499-521.
3. Markey CN, Markey PM. A correlational and experimental examination of reality television viewing and interest in cosmetic surgery. Body Image. 2010;7(2):165-71.
4. Swami V, Chamorro-Premuzic T, Bridges S, Furnham A. Acceptance of cosmetic surgery: Personality and individual difference predictors. Body Image. 2009;6:7-13.
5. Sarwer DB, Magee L, Clark V. What is beauty? Physical appearance and cosmetic medical treatments: Physiological and sociocultural influences. J Cosmet Dermatol. 2003;2:29-39.
6. Ching S, Thoma A, McCabe R, Antony M. Measuring outcomes in aesthetic surgery. Plast Reconstr Surg. 2003;111:468-80.
7. Harter S. Causes, correlates, and the functional role of global self-worth: A life span perspective. In: J Kollingian, R Sternberg (Eds). Perceptions of Competence and Incompetence across the Life-span. New Haven, CT: Yale University Press. 1989; pp. 67-97.
8. Harter S. The development of self-esteem. In: MH Kernis (Ed), Self-esteem Issues and Answers: A Sourcebook of Current Perspectives. New York: Psychology Press. 2006; pp. 144-50.

CHAPTER 8

Psychology of an Aesthetic Patient

Manjot Marwah Sharma, Venkataram Mysore

> **Key Messages**
> - Skin is the outermost and the most visible organ of the body.
> - Skin and mind are closely connected and hence play a major role in creating self-image and self-esteem of a person.
> - Increasing awareness due to globalization and changing patterns of beauty standards about body image and appearance has led to a boom in aesthetic practice.
> - Often, these standards create unrealistic expectations and beliefs in patients and tend to develop body dysmorphophobia, and hence proper psychological assessment and counseling are needed prior to procedures.

INTRODUCTION

Skin is the outermost and the largest organ of the body which has functions of protecting, eliminating waste, regulating body temperature, and many more. The skin, along with the hair, nails, sebaceous glands, and sweat glands, forms an integumentary system (meaning: outer covering). As we know, the skin along with its appendages plays a vital role in maintaining a healthy body and also plays a crucial role in emotional and mental health. It plays a role in an individual's personal relationships and communications to workspace success. In the current scenario of pursuit of beauty and technological developments in the field of aesthetic medicine, there are a lot of options and treatments available to change or better one's appearance. Additionally, due to the excessive amount of focus and emphasis put by the society on what is perceived as ideal beauty, via advertisements of beauty products, movies, or social media, there has been an exponential growth in the demand for aesthetic procedures worldwide. This has also led to many people being subjected to societal pressure to reach unreachable standards of physical beauty.

If this desire to achieve higher beauty standards increases, it may be associated with underlying components of stress, depression, or obsession. Such patients are likely to approach for aesthetic treatments for correction and despite treatment may still be dissatisfied and depressed or even obsessed. Clinical studies have shown that 20-48% of patients seeking aesthetic treatments fulfill the diagnostic criteria for psychiatric diagnosis. Cosmetic psychodermatology is a new aspect in cosmetic practice. Hence, understanding and evaluation of psychology of an aesthetic patient should play a major part in the training of an aesthetician to avoid dire consequences. It is the physician's responsibility to comprehensively assess such patients with underlying psychological issues, and also understanding the degree of changes will allow a reasonable approach to selecting the patient for procedures and avoid dire consequences in patients who need counseling or treatment by a psychiatrist or rarely themselves become the psychotherapist.

Changing trends: Common procedures and indications in aesthetic practice are shown in **Table 1**. The statistics of the changing trend are as follows:
- Dermatologic surgeons performed nearly 14 million procedures in 2019 [American Society for Dermatologic Surgery (ASDS)]
- 8.9 million cosmetic treatments—injectable wrinkle relaxers and soft-tissue fillers, laser/light/energy-based procedures, and body sculpting

Table 1: Common procedures and indications in aesthetic practice.

Indication	Procedure
Aging changes	BTX, fillers, peels, lasers, face lifts, fat transfer, threads
Pigmentary problems	Peels, lasers
Baldness	PRP, hair transplantation
Fat deposits	Liposuction
Hair excess	Laser hair removal
Stretch marks	Lasers, other less established treatment

(BTX: botulinum toxin; PRP: platelet-rich plasma)

- Eleven percent more cosmetic procedures in 2018 and a 78% increase since 2012. Body treatments increased by 62% over 2018.

Factors influencing increased demand for aesthetic procedures:
- Increased longevity
- Changing standard and attitudes (e.g., Korean glass skin)
- Social media influence
- Increased awareness
- Increased affordability
- Newer treatments
- Demand for simple and safe treatments; weekend/lunchtime treatments

Paradoxically, coinciding with this demand for procedures, there is an increasing fear of side effects and demand for simpler and safer procedures, the so-called lunchtime procedures. Often in the same patient, one sees an obsessive urge for procedure and also a paranoid fear of side effect—the twin demand of providing "guaranteed efficacy with absolutely no side effects" is one of the challenges of aesthetic practice.

DISEASE DERMATOLOGY VERSUS DESIRE DERMATOLOGY

As a result, dermatology is changing from disease-oriented specialty to a desire-satisfying specialty, where a patient demands a procedure for a perceived problem. This has led to a debate as to whether such patients are indeed patients or should there be another term such as clients.

Characteristics of aesthetic or desire dermatology are as follows:
- Emphasis on concise and cohesive treatment
- Emphasis on comfort
- Emphasis on clear and consistent results
- Emphasis on complete safety
- Emphasis on patient/client satisfaction

The difference between a dermatology patient and an aesthetic patient is given in **Table 2**.

Table 2: Aesthetic patient versus a conventional dermatological patient.	
Dermatological patient	**Aesthetic patient**
Has a disease	Has a desire
Mostly needs medical treatment; occasional surgical treatment	Mostly needs a procedural treatment
Fear of consequences of disease, fear of infection, fear of spread	Well aware; often has read well; knows often what treatment is needed
Accepts treatments willingly	Wants options—safe options
Easier to counsel about side effects	Paranoid about side effects
Respectful toward doctor; doctor is dominant	Demands an equal relationship
Easier to handle if there is a side effect	Demanding; can be aggressive, more likely for a medicolegal situation

TYPES OF PATIENTS AND THEIR PSYCHOLOGICAL EXPECTATIONS

In an aesthetic clinic, there are different types of patients. They are comprised of different age groups, different social backgrounds, and different financial status. Each patient comes with specific complaints and specific expectations. **Flowchart 1** simplifies and divides these patients as per their approach to their problems.

Depending on their expectations, the physician can get a clue to the psychology of the patient. Patients with unrealistic expectations are one of the warning signs of an underlying psychiatric disorder. Patients of the type 1 group are the best candidates. The type 2 patients usually have an insight and on adequate counseling they may decrease their expectations and willingly accept them; however, a detailed evaluation is advised in them. Type 3 and 4 patients also need careful assessment to identify an underlying psychiatric component if present. Most cases of body dysmorphic syndrome fall in type 3 category; such patients will never be satisfied with the surgery and get repeated surgeries. They will benefit only with psychiatric interventions. In dermatologic aesthetic surgery, most patients come for minor treatments.

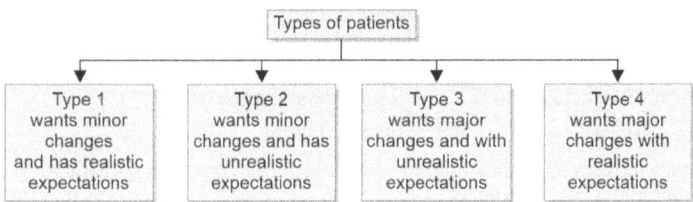

Flowchart 1: Types of expectations and psychological needs of different patients.

Assessment of the Patient's Psychology

In 1818, Heinroth described the term "psychosomatic" referring to the influence the mind has on the body. Hence, examining an individual's mind is as important as examining the physical body. The easiest way for a physician of a nonpsychiatric background to assess the psychology or thinking of the patient is via a good doctor–patient relationship. This is easier said than done. Despite the best medical education and training, good communication and interpersonal skills may not come naturally to healthcare providers or even with great experience and observation. Only a physician with good communication skills can have a successful psychologically based aesthetic practice.

The most important thing while evaluating a patient's psychology is to give the patient time. A minimum of 15 minutes per consultation is a must. It is often worthwhile to give a questionnaire asking the patient to fill. A counselor or a junior doctor can also screen the patient first. The following points give a stepwise guideline on evaluating a patient's psychology when he enters an aesthetic clinic.

- *General observation*: Assessment of the patient should start from the minute the patient enters the clinic. Subtle signs like: Who is accompanying the patient? Is the patient's dressing sense provocative or subtle? Is the patient maintaining eye contact? Who is talking more during the visit, the patient or the accompanying person? Does the patient's tone seem overexcited or monotonous? Is the patient continuously fidgeting with his/her hair or looking at the mirror frequently?
- Being anxious, nervous, and self-conscious is a normal feeling while visiting a doctor, and hence, it is important to make the patient feel comfortable during his visit. Anxiety may mask any underlying expression or behavior of the patient. Occasionally, a second visit may be required in overanxious patients.

- *Clinical observation*: Notice if the patient has exaggerated frown lines or glabellar lines, indicating stress. Any sign of a past cosmetic procedure carried out? Early signs of aging? Any sign of depression, such as hesitation marks?
- *Ambience*: To make the patient comfortable, greet the patients with their name and get them seated comfortably. This helps in relieving the initial anxiety too. Notice if the patient is quite most of the time or talkative, reluctant in mentioning the complaints, or overzealous and demanding as these can be warning signs.
- *Questioning*: Questions should be open ended so that the answers can be more elaborative and informative. Ask the patient what are his concerns, what is bothering him, how much is it bothering. The reason behind getting the surgery? If anyone else told them to get the surgery? For how long have they wanted to get this surgery?
- Concentrate on one target and discuss upon that to know the expectation. Ask details about the expectations. To understand his expectations, ask what and how much would satisfy him. Is there any minimum that he expects? Show him photos of what results can be achieved and then ask whether will he be happy if such results are achieved.
- *Social history*: History of any sleep disturbances, alcohol consumption or smoking, appetite loss, and weight gain gives a hint about the physical and mental well-being. Family history regarding relations may be asked indirectly, such as recent divorce or marriage, which gives a hint on interpersonal relationships. The patient's work type tells about their job satisfaction. Any hesitation to answer a question may also indicate a stress factor and should be noted.

Understanding the Root Cause Behind a Particular Psychological Behavior

Not all patients who ask for an aesthetic procedure necessarily have an underlying psychological issue. However, all patients do have an underlying emotion or motive behind getting an aesthetic surgery. Most of the reasons are purely physiological or due to an "ideal" self-image built by the person; we rarely encounter patients with psychosomatic causes asking for a surgery. These are the patients that need to be segregated.

- *"IDEAL" self-image*: Every decision an individual takes—his choice of clothes or house or car—is based on a self-image that he considers ideal for him. Similarly, patients usually have an ideal image in their mind when they approach for an aesthetic procedure. There is a goal, an ideal self-image they imagine; this determines the patient's behavior and their obsession and demands of different aesthetic procedures. For example, a perfectly good-looking male patient may demand for a cleft in the chin, even when it is not required, only because he sees his ideal self-image with a cleft in the chin. This is the most common reason patients get cosmetic surgery and if the patient has realistic expectations and is self-motivated, the procedure is going to benefit the patient not only physically, but also emotionally.
- *Psychosomatic causes*: One-third of the patients visiting a dermatologist have associated emotional and psychosomatic factors. Only treating the physical aspect in these patients is not going to yield any results; the psychosomatic factor needs to be resolved too. The most common presentation of these factors seen in an aesthetic clinic is in cases of body dysmorphic disorder (BDD) and depression.

Body Dysmorphic Disorder

Body dysmorphic disorder has been defined as a preoccupation with an imagined or a slight defect in appearance that leads to significant impairment in functioning, which usually starts during adolescence, at around 16 years of age. It has been reclassified and considered as a type of obsessive-compulsive disorder (OCD). **Table 3** gives a list of screening questions to be asked during history taking.

After the screening, BDD can be confirmed via a simple tool—visual analog scale (VAS). The doctor and patient independently rate disfigurement and record severity on the optical VAS using values between 0 and 10 (with 0 meaning "no disfigurement" and 10 meaning "most severe disfigurement"). When a discrepancy of more than 4 points on the VAS occurs, BDD is highly suspicious.

Harth et al. described a subtype of BDD known as botulinophilia, characterized by persistent demands of botox injections to treat hyperhidrosis despite absence of syndromes.

Table 3: Screening questions in BDD.

1. Do you believe that a part of your body is abnormal?
2. Have you ever been very concerned about your appearance?
3. Do you often and carefully view yourself in the mirror? How much time do you spend doing so?
4. Do you attempt to hide your defect with your hands, cosmetics, or clothes?
5. Does your preoccupation with appearance have affected your life in the areas of your profession, social contacts, and partnerships?
6. Have you neglected normal activities because of the defect?

If the answer to these five questions is "yes", it is highly likely that the patient has BDD, and elective aesthetic surgery should not be performed

Etiology

The cellular physiopathology has been explained in detail by the neuro-immuno-cutaneous-endocrine (NICE) model. This model explains how abnormal serotonin and dopamine play a role in BDD. The psyche behind BDD includes cognitive-behavioral factors, cognitive factors such as unrealistic ideas about the "ideal" self-image with respect to symmetry and perfection in looks. There may also be obsession about a particular part of the body, such as nose or hair. Repeatedly looking in the mirror or fidgeting with hair is a type of maladaptive behavior which develops as a result of these cognitive factors. Poot et al. have tried to simplify the factors behind psychosomatic disorders in **Figure 1**.

Interpersonal relationships—rejection or neglectful nature of family—may lead to BDD in the patients. Teasing in schools may lead to BDD in young adolescents too. Careful social history taking is important in such cases.

Studies have proven that 9-15% of the patients visiting a dermatologist for aesthetic procedures suffer from BDD. This emphasizes the need for aestheticians to be aware of this condition and its presentation in the cosmetic population.

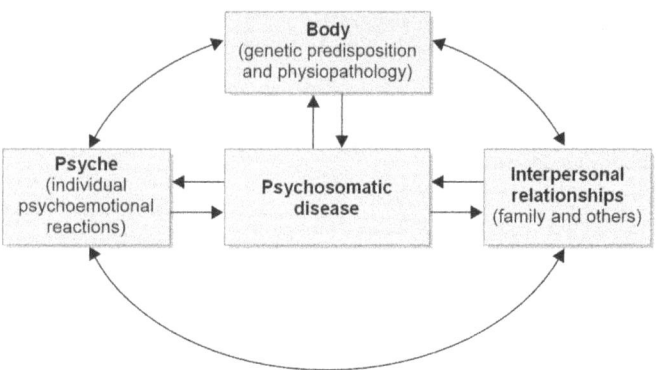

Fig. 1: Complexity and circularity in psychodermatology.

INTERVENTION AND DECISION TO DO THE PROCEDURE

An ideal case to perform a procedure is the one with no obvious psychopathology, clearly defined areas of dissatisfaction, realistic expectations, and who is self-motivated. Contradictorily, aesthetic procedures should be avoided in patients with major depression, signs of self-mutilation, troubled or agitated on day of surgery, or on psychotics. Depending on the assessment of the patient, if the physician feels that there are no psychosomatic factors behind the patient's demand for the surgery, he should go ahead. Borderline cases or mild cases of OCD or BDD also benefit with cosmetic procedures or a combination of psychiatric and cosmetic treatment. The author is aware of a young man wanting beard hair transplantation and was deeply disturbed despite having a reasonable beard. After psychiatric consultation, he was transplanted with good result both for the beard and for his psyche. This, however, is not true of all BDD patients—BDD patients believe that they have a "defective appearance" and despite doing a corrective surgery they will feel that it still looks defective; hence, they are always dissatisfied. They usually have a tendency to get multiple surgeries. Such patients also refuse to get psychiatric help initially. Counseling and communication skills are of utmost importance at such instances. It is the dermatologist's responsibility to act like a psychotherapist and explain the complexity of the condition to the patient. It is only after the patient has insight will he be willing to accept change. The dermatologists should work in a formalized collaboration with a psychiatrist, so it is easier for the patient to open up to psychiatric therapy without much resistance. Occasionally, a dermatologist may also have to prescribe selective serotonin reuptake inhibitors, such as fluoxetine, sertraline, or escitalopram, in case the patient is extremely reluctant to visit a psychiatrist, which is frequently the case.

Doing a procedure on a patient with BDD may have dire consequences too, as patients may occasionally turn violent. There are two cases of murder of surgeons by patients showing symptoms of BDD. Surveys have shown that 29% of aesthetic surgeons have been threatened legally by BDD patients. This is, therefore, one area which needs utmost consideration and deliberation by the dermatologist while deciding the procedure.

WARNING SIGNS FOR WHEN NOT TO DO PROCEDURES

It is important for a dermatologist, not just to know when to do, how to do, but also when not to do. The following tips can be of help in identifying such patients:
- A patient who is obsessively concerned
- A patient who wants 100% guarantee
- A patient who wants absolute safety
- A patient who demands multiple procedures
- *A patient who says*: I want to look like that person or that film star
- A patient who has visited several doctors for the same indication previously
- A patient who comes for the same problem repeatedly without ever deciding

Some personal examples of patients encountered by the author, to explain such patients, are given in the following text:
- A young girl was brought by the father for hair loss who was demanding hair transplantation but was found to have a headful of hair, and attempts to convince her otherwise failed. A biopsy as well as a scan was done to show that everything was normal, but she refused to agree. One day, she was brought in an "emergency" to show that she had lost 90% of hair whereas she was found to have full head. At this stage, a psychiatric component was suspected and she was asked to be shown to the psychiatrist. The father who was a doctor agreed, only to come back a week later, asking that the

drugs prescribed by the psychiatrist be given on a dermatologist's prescription so that they do not appear psychiatric. After checking with a psychiatrist, a prescription was given, but this request was repeated multiple times, till finally the author refused to give any further prescriptions till a psychiatrist gives his opinion. The psychiatrist intervened and gave a final diagnosis of schizophrenia; the father knew it all along but only had refused to accept it.
- A patient who came for laser for scars, followed by augmentation of lips, then wanted dimple creation and nose correction, all because she was trying to be a model. History of repeated surgeries hinted toward BDD.
- A patient was obsessed about donor scar after hair transplantation (strip surgery). He kept calling and questioning about the scar. Eventually, the patient was not considered a good candidate due to unrealistic expectations.
- A 34-year-old woman married for 7 years was obsessed about getting a lower hairline. On inquiry, she revealed that she wanted to enhance her beauty as she felt her husband was not paying her attention after her delivery. The patient was referred for counseling.

CONCLUSION

Only a psychologically fit patient will be satisfied by an aesthetic surgery. The aesthetic dermatologist should not be trained only in aesthetics but also in psychotherapy and should know the basics of pharmacology behind psychology. The judgment of taking a decision in such patients depends purely on the physician's knowledge and experience in dealing with psychological conditions.

Tips for practice
- Establish rapport with the patient—understand not only his indications but also reasons for indications.
- Be empathetic; spend time with the patient—avoid doctor's ego.
- Know when to do, how to do, and also when not to do.
- Learn to say no.
- Always underpromise but overdeliver.
- If there is a side effect, be prepared for an aggressive reaction.

FURTHER READINGS

1. Elsaie ML. Psychological approach in cosmetic dermatology for optimum patient satisfaction. Indian J Dermatol. 2010;55(2):127-9.
2. Gupta MA, Gupta AK. Psychodermatology: an update. J Am Acad Dermatol. 1996;34:1030-46.
3. Harth W, Lines R. Botulinophilia: Contraindication for therapy with botulinum toxin. Int J Clin Pharmacol Ther. 2001;39:460.
4. Koblenzer CS. Psychocutaneous Disease. Orlando, FL: Grune & Stratton; 1987.
5. Napoleon A. The presentation of personalities in plastic surgery. Ann Plast Surg. 1993;31:193.
6. O'Sullivan RL, Lipper G, Lerner EA. The neuroimmuno-cutaneous-endocrine network: relationship of mind and skin. Arch Dermatol. 1998;134:1431-5.
7. Phillips KA, Dufresne RG. Body dysmorphic disorder. A guide for dermatologists and cosmetic surgeons. Am J Clin Dermatol. 2000;1:235-43.
8. Phillips KA, McElroy SL, Hudson JI, Pope HG. Body dysmorphic disorder: An obsessive-compulsive spectrum disorder, a form of affective spectrum disorder, or both? J Clin Psychiatry. 1995;56:41.
9. Phillips KA. Body dysmorphic disorder: The distress of imagined ugliness. Am J Psychiatry. 1991;148:1138.
10. Poot F, Sampogna F, Onnis L. Basic knowledge in psychodermatology. J Eur Acad Dermatol Venereol. 2007;21:227-34.
11. Sarwer DB, Gibbons LM, Crerand CE. Treating body dysmorphic disorder with cognitive-behavior therapy. Psychiatr Ann. 2004;34:934.
12. Sarwer DB. Awareness and identification of body dysmorphic disorder by aesthetic surgeons: Results of a survey of American Society for Aesthetic Plastic Surgery members. Aesthetic Surg J. 2002;22:531.
13. Tory HE. Self-discrepancy: A theory relating self and affect. Psychol Rev. 1987;94(3):319-40.
14. Uzun O, Basoglu C, Akar A, Cansever A, Ozşahin A, Cetin M, et al. Body dysmorphic disorder in patients with acne. Compr Psychiatry. 2003;44:415.
15. Walker C, Papadopoulos L. The psychological impact of skin disorders. New York: Cambridge University Press; 2005.
16. Yazel L. The serial-surgery murder. Glamour. 1999;108-14.
17. Jafferany M, Salimi S, Mkhoyan R, Kalashnikova N, Sadoughifar R, Jorgaqi E. Psychological aspects of aesthetic and cosmetic surgery: clinical and therapeutic implications. Dermatol Ther. 2020;33(4):e13727.

CHAPTER 9

Dermatological and Aesthetic Issues in Adolescents

Tarun Narang, Shikha Shah

> **Key Messages**
> - Adolescence is a unique and crucial stage in human development.
> - Dermatological, psychological, and aesthetic issues are fairly common during this transitional period.
> - A comprehensive approach is very essential to address various issues in adolescents.

INTRODUCTION

Adolescence is defined by the World Health Organization (WHO) as "the phase of life between childhood and adulthood, from ages 10 to 19 years." Adolescence is a unique and crucial stage in human development, experienced in the form of a rapid physical, cognitive as well as psychosocial growth. Dermatological issues are fairly common during this period, with a prevalence of around 15-20% in various studies. The vulnerability of the psyche along with physiological changes occurring in the skin and adnexa during puberty result in a myriad of aesthetic concerns in this age group.

ADOLESCENT DERMATOLOGY

There is increased awareness on the subject that this "transitional" turmoil period comes with a special set of cosmetic issues. Although any dermatosis can have its presentation or temporal continuation during adolescence, certain dermatology issues remain more

> **BOX 1: Various dermatological and aesthetic concerns in adolescents.**
>
> *Dermatologic and aesthetic concerns in adolescents:*
> - *Dermatoses related with pathophysiological changes in hormonal and adnexal milieu*: Acne, rosacea, seborrheic dermatitis, Fox–Fordyce disease, hidradenitis suppurativa, and manifestations of insulin resistance/polycystic ovarian syndrome
> - *Dermatoses related with the changes in physical appearance*: Striae, frictional intertrigo related with obesity, frequent indulgence in cosmetics leading to allergic and/or pigmented contact dermatitis
> - *Psychosexual dermatoses related to environmental stressors*: Body dysmorphic disorder related to facial features, appearance of genitals and secondary sexual characters, trichotillomania, and acne excoriee
> - *Dermatoses related with psychosexual changes*: Risk-taking behavior and susceptibility to sexually transmitted infections, particularly during late adolescence
> - *Miscellaneous*: Various infections, eczemas particularly atopic dermatitis, hair fall, and dyspigmentation, which may start or continue to occur in adolescence

prevalent than others in adolescence. **Box 1** aims to summarize some of these most important dermatoses with unique repercussions on adolescence.

ACNE

Acne is the archetypal example of dermatological and aesthetic concern in adolescents. Acne and its sequelae (pigmentation and scarring) pose significant physical and psychosocial distress in this age group due to its troublesome symptoms and concerns about appearance. Earlier onset of severe variants can lead to significant scarring. This may lead to frustration with treatment options, social withdrawal, decreased self-esteem, anxiety, and even depression. Acne excoriee is also not uncommon. Treatment of acne itself may cause local irritation and intolerance, further impairing the functioning. Assessment tools such as Acne-Q, Comp-AQ, and Cardiff Acne Disability Index (CADI) may be useful to ascertain the impairment in life quality, especially as PROMs (patient-reported outcome measures). There are few Indian studies, which have measured the burden of acne in adolescence, with mean DLQI score of 6.91 and mean CADI score was 5.2, with greater correlation with late adolescent age group.

ATOPIC DERMATITIS

Atopic dermatitis (AD) is highly prevalent in adolescents. The special issues in this age group include the embarrassment of lesions and/or their sequelae on visible sites especially the face, constant scratching that hinders sleep and academic performance, dysfunctional social relationships with peers and frustration with the disease and its treatment. AD in adolescence is significantly associated with anxiety, sleep disorders, depression, conduct, and behavioral problems and attention-deficit hyperactivity disorder. A holistic approach must include evaluation of psychological well-being in this period, along with encouragement to self-care and continue applying moisturizers along with medications on a regular basis.

HAIR LOSS

Alopecia areata, early onset of androgenetic alopecia, and telogen effluvium are some of the most common causes of hair loss reported in adolescents. Alopecia areata occurs less frequently than in children, but greatly impairs the life quality in adolescence. Telogen effluvium is very common and often related to nutrition and acute stressors. There can be tremendous amount of stress generated with the apprehension of "going bald," creating a vicious cycle of stress and hair fall. Iron deficiency anemia, particularly around menarche should be investigated, along with the other routine tests. With the rising trend of metabolic syndrome and lifestyle changes, androgenetic alopecia/patterned hair loss is also seen as early as 15 years of age. Hair disorders warrant appropriate workup and patient counseling to mitigate stress.

DYSPIGMENTATION

Disorders of hypo- and hyperpigmentation often affect the social life of adolescents. Vitiligo and pityriasis alba are common disorders of hypopigmentation seen in this age group, the former being more debilitating in terms of associated stigma. The social concern of marriage suitability around late adolescence puts the patients and their family in stress. Hyperpigmentation is also common, and concerns about skin tone, tanning, and freckling are often seen due to sun exposure. Overuse of cosmetic products is also common, sometimes leading to allergic/pigmented contact dermatitis.

BODY DYSMORPHIC DISORDER

Body dysmorphic disorder (BDD) falls within the spectrum of obsessive–compulsive and related disorders in which patients have an "impairing preoccupation with a minor or perceived defect of their physical appearance." The prevalence of BDD is 4.9–36%, which is much higher compared to 1.7–2.4% in the general population. BDD usually has its onset in adolescence, with a reported prevalence of 1.7–3.3% in some studies. Symptoms may pertain to skin (acne, wrinkles, etc.), hair (loss, thinning, balding, etc.), and/or nose (misshapen or size). Repeated mirror examinations, compulsive skin picking, and constant efforts to hide the perceived defects is often seen. BDD in adolescents is usually more severe than the adult counterpart, associated with social withdrawal, experience academic difficulties, and go doctor shopping for their relentless and sometimes even delusional self-derogatory perception, asking for multiple treatments and procedures. There are available screening tools such as the BDD questionnaire and the body image questionnaire having a series of yes-or-no questions about appearance preoccupation, distress, and impairment. These cases are often missed and passed off as a normal worry of teenagers for appearance. Appropriate counseling and liaison with behavioral therapies are crucial as BDD is associated with severe depression, even suicide.

SOCIAL MEDIA: THE DOUBLE-EDGED SWORD

The impact of social media on adolescent health is tremendous. The "aesthetic" awakening of adolescence is on the rise with lifestyle changes. The tremendous amount of (mis)information is readily accessible within seconds, including "quick tips," "remedies," and "hacks," of the so-called pimples, marks, stretch marks, and the quintessential "glow." Apart from the cosmetic hoax, internet is often flooded with treatment suggestions for rashes and itching. As per a recent survey, these terms have been the most "googled" searches on the internet and adolescence accessing this information way more than others can be a possible conjecture. It poses significant psychosocial impact on "self-esteem" and "perception of self," two of the most common psychological domains affected in adolescent dermatoses. Social media also contributes to the "unrealistic expectations" that patients often present with. Although there are many fallacies, social media may be a useful tool in patient outreach and support groups as well as in therapeutic patient education, particularly in diseases such as AD.

Social media "trends" have also led to some new disease entities called as "digital dermatoses." These are the consequences of risk-taking "challenges" taken up on social media with unintentional self-inflicted self-harm by not realizing the nature of their actions. Examples include ice bucket challenge which may inadvertently cause violaceous edematous plaques, the fire challenge leafing to burns or the snapchat filters which may reinforce the dysmorphophobias in teens. Social media trends are constantly evolving; hence, physicians need to stay updated to avoid potential misdiagnoses.

SELF-INDUCED DERMATOSES

Self-inflicted disorders are fairly common in adolescence but their exact incidence is not known in Indian settings. These include "Skin-picking disorders" (SPD) (including dermatillomania, psychogenic excoriations, acne excoriée), trichotillomania (TTM), onychotillomania, onychophagia and dermatitis artefacta (DA). There can be some primary/secondary again as well as intentional factitious disorders such as Munchausen syndrome. There can be underlying stressors of primary skin disease (e.g., in acne excoriee), or stressors beyond the skin such as family conflict, interpersonal relationships, peer pressure, etc., which lead to these habitual picking disorders. Patients present with a wise array of sometimes bizarre morphologies pose a diagnostic challenge. It is important to address the underlying psyche simultaneously.

Table 1: Quality of life domains affected in adolescent dermatoses.

Domain	Outcomes
Appearance	Preoccupation with looks, constant try for concealing their defects/skin tone
Social	Isolation, avoidance of family/friends, limitation of engagements/activities
Activities of daily life	Change in self-care, difficulty in concentrating for daily chores, sleep disturbances, changes in eating patterns
Emotional/psychological	Feeling conscious about self, low confidence and self-esteem, embarrassed or frustrated about the disease, anxiety, depression, fear of stigma
Physical	Inability to participate in exercise, outdoor activities/sports
Academic	Impaired scholastic performance, absent days from school/college
Treatment burden	Treatments may be found inconvenient, adverse effects
Sexual	Late adolescent period with affected sexual relationships, insecurity and fears about sexual health, concerns for appearance if dermatoses affect genitalia

BURDEN OF THE DISEASE AND IMPACT ON QUALITY OF LIFE

The burden of cosmesis in adolescence is enormous and **Table 1** aims to briefly summarize the domains of life quality impaired by various dermatoses.

ASSESSMENT OF LIFE QUALITY IN ADOLESCENTS

The conventional tools for quality of life (QoL) assessment may not do justice in adolescents, since subjective perceptions and influence of peers are of higher significance than actual objective disease in most situations. The Children's Dermatology Life Quality Index (CDLQI) is meant for children aged 4–16 years, which still does not cater to all aspects in teens. Skindex-Teen and T-QoL (Teen QoL) are designed for adolescents. The Skindex-Teen has been derived from preexisting adult questionnaire, while T-QoL has been derived after psychometric analysis after studying teens with different dermatoses. The latter includes domains on self-image, physical well-being and future aspirations, psychological impact and relationships. Other than these, screening questionnaires for anxiety and depression (e.g., PHQ-9) may also be employed, like the PHQ-9 scale.

MANAGEMENT ASPECTS

Adolescent Healthcare Set-up

Special clinics or a setup designed for addressing adolescent issues in dermatology is ideal. Some countries have Teenage and Young Adult (TYA) skin clinics for the same. In clinical practice, approach called "THRxEADS (T for Transition, H for Home, Rx for Medication and Treatment, E for Education and Eating, A for Activities and Affect, D for Drugs and S for Sexuality)", may be used as a comprehensive tool to address various aspects in adolescent health. The patient needs addressal as a whole in order to manage these dermatoses.

Aspects in management include:
- *Treatment of underlying dermatological disease*: The underlying disease needs to be managed as per severity and standard practice and/or guidelines. Adequate treatment of the disease can bring down the secondary psychological consequences.
- *Psychotherapy*: Habit reversal and cognitive behavioral therapy are important aspects of management, particularly in self-inflicted dermatoses. Liaison with psychiatry is imperative.
- *Family counseling*: Conflict resolution and managing "the greater patient" is crucial, with family members involved actively in the disease management and stress mitigation.
- Adoption of a multidisciplinary approach involving collaboration with experts from endocrinology, gynecology, and psychology is crucial for comprehensive management.

CONCLUSION

Just like children, adolescents are also not small adults. There are many dermatological and aesthetic issues in this age group that warrant addressal to the psyche in conjunction with therapy. Acne, pigmentary disorders, atopic dermatitis, body dysmorphia, etc., significantly impair the QoL, especially in terms of self-esteem, warranting an approach beyond the skin.

FURTHER READINGS

1. Satish N, Dakshinamoorthy A, Srikanth S. A study of the pattern of dermatoses in adolescent patients in South India. Int J Dermatol. 2022;61:299-305.
2. Layton AM, Ravenscroft J. Adolescent acne vulgaris: current and emerging treatments. Lancet Child Adolesc Health. 2023;7:136-44.
3. Hornsey S, Stuart B, Muller I, Layton AM, Morrison L, King J, et al. Patient-reported outcome measures for acne: a mixed-methods validation study (acne PROMs). BMJ Open. 2021;11:e034047.
4. Durai PC, Nair DG. Acne vulgaris and quality of life among young adults in South India. Indian J Dermatol. 2015;60:33-40.
5. Xie QW, Dai X, Tang X, Chan CHY, Chan CLW. Risk of mental disorders in children and adolescents with atopic dermatitis: A systematic review and meta-analysis. Front Psychol. 2019;10:1773.
6. Bedocs LA, Bruckner AL. Adolescent hair loss. Curr Opin Pediatr. 2008;20: 431-5.
7. Griggs J, Burroway B, Tosti A. Pediatric androgenetic alopecia: A review. J Am Acad Dermatol. 2021;85:1267-73.
8. Herbst I, Jemec GBE. Body dysmorphic disorder in dermatology: A systematic review. Psychiatr Q. 2020;91:1003-10.
9. Dennin MH, Lee MS. Body dysmorphic disorder in pediatric dermatology. Pediatr Dermatol. 2018;35:868-74.
10. Rieder EA, Andriessen A, Cutler V, Gonzalez ME, Greenberg JL, Lio P, et al. Dermatology in contemporary times: Building awareness of social media's association with adolescent skin disease and mental health. J Drugs Dermatol. 2023;22:817-25.
11. Kamiński M, Tizek L, Zink A. 'Dr. Google, what is that on my skin?'-internet searches related to skin problems: Google Trends Data from 2004 to 2019. Int J Environ Res Public Health. 2021;18:2541.
12. Young TK, Oza VS. Digital dermatoses: skin disorders engendered by social media in tweens and teens. Curr Opin Pediatr. 2021;33:373-9.
13. Gupta MA, Gupta AK. Self-induced dermatoses: A great imitator. Clin Dermatol. 2019;37:268-277.
14. Basra MKA, Salek MS, Fenech D, Finlay AY. Conceptualization, development and validation of T-QoL© (Teenagers' Quality of Life): a patient-focused measure to assess quality of life of adolescents with skin diseases. Br J Dermatol. 2018;178:161-75.
15. De Vere Hunt IJ, Howard E, McPherson T. The impact of chronic skin disease in adolescence and the need for specialist adolescent services. Clin Exp Dermatol. 2020;45:5-9.
16. McPherson T, Ravenscroft J, Ali R, Barlow R, Beattie P, Bewley A, et al. British Society for Paediatric and Adolescent Dermatology (BSPAD) assessment and support of mental health in children and young people (CYP) with skin conditions: A multi-disciplinary expert consensus statement and recommendations. Br J Dermatol. 2023;189(4):459-66.

CHAPTER 10

Psychological and Neuropsychiatric Complications of HIV and STD

Rakesh Bharti, Satnam Singh Palia

> **Key Messages**
> - Sexually transmitted disease (STD)—patients are not only suffering physically but mentally too.
> - The mental agony is very painful in chronic and life-compromising ailments such as HIV and leads to psychiatric comorbidities.
> - In a good number of patients, the psychiatric morbidity alone producing symptoms without physical illness.
> - The STD specialists need to be aware of such psychological comorbidities for comprehensive treatment.

INTRODUCTION

The disease which are transmitted sexually, including human immunodeficiency virus (HIV), leave an indelible mark on the minds of the sufferers besides the physical disturbances. In this chapter authors will try to explore the effects of STD's on psyche of a person.

HIV/AIDS (ACQUIRED IMMUNODEFICIENCY SYNDROME)

It has been more than three decades ever since the first patient of HIV was reported and since then much water has flown in various rivers of the world. Despite much passage of time and awareness campaigns of large scale and acquired immunodeficiency syndrome (AIDS) being considered a manageable chronic disease rather than a certificate of a certain death, the diagnosis of it send shivers down the spine of majority people.

Both the diagnosis with the disease and the mortality associated with it, have major consequences for the psychological and social functioning of individuals and their communities. It is known that the HIV infection affects the brain at an early stage and the disease has a chronic progressive course associated with a wide range of psychiatric consequences. Even so, many patients with AIDS manage to lead relatively normal lives for substantial periods. Highly active antiretroviral therapy (HAART) has led to a reduction in HIV-related morbidity and mortality to an improved life expectancy. Hence, it is more likely to encounter patients with psychiatric manifestations of the disease.

Following neuropsychological events would be observed as the disease progresses:

- *HIV—early stage—asymptomatic infection*: There are no early neuropsychological deficits.
- *HIV—intermediate stage 6-18 months)*: Before the clinical AIDS develops, there is a marked increase in the prevalence of major depression, mania, dementia, and delirium.
- *HIV—late stage*: Significant cognitive decline or AIDS— associated dementia.

It is observed that in the richer nations, the picture is one of a chronic but treatable disease, where the main problems are the side effects of the complex drug regimens, drug resistance, and the psychological problems of coping with a chronic disease, whereas in the poorer developing nations, large number of people are still subject to severe neuropsychiatric complications, associated mood disorders, psychosis, and AIDS dementia in the years before their death. In the developed world, HIV is still associated with the increased rates of psychiatric morbidity but the severe life-threatening organic picture (AIDS dementia) is thankfully now much less frequent.

There could be several consequences psychologically such as reactions to testing, psychiatric problems, suicide, deliberate self-harm, neuropsychiatric disorders, social consequences, and ethical problems along with problems in relation to illicit drug use. The following are the contexts in which psychiatric problems may arise.

Whenever someone, especially a person of LGBTQ+ community, is asked to take the diagnostic test, the consequences are of panic, anxiety, and fear. Those having a psychotic personality may suffer

from delusions, whereas those who are neurotic in nature may become hypochondriacal.
- Posttest stress and anxiety, which may precipitate adjustment or psychiatric disorder
- Living with infection, resulting in stressful life events
- HIV infection directly infecting the brain cells (neurons) causing neuropsychiatric symptoms
- Antiretroviral (ARV) medications may cause psychiatric symptoms, e.g., azidothymidine (AZT) may precipitate a major depressive episode whilst isoniazid prophylaxis has been known to precipitate psychosis.

CLINICAL PSYCHIATRIC PRESENTATIONS

- Acute psychological reactions
- Longer-term psychiatric disorders
- HIV-associated cognitive disorders

Acute psychological reactions: Whenever a patient is handed over a HIV positive report, then the chances of him/her reacting by way of shock, anger, denial, or depression results. Shock may manifest in the form of escapism and taking shelter of drugs/alcohol, aloofness and even loss of sleep. This phase may be stretched to long duration, especially if proper counseling is not offered. The other reaction of depression can sometimes be severe enough to lead to suicidal thoughts.

The psychological distress diminishes in most cases by ten weeks after notification. Pre- and post-test counseling should help abate these psychological problems.

- *Longer-term psychiatric disorders*:
  - *Depression*: The depressive spectrum disorders are most common (35.6%).

    15% ARV-naive patients may even have pain and complaints of fatigue and loss of sleep, besides having mood swings. These can usually be treated with selective serotonin reuptake inhibitors (SSRIs).
  - *Disorders*: 4–19% of patients, in the context of adjustment disorders, including generalized anxiety disorder (GAD), panic disorder, post-traumatic stress disorder (PTSD), and obsessive compulsive disorder (OCD)—repeated bodily scrutiny for evidence of progression of disease. Ruminations may center on death and dying or to recollect past sexual partners to

whom infection may have been transmitted. Management should be through psychotropic medication (see in the following text) and or specific psychological therapy through cognitive behavior therapy (CBT) modules.
  - *Psychoses*: Not infrequent, incidence less than depression. Thoughts of death and dying constantly haunt such patients. HIV patients suffers less commonly with psychosis. They, however, can have more of maniac symptoms.
  Treatment to include low-dose risperidone or any other atypical antipsychotic (olanzapine, quetiapine, and clozapine) remain watchful of any emerging extrapyramidal side effects. Manic symptoms would respond to mood stabilizers, especially lithium. Sodium valproate may increase viral replication and reduce white cell count (WCC).
  - *Suicide*: There is a 30% increased risk of suicide in individuals who are HIV positive (suicidal ideation along with suicidal attempts). High risk times include, at diagnosis, at the death of an HIV-positive friend as the individual experiences deterioration in physical health.
- *HIV-associated cognitive disorders*: Generally, three categories are acknowledged:
  i. HIV-associated dementia (HAD) increasing forgetfulness
  ii. Minor cognitive-motor disorder (MCMD)
  iii. Neuropsychological impairment including delirium

HIV-associated dementia is a relatively common outcome in full-blown AIDS. The mean survival after diagnosis with HAD is 6 months. It presents earlier with minor cognitive slowing and memory deficits as well as motor slowing and subtle in coordination. In later stages, there is a full-blown clinical dementia syndrome picture with deficits in cognitive (including amnesia and mutism), motor (tremor, ataxia, choreoathetosis, spasticity, and myoclonus) and affective (depression, apathy, agitation, disinhibition, and mania). The cognitive decline may be assessed using the HIV dementia scale. Reverse transcriptase inhibitors (AZT) may delay HAD progression.

MANAGEMENT OF PSYCHIATRIC DISORDERS

Management should include alterations in sexual practices, control of risk-taking behavior in drug addicts and children born to infected mothers.

When the presentation is not of organic origin, psychotropic medication would be the primary treatment. Please follow the principles of:
- Start with a low dose and titrate according to tolerability and response.
- Choose the simplest dosing regimen possible.
- Choose a drug with the fewest side-effects/drug interactions.

Depression and stress-related mood disorders: Need treatment with a trial of SSRI-antidepressant as side effects profile is better with such patients. First-line agents are SSRIs, especially citalopram and can be tricyclic antidepressants but watch for side effects. Alternative could be a trial of mirtazapine.

Bipolar affective disorder or mania: Patient may be sensitive to lithium as a mood stabilizer. Alternative is valproate or lamotrigine or gabapentin. Avoid carbamazepine as it has drug interaction with antiretroviral agents such as ritonavir as well as risk of neutropenia.

Anxiety disorders: A short-term use of benzodiazepines in an acute crisis but risk of misuse and dependence and drug interactions needs to be monitored. SSRIs and other antidepressants, e.g., buspirone may be useful.

Obviously, there is need for psychological therapy on cognitive behavior therapy (CBT) lines and stress management.

Psychosis: Atypicals are usually used first line, e.g., risperidone, which is widely used and is safe. Alternative could be small doses of clozapine but needs blood monitoring. These patients are more susceptible to extrapyramidal side effects, neuromalignant syndrome, and tardive dyskinesia.

Delirium: Organic causes should be identified and treated. Short-term symptomatic treatment may include low-dose atypicals such as risperidone, olanzapine, quetiapine, or ziprasidone. The concomitant short use of short-acting benzodiazepine such as lorazepam may also be helpful.

Neurocognitive disorders: Mild forgetfulness to severe and debilitating dementia may respond to a combination of therapy with antiretroviral therapy with a judicious short-term use of antipsychotic such as risperidone.

Drug interactions: Certain psychotropics (potent enzyme inducers) are contraindicated with antiretroviral agents of all classes as they can compromise antiretroviral therapy and they include carbamazepine, phenobarbital, phenytoin, primidone, and St. John's Wort.

SEXUALLY TRANSMITTED DISEASES

The major focus here is neurosyphilis; historically known as general paresis of the insane (GPI or dementia paralytica) or Cupid's disease.

STDs affect psyche of males (30-50 years of age) more frequently, and they may have mood swings and impaired intellect.

The presentation could be as follows:
- A simple dementing form
- A grandiose form involving euphoria, irritability, grandiose manner and delusions, with hypomanic or manic features
- A depressive form with low mood, melancholic delusions, suicidal thoughts, and retardation
- A paranoid schizophreniform and neurasthenic presentation.

Neurological features such as Argyll Robertson pupils, tremor, ataxia, dysarthria, myoclonus, hyperreflexia, spasticity, and extrapyramidal signs are also usually present.

Management

Whereas depression is best tackled with antidepressants, psychotropic drugs are mainly required to control agitation, delusions, and hallucinations.

Venereological Hypochondriasis

There is persistent preoccupation with the fear or conviction of suffering from a serious physical illness due to STDs without sufficient physical findings. This is one of the common presentations in STD clinics and dermatological consultations. This conviction and preoccupation with fear of illness persists despite negative medical diagnostic tests and assurance from the physician about the absence of somatic illness. The symptoms cannot be better explained by other primary psychiatric disorders such as anxiety, panic, compulsive, or depressive disorder. AIDS phobia, syphilis phobia, venereophobia, and *Candida* phobia are the usual conditions presenting as venereological hypochondriasis.

They may present with different bodily symptoms, especially related to general health, skin, and genitalia. It is very difficult to convince and treat even though evidences exist against the presence of the disease and doctor shopping very common.

Management

Tricyclic antidepressants, SSRIs, or neuroleptics may be often helpful.

Useful Psychological Procedures

The following psychological techniques are useful in the management of STD-related psychiatric comorbidities—psychoeducation, CBT, relaxation therapies, mindfulness-based cognitive therapy, hypnotherapy, family therapy, group therapy, and physical exercises.

They can be used as monotherapy or as an adjuvant along with psychopharmacotherapy depending upon the clinical situation.

CONCLUSION

Psychological evaluation and treatment is very essential in STD patients as a large number of patients are suffering from minor to major psychiatric comorbidities. Even persons who are absolutely normal and no evidence of any STDs suffer from hypochondriasis and somatoform disorders due an accidental extra marital or pre marital sexual exposure. All healthcare professionals dealing with STDs should be aware of this important area and arrange facilities for providing psychological care and treatment.

FURTHER READINGS

1. Frost DP. Recognition of hypochondriasis in a clinic for sexually transmitted disease. Genitourin Med. 1985;61:133-7.
2. Safdar S, Kosakowska-Berezecka N. Psychology of Gender through the Lens of Culture: Theories and Applications. New York: Springer; 2015.
3. Sepkowitz KA. One disease, two epidemics: AIDS. N Engl J Med. 2006;354: 2411-4.
4. Sutton S, Baum A, Johnston M. The SAGE Handbook of Health Psychology. New Delhi: Sage Publication; 2004.
5. Nebhinani N, Mattoo SK, Wanchu A. Psychiatric morbidity in HIV-positive subjects: a study from India. J Psychosom Res. 2011;70(5):449-54.
6. Tamminga CA. HIV and AIDS. Am J Psychiatry. 2006;163(8):1322.
7. Lyketsos CG, Hutton H, Fishman M, Schwartz J, Treisman GJ. Psychiatric morbidity on entry to an HIV primary care clinic. AIDS. 1996;10(9):1033-9.

CHAPTER 11

Psyche and Genitals: Conspicuous Associations in Psychodermatologic Perspective

Bishurul Hafi NA, Uvais NA

> **Key Messages**
> - This chapter delves into the connection between psychology and genitalia, a subject not previously explored with the respect it deserves.
> - It covers various topics such as anogenital itch, mucocutaneous skin syndrome, body dysmorphic disorder, small penis syndrome, among others.
> - These insights aid dermatologists in better comprehending and addressing psychogenic disorders related to the genitals.

INTRODUCTION

The intersection between our psyche and our genitals is a fascinating realm within the broader spectrum of psychodermatology. Our skin serves as a communicative canvas for our emotions, stressors, and psychological well-being. Despite being concealed beneath clothing, our genitals wield significant influence over our self-confidence and overall mental health.

Exploring this correlation unveils the intricate connections between our psyche and our most intimate body parts. It is a domain where psychological factors interlace with dermatological manifestations that impact not just physical health but also emotional and mental states. Moreover, different philosophies have contradicting concepts about sexuality. These significant differences might have impact on the people's perception of human sexuality and its effect on health.

Skin, as the organ of communication, interacts deeply with the human brain. The skin over genitals is densely innervated for the purpose of sexual pleasure. Sexual gratification during activities including solo performances, where one's skin over genitals gets stimulated by skin of his/her fingers, possess additive potential as explained in theories of masturbation addictions. The very superficial activities of the skin can potentiate dopaminergic surge in brain which signal positive reinforcement. On the contrary, inappropriate touch on genitals can cause sexual dysfunctions including erectile dysfunction and vaginismus. These examples highlight delicate nature of impact of genital skin over sexual life and general psychological health of a person, irrespective of gender. Moreover, the fact that sexuality is one of the basic needs for the survival of the species, if not individual, makes this topic extremely important. Unfortunately, interactions between psych and genitals have not been discussed properly in literature yet.

Psychodermatology, as an evolving field, recognizes the psychological implications of skin conditions, including those affecting the genital region. Understanding the psychological nuances tied to genital health and appearance is pivotal in comprehending the holistic impact on an individual's mental health and well-being. All psychodermatological disorders can be broadly classified into three main categories. According to the same categorization, disorders affecting psych and genitals can also be described generally, as given below:

- *Primary psychogenital disorders*: These are the primary psychiatric disorders related with genitals, e.g., delusion of parasitosis, factitious disorders, and body dysmorphic disorders.
- *Psychological comorbidities secondary to genital dermatoses*: Normal or abnormal findings on genitals eliciting strong emotional response to the patient, irrespective of the etiopathogenesis, e.g., depression, anxiety, and venereophobia secondary to symptomatic or asymptomatic dermatoses.
- *Psychophysiologic disorders involving genitals*: There are several genital dermatoses aggravated by stress, e.g., psoriasis, lichen planus, balanitis, and vulvitis.
- *Miscellaneous*: Medication-induced adverse effects manifesting on genitals, genital mutilation-associated psychologic comorbidities, culture-bound syndromes involving genitals (e.g., dhat syndrome, koro syndrome), mucocutaneous pain syndrome (e.g., scrotodynia, vulvodynia, anodynia).

Being proposed a provisional classification, we would like to elaborate on certain conditions, which are closely related with psych and genitals.

ANOGENITAL ITCH

It is defined as intense itching, acute or chronic, affecting the anal, perianal, perineal, and genital skin, which is a dominant problem in the course of various cutaneous and systemic conditions. As a cause of chronic pruritus, genital itch affects quality of life badly and is a very annoying symptom dermatologists face difficulty to treat. Causes of genital itch range from psychogenic to neoplasm **(Table 1)**. While etiology-specific treatment remains the cornerstone of management, many cases turn out to be idiopathic or psychogenic which are very resistant to conventional treatment protocols in both genders. Probably, neither psychogenic nor organic pruritus exists in a pure form, and both are always in coexistence. Being an

Table 1: Common causes for anogenital itch.

Acute anogenital pruritus	Chronic anogenital pruritus
Infections:	*Dermatoses*: Seborrheic dermatitis, psoriasis, atopic dermatitis, lichen sclerosus, lichen planus, plasma cell vulvitis/balanitis, papular acantholytic dyskeratosis, dermatographism, atrophic vulvovaginitis
• *Fungal*: Dermatophytoses, *Candida*	
• *Bacterial*: Corynebacterium minutissimum, Staphylococcus aureus, group A *Streptococcus*	
• *Bacterial vaginosis*: Gardnerella vaginalis, Mobiluncus species, Bacteroides species, Mycoplasma hominis, anaerobic gram-positive cocci	*Neoplasms*:
	• Extramammary Paget's disease, Bowen's disease, Erythroplasia of Queyrat, syringomas, Hidradenoma papilliferum, Langerhans cell histiocytosis, and basal cell carcinomas
• *Viral*: Herpes simplex virus, Human papilloma virus, Molluscum contagiosum	
• *Parasitic*: Trichomonas vaginalis	
• *Infestation*: Scabies, Phthirus pubis, Pin worms	• Idiopathic pruritus (lichen simplex chronicus, neurodermatitis, essential pruritus, pruritus vulvae, pruritus ani, pruritus scroti)
• *Contact dermatitis*: Irritant allergic (common agents include local anesthetics, medicaments, perfumes, cleansers, condoms, garments, sweat, urine, and feces)	• Psychogenic

Source: Swamiappan M. Anogenital pruritus: An overview. J Clin Diagn Res. 2016;10(4):WE01-3.

area of constant occlusion and close contact with cloth materials, mechanical stimuli seem to play an important role in genital itch. In a study from Ikoma's group, researchers could elicit mechanically evoked "pure itch" without nociceptive sensations which could be very addictive in nature. But as we know itch is a multidimensional sensation that involves discriminative sensory, cognitive, and emotional components. Itch sensation is not perceived similarly in brain (even in same person in different contexts!), which is subject to innumerable psychosocial factors. Pruritus and psyche are intricately and reciprocally related, with psychophysiological evidence and psychopathological explanations helping us to understand their complex association. Not only can a person's psychological status aggravate pruritus, but pruritus and scratching genitals can also severely affect the person's psychological status and self-image which in turn exacerbates the morbidity. As of now, genital itch has no established relationship with any personality traits. Idiopathic itch is considered as the psychopathology of most cases. Diagnosis of psychogenic itch must be made after excluding all organic causes and the diagnostic criteria for functional itch disorders proposed by the French psychodermatology group can be utilized **(Box 1)**. A psychogenic origin of itching has been found in 2% of patients with chronic pruritus; these cases need to be treated with psychotherapy and antidepressants. Other cases have to be treated as per the etiology.

BOX 1: French psychodermatology group's diagnostic criteria for functional itch disorder.

Three compulsory criteria:
1. Localized or generalized pruritus sine materia (without primary skin lesion)
2. Chronic pruritus (>6 weeks)
3. No somatic cause

Three of seven optional criteria:
1. A chronological relationship of pruritus with one or several life events that could have psychological repercussions
2. Variations in intensity associated with stress
3. Nocturnal variations
4. Predominance during rest or inaction
5. Associated psychological disorder
6. Pruritus that could be improved by psychotropic drugs
7. Pruritus that could be improved by psychotherapies

MUCOCUTANEOUS PAIN SYNDROMES

Mucocutaneous pain syndromes are a group of chronic, focal pain syndromes that mainly affects the urogenital region as well as the oral cavity. The "dynias" that affect the urogenital region are vulvodynia, penodynia, orchidynia, prostatodynia, coccygodynia, and proctodynia. The common presenting complaint in all these regional pain syndromes is severe burning sensation confined to the involved region. These are complex regional pain syndromes which can be highly debilitating and frustrating to the patients and at the same time challenging to the treating physician.

Vulvodynia is defined as chronic burning and/or pain in the vulva without any evidence of organic pathology. Pain can be neuropathic in nature without any provoking stimulus or can be provoked by coitus. The neuropathic or dysesthetic vulvodynia is poorly localized and is more common in elderly females. Vulvodynia provoked by coitus also known as vulvar vestibulitis syndrome is seen in nulliparous females of early reproductive age following pressure within the vulvar vestibule and the pain is restricted to the vestibule. Though the etiology of vulvodynia is not clearly understood, increased innervation of the vestibule is considered to have a role. Dyspareunia and vulvar pruritus may be associated symptoms and often can lead to sexual dysfunction.

Though in primary vulvodynia, no objective findings are seen except vulval erythema, a detailed history and physical examination followed by relevant investigation should be carried out to rule out any secondary causes of vulvodynia in suspected patients. Certain causes of secondary vulvodynia include candidiasis, atopy, dermatographism, irritant contact dermatitis, and rarely, carcinoma.

Treatment modalities for primary vulvodynia include tricyclic antidepressants, gabapentin, pelvic floor rehabilitation combined with surface electromyography, interferon alpha, estrogen creams, and surgery. The role of patient education and psychological support cannot be overemphasized. In recalcitrant cases, assistance of psychiatrists as well as pain management specialists should be sought.

PERSISTENT GENITAL AROUSAL DISORDER

Persistent genital arousal (PGAD) is a syndrome of unprovoked sexual arousal/orgasm of uncertain cause primarily reported in female patients. A largely underrecognized condition characterized by persistent, unwanted genital arousal (sensations, sensitivity, and vasocongestion) in the absence of subjective/cognitive arousal and sexual desire. PGAD is a distressing condition that is associated with a significant negative impacts on psychosocial and daily functioning. It was thought to be a psychological disorder until recently. Caroline et al. put forward a theoretical model which conceptualized PGAD as an overarching nosology of genitopelvic dysesthesia. They proposed a model of genitopelvic dysesthesias, with subcategories of unpleasant sensations that are based on patients' primary complaint: arousal, arousal and pain, or pain (and other sensations). Another recent work by Anne Louise et al., observed PGAD symptoms are due to unprovoked firing of C-fibers in the regional special sensory neurons that subserve sexual arousal with some PGAD symptoms sharing same pathophysiologic mechanisms with neuropathic pain and itch. They observed a strong association of PGAD with Tarlov cysts and sensory polyneuropathy. As treatment strategies validation, psychoeducation, identification of triggers, distraction techniques, and pelvic massage to decrease the pelvic floor tension have been attempted. In addition, use of antidepressants, olanzapine, risperidone, carbamazepine, valproic acid, opioid agonist tramadol, varenicline, duloxetine, and pregabalin are tried.

BODY DYSMORPHIC DISORDER AND GENITALS

Body dysmorphic disorder (BDD) is defined by a preoccupation with a perceived defect or problem with physical appearance. The defect in appearance is either imagined or minor, and distress about it results in impaired functioning. Most people with BDD have several body image concerns. BDD is associated with depression, suicidal ideation, completed suicide as well as impaired functioning in multiple domains. Although BDD is more common in women, men with BDD have more concerns regarding genitals. They often make repeated medical visits seeking cure to their perceived defect, most related with penile size, or undergo treatments with vacuum pumps, penile stretching devices or even surgeries, or indulge in self-activities such as jelqing, a massage technique intended to lengthen or enhance the shape of the erect penis. Idea about this condition is necessary for dermatologists since aggressive treatment of BDD patients for subjective problems may be highly counterproductive and may invite legal liabilities.

Growth of cosmetic gynecology has created exponential increase of genital-associated BDD in women. Demand for cosmetic labioplasty has increased enormously in many developed countries. BDD is a strong contraindication for corrective surgery in women too for essentially ethical reasons: firstly, BDD undermines autonomy to such an extent that the person wanting cosmetic surgery does not have the capacity to make a valid informed choice, because their perception of reality is so skewed; and secondly, that surgery will do more harm than good, because the fixation of one aspect of bodily experience will soon be replaced by another one, leading to more distress, not less.

Even though treatment of BDD of genitals have not been researched extensively, anecdotal reports support cognitive behavioral therapy (CBT) as an effective treatment modality.[24] CBT for BDD consists of exposure, ritual prevention, mirror retraining, mindfulness, and cognitive restructuring. Mirror retraining, a key component of CBT for BDD, entails standing undressed at a distance from the mirror and scanning the body from head to toe without focusing on the area of concern, which is genital in this case. The rationale is to help patients to see their bodies as other men would see them. Another component in therapy is to create a list of situations that create BDD-related anxiety for them and expose them to those situations. They then learn to expose themselves to those situations, some of which may have been avoided consistently over time, and to handle those situations without engaging in overlearned habits.

SMALL PENIS SYNDROME

It was first published by Murtagh in 1989 while Wylie and Eardley modified the concept after 20 years. It is defined as "an anxiety about the genitals being observed, directly or indirectly (when clothed), because of concern that the flaccid penis length and/or its girth is less than the normal for an adult male, despite evidence from a clinical examination to counter this." It is an independent diagnosis outside BDD definition and both can be differentiated using a validated screening scale developed by Veale et al. by assessing distress, appearance preoccupation, checking and avoidance behavior, impact on occupation, social life, sexuality, and partner relationship. BDD could be considered a more serious form of small penis syndrome (SPS) with psychiatric comorbidities and in some cases, even delusional aspects. Not all men with SPS have symptoms of BDD. A thorough assessment and diagnosis to differentiate between SPS and BDD is required to determine which treatment is needed. In about two thirds of men with SPS, concerns originate during childhood. Comparing one's penis with others and those in erotic images, being bullied or having heard negative remarks about penis size are some reasons for developing insecurity in child's mind. Even the habit of observing penis by looking down instead of looking at it in a mirror makes the penis seem smaller. Obsessive-compulsive disorder, social phobia, anxiety, depression, and possibly personality disorders can be comorbid conditions. They also might contribute to the development of penile size dissatisfaction. Sexual dysfunction might be a result of SPS and contributing to it. We must approach patients with SPS seriously by taking good psychologic history and thorough physical examination. Prompt referral to mental health professionals or sexologists may be needed.

VENEREOPHOBIA

Venereophobia is defined as excessive and obsessive thoughts about sexually transmitted infections possibly triggered by single or multiple episodes of sexual encounters, not necessarily be intercourse proper. Emergence of venereophobia can be paralleled to propaganda war against venereal diseases, which was effective in advocating safe sex practices to a certain level, but in turn led to the growth of venereophobia through panic mood associated with it. Exact burden of the disease is not known since large-scale studies have not been done yet. In an Indian study, venereophobia was seen in 13% of patients attending a psychosexual clinic. It has been reported more in males probably due to easy visibility of male genitalia, increased symptoms among males, paucity of female patients declaring sexual encounters. In some studies on cutaneous manifestation among psychiatric patients, venereophobia was seen in 1–4%. In a study by Wang et al., they have shown that in symptom check list (SCL)-90, the scores of somatization, obsessive-compulsive, interpersonal sensitivity, depression, anxiety, phobic anxiety, and paranoid ideation are obviously higher among venereophobia patients than healthy people. Some of the presenting complaints in venereophobia are spermatorrhea, pearly penile papules, sticky meatus, threads in urine, phosphaturia, hyperpigmentation of median raphe penis and scrotum, fox Fordyce spots, sebaceous hyperplasia, smegma, prominent veins, Bier's spots, skin tag, congenital and acquired melanocytic nevi, angioma, angiokeratoma, etc. A detailed psychiatric evaluation is needed to understand the psychopathology better and a liaison approach provides significant improvement in such cases. In severe cases with psychological comorbidities, pharmacotherapy might be needed.

GENITAL DERMATILLOMANIA

Dermatillomania is a skin picking disorder (SPD) that is defined as repetitive scratching, rubbing, digging, picking or squeezing of the skin resulting in visible damage and impairment in social functioning. SPD is more common in females with a female-to-male ratio of approximately 8:1 mostly in age group between 15 and 45 years. Clinical manifestations include excoriation and polymorphic lesions of varying sizes with a wide variation in severity and extent due to different stages of healing. The most commonly affected sites are the face, scalp, shoulders, and back, but genital region can also be affected. Dermatillomania is also commonly associated with other major psychiatric disorders such as depression (42%), obsessive-compulsive disorder (40%), bipolar disorder (38%), etc. CBT, habit reversal therapies, and pharmacotherapy [selective serotonin reuptake inhibitors (SSRIs)]might be required in severe cases.

PSYCHOLOGICAL EFFECTS OF GENITAL MUTILATION

This is particularly common among females of African ethnic groups. Female genital mutilation (FGM) "comprises all procedures involving the partial or total removal of the external female genitalia or other injury to the female genital organs whether for cultural, religious, or other nontherapeutic reasons." Though FGM is considered as a violation of human rights, and outlawed in many countries, it is still performed in a large part of Africa, particularly in Eastern regions. Research suggests that FGM is associated with a wide range of long-term health and psychological problems with about a sixth reporting scores above the threshold for posttraumatic stress disease (PTSD) and a third reporting severe levels of depression or anxiety.

Prevalence of male genital mutilation (MGM) is lesser compared to FGM due to lack of cultural factors promoting it. Genital self-mutilation (GSM) in males are reported in many psychological conditions. Some of the risk factors for this act are: presence of religious delusions, command hallucinations, low self-esteem and feelings of guilt associated with sexual offences, failures in the male role, problems in the early developmental period, such as experiencing difficulties in male identification and persistence of incestuous desires, depression and having a history of GSM. The eponym Klingsor syndrome, which involves the presence of religious delusions, is proposed for GSM. In a study by Veeder et al., common psychiatric disorders associated with GSM included schizophrenia spectrum (49%), substance use (18.5%), personality (15.9%), and gender dysphoric disorders (15.3%). Further analyses revealed that schizophrenia spectrum disorders occurred significantly more often among autoamputates as compared with self-castrators or mutilators. Gender dysphoria occurred significantly more often among self-castrators than autoamputates. Another study by Martin et al. described schizophrenia and affective psychosis as the most frequent diagnoses while alcohol intoxication was diagnosed in about one-fourth of the cases published.

DISORDERS OF SEX DEVELOPMENT

Disorders of sex development (DSD) are a group of congenital medical conditions due to discrepancy of chromosomal, gonadal, or anatomic sex, which affect the whole life span. It is estimated to occur in one of every 4,500–5,000 births. This condition has serious effects on all three components of psychosexual development, i.e., gender identity, gender role, and sexual orientation. Gender dissatisfaction is higher prevalent among people with DSD than general population. It must be diagnosed early and managed by a multidisciplinary team.

POSTORGASMIC ILLNESS SYNDROME

Postorgasmic illness syndrome (POIS) is a rare disorder characterized by flu-like and allergic-type symptoms that occur soon after ejaculation. This allergic reaction to semen occurs after intercourse, masturbation, or spontaneous ejaculation and can last up to 2–7 days. It has a chronic course with primary pattern occurring in adolescence and a secondary acquired pattern with a later onset. Being underreported or underdiagnosed, data on its incidence and prevalence is scarce. The pattern of symptoms suggests an allergic or autoimmune etiology. However, there is no consensus on exact etiopathogenesis or management. Men suffering from POIS have a significant emotional trauma and a poor quality of life. Treatment recommendations have included antihistamines, benzodiazepines, SSRIs, and CNS stimulants.

SEMEN CONTACT ALLERGY

A female counterpart of POIS is semen contact allergy. Around 40% of affected women present with allergic symptoms, usually localized contact urticarial like, after first sexual intercourse itself. There is a strong prevalence of atopy in the family of affected individuals. The localized form of semen contact allergy presents as severe burning, itching, edema, redness, or even blistering on the vulvovaginal area. The systemic form is characterized by urticaria, angioedema, and respiratory or gastrointestinal symptoms. After the initial onset, symptoms usually arise with all subsequent exposures and it may even increase in severity with repeated exposures. A skin prick test with the partner's seminal fluid may help in the diagnosis. Semen contact allergy is not a cause of primary infertility and artificial insemination with washed spermatozoa is generally very well-tolerated. However, semen contact allergy may pose significant stress to the couples and may lead to sexual dysfunction. Taking oral antihistamines 30–60 minutes before the intercourse may help to alleviate the symptoms, and barrier contraceptive like condoms helps to prevent the occurrence. Desensitization via intravaginal graded challenge with seminal fluid may work as a specific management of semen contact allergy.

KORO SYNDROME

Koro syndrome, which is traditionally considered as a culture bound syndrome, is a psychiatric disorder characterized, in its typical form, by acute and intense anxiety, with complaints in men of a shrinking penis or fear of its retraction into the abdomen and resultant death. The origin of the word, "koro," is connected to the Malaysian term for the retracting of a turtle's head. The first descriptions of koro-like symptoms (with some similarity to panic disorder symptomatology) can be found in ancient Chinese medical records that are over 2,000 years old. Although koro is often thought to be a disorder associated with Asian populations, multiple cases reported from Western countries highlight the association of the condition with psychiatric comorbidities such as schizophrenia, obsessive-compulsive disorder, beyond cultural contexts. The clinical course of culture-bound koro syndrome is usually self-limited, but in some cases, it can be transient or take on a chronic or recurrent form, lasting from days to weeks, months or even years. Koro-affected individuals may have conflicting feelings about sexuality and sexual identity. Reassurance, psychotherapy, and pharmacotherapy might be required according to the severity of the symptoms.

DHAT SYNDROME

Discussion of psych and genitals is never complete without mentioning dhat syndrome in Indian context. Dhat syndrome is a culture-bound syndrome (CBS) more commonly reported among young males from low-to-medium socioeconomic background. It is a "semen loss"-related psychological distress seen mainly in Indian subcontinent. Semen was glorified in the past as most perfected component of food by Aristotle and as equivalent to 40 ounce blood by Andrew Tissot. In Indian mythology too, it was regarded as most powerful and perfect bodily substance which guarantee health and longevity. This exalted ideation about the importance of semen has led to undue mental pressure in preserving it, resulting in many psychological comorbidities. Dhat syndrome is a poorly defined condition characterized by vague symptoms such as fatigue, weakness, anxiety, loss of appetite, and guilt attributed to semen loss through nocturnal emissions, urine, and masturbation. In this syndrome, hypochondriacal, anxiety, and depressive symptoms become subsumed in the major visible "pathology" of semen loss. Diagnosis of the syndrome is limited by the absence of a clear definition. A wide range of presenting symptoms adds to the confusion in diagnosing it properly and in prevalence studies. CBT is the cornerstone treatment with SSRIs if needed according to the severity of the symptoms.

CONCLUSION

Human genitals play complex interaction with mind. Any real or perceived defect in the interplay can create tremendous sufferings for the patient, almost destroying confidence and self-esteem. It will have massive repercussion on their intimate and sexual life too. With these points in mind, we dermatologists should master the condition related with same beyond the formal syllabus of sexually transmitted diseases. However, this article might not have enlisted all the related conditions and further studies are required for a better understanding of the relationship between mind and genitals.

FURTHER READINGS

1. Chakraborty K, Thakurata RG. Indian concepts on sexuality. Indian J Psychiatry. 2013;55(Suppl 2):S250-5.
2. Goodman A. Sexual addiction. In: Lowinson JH, Ruiz R, Millman RB, Langrod JG (Eds). Substance abuse: A comprehensive textbook. Baltimore MD: William & Wilkins; 1997. pp. 340-54.
3. Koo JY, Lee CS. General approach to evaluating psychodermatological disorders. In: Koo JY, Lee CS (Eds). Psychocutaneous medicine. New York: Marcel Dekker Inc.; 2003. pp. 1-29.
4. Swamiappan M. Anogenital Pruritus: An Overview. J Clin Diagn Res. 2016; 10(4):WE01-WE3.
5. Fukuoka M, Miyachi Y, Ikoma A. Mechanically evoked itch in humans. Pain. 2013;154:897-904.
6. Yosipovitch G, Samuel LS. Dermatol Ther. 2008;21(1):32-41.
7. Tey HL, Wallengren J, Yosipovitch G. Psychosomatic factors in pruritus. Clin Dermatol. 2013;31(1):31-40.
8. Misery L, Alexander S, Dutray S, Chastaing M, Chastaing M, Consoli SG, Audra H, et al. Functional itch disorder or psychogenic pruritus: suggested diagnosis criteria from the French psychodermatology group. Acta Derm Venereol. 2007;87:341-4.
9. Ball SL, Howes C, Affleck AG. Functional symptoms in dermatology: Part 1. 2020;45:15-9.
10. Wesselmann U, Reich SG. The dynias. Semin Neurol. 1996;16:63-74.
11. Lotery HE, McClure N, Galask RP. Vulvodynia. Lancet. 2004;363:1058-60.
12. Welsh BM, Berzins KN, Cook KA, Fairley CK. Management of common vulval conditions. Med J Aust. 2003;178:391-5.
13. Tympanidis P, Terenghi G, Dowd P. Increased innervation of the vulval vestibule in patients with vulvodynia. Br J Dermatol. 2003;148:1021-7.
14. Sadownik LA. Clinical profile of vulvodynia patients. A prospective study of 300 patients. J Reprod Med. 2000;45:679-84.
15. O'Hare PM, Sherertz EF. Vulvodynia: a dermatologist's perspective with emphasis on an irritant contact dermatitis component. J Womens Health Gend Based Med. 2000;9:565-9.
16. Fischer M, Marsch WC. Vulvodynia: an indicator or even an early symptom of vulvar cancer. Cutis. 2001;67:235-8.
17. Edwards L. New concepts in vulvodynia. Am J Obstet Gynecol. 2003;189: S24-30.

18. Jackowich RA, Pukall CF. Persistent Genital Arousal Disorder: a Biopsychosocial Framework. Curr Sex Health Rep. 2020;12:127-35.
19. Pukall CF, Jackowich R, Mooney K, Chamberlain SM. Genital sensations in persistent genital arousal disorder: A case for an overarching nosology of genitopelvic dysesthesias? Sex Med Rev. 2019;7:2-12.
20. Oaklander AL, Sharma S, Kessler K, Price BH. Persistent genital arousal disorder: a special sense neuropathy. Pain Rep. 2020;5(1):e801.
21. Phillips KA, Diaz SF. Gender differences in body dysmorphic disorder. J Nerv Ment Dis. 1997;185:570-7.
22. Veale D, Miles S, Read J, Troglia A, Wylie K, Muir G. Sexual functioning and behavior of men with body dysmorphic disorder concerning penis size compared with men anxious about penis size and with controls: a cohort study. Sex Med. 2015;3:147-55.
23. Deans R, Liao LM, Crouch NS, Creighton SM. Why are women referred for female genital cosmetic surgery? Med J Aust. 2011;195:99.
24. Claiborn J, Pedrick C. The BDD work book: overcome body dysmorphic disorder and end body image obsessions. Oakland: New Harbinger Publications, Inc.; (2002).
25. Wilhelm S, Phillips KA, Steketee G. Cognitive-behavioral therapy for body dysmorphic disorder: a treatment manual. New York: Guilford Press; 2013.
26. Mansfield AK. Genital manifestations of body dysmorphic disorder in men: a review. Fertil Steril. 2020;1:16-20.
27. Pastoor H, Gregory A. Penile size dissatisfaction. J Sex Med. 2020;1:1-5.
28. Wylie KR, Eardley I. Penile size and the "small penis syndrome". BJU Int. 2007;99:1449-55.
29. Veale D, Miles S, Read J, Fiorito C, Wylie K, Miles S, et al. Penile Dysmorphic Disorder: Development of a Screening Scale. Arch Sex Behav. 2015;44:2311-21.
30. Verma KK, Khaitan BK, Singh OP. The frequency of sexual dysfunctions in patients attending a sex therapy clinic in North India. Arch Sex Behave. 1998;27(3):309-14.
31. Mahajan BB, Shishank M. An approach to venereophobia in males. Indian J Sex Transm Dis AIDS. 2017;38(1):103-6.
32. Maheshwaran P. A study of cutaneous manifestations of patients with psychiatric disorder. J Evol Med Dent Sci. 2016;5(13):564-6.
33. Wan-juan W, Hong-min L, Wen-yu G. Analysis on the psychological state of patients suffered from venereal hypochondriasis. Chinese Med Ethics. 2007;4:R395.
34. Arnold LM, Auchenbach MB, McElroy SL. Psychogenic excoriation. Clinical features, proposed diagnostic criteria, epidemiology and approaches to treatment. CNS Drugs. 2001;15:351-9.
35. Keuthen NJ, Koran LM, Aboujaoude E, Large MD, Serpe RT. The prevalence of pathologic skin picking in US adults. Compr Psychiatry. 2010;51:183-6.
36. Neziroglu F, Rabinowitz D, Breytman A, Jacofsky M. Skin picking phenomenology and severity comparison. Prim Care Companion J Clin Psychiatry. 2008;10:306-12.
37. Alexandrov P, Tan WP, Elterman L. Genital Dermatillomania. Curr Urol. 2017;11(1):54-6.

38. Odlaug BL, Grant JE. Clinical characteristics and medical complications of pathologic skin picking. Gen Hosp Psychiatry. 2008;30:61-6.
39. World Health Organization. (2001). Female Genital Mutilation: Integrating the Prevention and the Management of the Health Complications into the Curricula of Nursing and Midwifery. [online] Available from https://www.who.int/publications/i/item/WHO-RHR-01.16. [Last accessed January, 2024].
40. Knipscheer J, Vloeberghs E, van der Kwaak A, van den Muijsenbergh M. Mental health problems associated with female genital mutilation. BJ Psych Bull. 2015;39(6):273-7.
41. Ozan E, Deveci E, Oral M, Yazici E, Kirpinar I. Male genital self-mutilation as a psychotic solution. Isr J Psychiatry Relat Sci. 2010;47(4):297-303.
42. Veeder TA, Leo RJ. Male genital self-mutilation: a systematic review of psychiatric disorders and psychosocial factors. Gen Hosp Psychiatry. 2017;44:43-50.
43. Martin T, Gattaz WF. Psychiatric aspects of male genital self-mutilation. Psychopathology. 1991;24(3):170-8.
44. Hullmann SE, Fedele DA, Wolfe-Christensen C, Mullins LL, Wisniewski AB. Differences in adjustment by child developmental stage among caregivers of children with disorders of sex development. Int J Pediatr Endocrinol. 2011;2011:16.
45. Özbaran B, Özen S, Gökşen D, Korkmaz O, Onay H, Özkınay F, et al. Psychiatric approaches for disorders of sex development: experience of a multidisciplinary team. J Clin Res Pediatr Endocrinol. 2013;5(4):229-35.
46. Paulos MR, Avelliino GJ. Post-orgasmic illness syndrome: history and current perspectives. Fertil Steril. 2020;113:13-5.
47. Sublett JW, Bernstein JA. Seminal plasma hypersensitivity reactions: an updated review. Mt Sinai J Med. 2011;78:803-9.
48. Bernstein JA. Human seminal plasma hypersensitivity: an under-recognized women's health issue. Postgrad Med. 2011;123:120-5.
49. Ntouros E, Ntoumanis A, Bozikas VP, Donias S, Giouzepas I, Garyfalos G. Koro-like symptoms in two Greek men. BMJ Case Rep. 2010;2010:bcr08.2008.0679.
50. Edwards JG. The koro pattern of depersonalization in an American schizophrenic patient. Am J Psychiatry. 1970;126:1171-3.
51. Silva L, Raposo-Lima C, Soares C, Cerqueira JJ, Morgado P. Koro syndrome in an obsessive compulsive disorder patient. Eur Psychiatry. 2016;33S:S496.
52. Prakash O. Lessons for postgraduate trainees about Dhat syndrome. Indian J Psychiatry. 2007;49(3):208-10.
53. Akhtar S. Four culture bound psychiatric syndromes in India. Int J Soc Psychiatry. 1988;34:70-4.
54. Deb KS, Balhara YP. Dhat syndrome: A review of the world literature. Indian J Psychol Med. 2013;35(4):326-31.

CHAPTER 12

Psychiatric Morbidities in Hansen's Disease

Minu Ulpurath, Abdul Latheef EN

> **Key Messages**
> - Hansen's disease is a major health problem in different parts of the world.
> - Social stigma associated with the disease is a significant issue.
> - Psychiatric morbidities are found to be higher in leprosy patients.
> - Comprehensive psychiatric care and public awareness are essential to tackle these.

INTRODUCTION

Hansen's disease continues to be a significant health problem in different parts of the world. It results from infection with bacteria—*Mycobacterium leprae*. It causes a chronic infection in human being that affects mainly peripheral nerves and skin and produces a spectrum of clinical manifestations. The social stigma associated with Hansen's disease produces immense psychosocial issues in these patients. They include social stigma, depressive disorder, anxiety disorder, stress, quality of life impairment, suicidal thoughts, and other morbidities.

Stigma is defined as "a strong feeling of disapproval that most people in a society have about something."

TYPES OF STIGMA

- *Perceived stigma*: An individual assumes that his disease will incite negative behavior from others.

- *Self-imposed stigma*: People affected with leprosy may become ashamed, because of local attitudes and deformity, and may isolate themselves from society.
- *Enacted stigma*: Negative actions conducted by others to the detriment of labeled individuals.
- *Institutional stigma*: Stigma or discrimination which is a part of institutional arrangements or policies.

CAUSES FOR STIGMA

- *Beliefs about the causation of leprosy*: Lack of knowledge about the etiology, modes of spread, and cure of the disease accounts for irrational behavior. Some communities believe that that leprosy is a judgment from God for wrongdoing either in this life or a previous life.
- *Lack of complete cure in the past*: Until 1940 there was no effective treatment or cure for leprosy, which resulted in the thought that it is an incurable disease, and it was considered like a death sentence.
- *Disability and deformity*: The most important reason for the stigma associated with Hansen's disease is the deformity and disability caused by the disease. In lepromatous leprosy, there is a characteristic facial appearance that marks out a patient as having the disease. It has been reported that greater the disability, greater the level of stigma.
- *Fear*: Fear is a major driving force of stigma. People fear that the disease is contagious. In the past, leprosy ran in families to the extent that many authorities considered it an inherited rather than an infectious disease.

EFFECTS OF STIGMA ON PATIENTS

Social Life

Leprosy and its stigma strongly affect a patient's life, marriage, employment, interpersonal relationships, leisure activities, and attendance at social and religious functions.

Effect on Treatment and Cure

Fear of stigma and the resulting discrimination discourage individuals and their families from seeking medical help. Stigma is a serious obstacle to case finding and to the effectiveness of treatment, which are the major concerns of disease control programs.

Gender Variations

Women are affected more by the stigma than men, suffering more of isolation and rejection and have more restrictions than men with the same level of disease.

As the people affected with this disease are rejected by the local community and their own family members, they are forced to stay in ashrams, Mandirs, and leprosy homes. As a result of these problems, the prevalence of various psychiatric disorders among these patients is higher than that among the general population. Besides this, the long duration of the illness and physical handicaps increase the risk of psychiatric morbidities.

Depressive Disorder

Depression is a mood disorder characterized by a persistently low mood, feeling of sadness and loss of interest. It is the most common psychiatric comorbidity seen in patients with Hansen's disease. The prevalence of depression varied in different settings and various countries.

The clinical features of depression include:
- Depressed mood
- Markedly diminished interest or pleasure in most or all activities
- Significant weight loss or weight gain
- Insomnia or hypersomnia
- Psychomotor retardation
- Fatigue or loss of energy
- Feelings of worthlessness or excessive guilt
- Diminished ability to think or concentrate
- Recurrent thoughts of death, or suicidal ideation, plan, or attempt

Anxiety Disorder

According to the American Psychological Association, "Anxiety is an emotion characterized by feelings of tension, worried thoughts and physical changes such as increased blood pressure."

Anxiety disorders are the second most frequently reported mental health condition in leprosy patients. The prevalence of anxiety disorders among leprosy-affected persons ranged from 10 to 20% in different studies.

Stress

According to Lazarus et al., *"Stress occurs when a person perceives the demands of environmental stimuli to be greater than their ability to meet, mitigate, or alter those demands."* In a study conducted by Leekassa et al. in Addis Ababa, the prevalence of psychological stress among people with leprosy was 52.4%.

Quality of Life Impairment

The World Health Organization (WHO) defines Quality of Life as individuals' perception of their position in life in the context of the culture and value systems in which they live and in relation to their goals, expectations, standards, and concerns. Individuals affected by leprosy had low quality of life scores in the physical and psychological health domains. Leprosy subjects are strongly affected not only by physical issues such as peripheral neuropathy but also by massive social exclusion that leads to quality of life impairment.

Suicidal Thoughts

Suicide, suicide attempts and suicidal thoughts are also present in leprosy-affected persons. According to Bharath et al., 33.3% of the investigated leprosy patients in Bengaluru dealt with suicidal thoughts, and 20% had attempted suicide.

Sleep Disturbances

Leprosy patients often suffer from sleep disturbances. The prevalence of insomnia in leprosy patients was found to be 50% in a study by Giesel et al. The frequency of Restless leg syndrome among leprosy patients was also found to be 25.4% when compared to the general population (8.8%).

Other Neuropsychiatric Conditions

Other conditions that were found in leprosy patients include dementia, delusional disorder, hypochondriacal disorder, adjustment disorders, substance-related disorders, somatic symptom disorder, somatoform disorders, and schizophrenia. A Taiwanese study found a high prevalence of dementia (45.7–50.4%) among leprosy patients. The prevalence of hypochondriacal disorder was found to be quite low in patients.

We conducted a study in the Department of Dermatology, Government Medical College, Kozhikode, Kerala, India to assess the psychiatric morbidities in leprosy patients (study just finished and is yet to be published). A total of 126 patients were included in the study. 38% of the study participants were depressed and 35.7% had anxiety, 30.2% had high stress, and 11.1% had extremely large impact on quality of life. Depression was found to be significantly associated with the WHO grade 2 disability, presence of motor weakness, face lesions, and trophic ulcer. Anxiety was found to be significantly associated with urban residence, long duration of illness, and the presence of face lesion. Mental stress of the patients was found to have statistically significant association with the WHO grade 2 disability, trophic ulcer, and the presence of face lesion. Quality of life impairment was found to be associated with the presence of motor weakness, the WHO grade 2 disability, and the presence of face lesion and trophic ulcer.

APPROACH TO PSYCHO SOCIAL ASPECTS OF LEPROSY

Efforts to address stigma and discrimination toward people affected by leprosy have focused on a number of areas. Here methods to address the patient' issues and public awareness programs has to be instituted simultaneously. The following strategies are helpful in attaining this goal.
- *Cognitive behavioral and information-based strategies*: Cognitive restructuring is one commonly used method in stigmatized person. Peer counseling and self-help groups can be effectively utilized in this area.
- Stress management, assertive training, and supportive counseling are useful in patient management.

- The stigmatizing context, by addressing community and social attitudes that have impact on the person and their family. For example, by enhancing personal contact between persons affected and community members through "contact events" or the production of videos and comics.
- Discriminatory laws, policies, and systems that may impact on them such as the use of nondiscriminatory terminology, integrated care, and mass media campaigns.
- Addressing economic and livelihood issues through practical interventions, such as microfinance.

Counseling and Psychoeducation in Leprosy

Psychoeducation is an intervention in the form of education and information that is given to participants with psychological distress such as depression or physical impairment.

Counseling is given for:
- Leprosy-affected person
- Family members
- *Community*: Group counseling

Appropriate time for counseling:
- Diagnosis of leprosy
- Irregularity in taking antileprosy treatment
- Developing reactions during therapy
- Poor compliance on self-care
- Developing deformity or disability during treatment or those noticing further deterioration in their condition ignoring advice disability or deformity
- Developing fear, frustration, inferiority complex, and confusion by patient
- Participation restriction/receiving ill treatment by others

Psychological Interventions

Studies have showed that psychological interventions can improve the mental well-being of leprosy-affected persons.
- *Jacobsons progressive muscle relaxation*: Relaxation has a significant psychological impact. Patient should be explained about how stress plays a role in aggravating the disease and how

relaxation will help. Procedure takes 30–40 minutes. There are two components, one is relaxing the muscles and second is tensing the muscles.
- *Cognitive behavior therapy*: In cognitive behavior therapy, the therapist and the client work together as a team and solve problems. This includes problem solving, cognitive restructuring, modeling, etc.
- *Hypnotherapy*: Hypnotherapy is used as an adjunctive procedure in various dermatological conditions. In a case report by Abdul Latheef et al., dramatic improvement was noted in two patients with erythema nodosum leprosum (ENL) and neuralgia with three sessions of hypnotherapy. Hypnosis is induced by means of relaxing suggestions nerves and skin. The probable mechanism involved in the relief of neuralgia in HD may be due to the analgesic effect of endogenous opioids released in the brain during hypnosis.
- *Reminiscence group therapy*: Group reminiscence therapy is a brief and structured intervention in which participants share their personal past events with peers. This approach involves recollection, review, and re-evaluation of past events. Reminiscence treatments usually last 6 weeks or longer, and include at least one or two sessions per week, each session lasting between 1 and 2 hours.

Role of Psychopharmacology

The psychotropic drugs should initially be started at a low dose, increased to therapeutic range, then tapered for termination of treatment as appropriate.
- *Antidepressants*: Selective serotonin reuptake inhibitors (SSRIs) should be started at low doses and titrated upward. Response to SSRIs usually takes 3–6 weeks. Tricyclic antidepressants (TCAs) are also used. Usually used SSRIs include Citalopram, Escitalopram, Fluoxetine, Fluvoxamine, Paroxetine sertraline, and Venlafaxine. TCAs include Amitriptyline, Clomipramine, Doxepin, Imipramine, Nortriptyline.
- *Anxiolytics*: Benzodiazepines are schedule intravenous (IV) controlled substances due to risks of potential abuse and addictive dependence. Alazopram, oxazepam, and lorazepam are

short-acting benzodiazepines and clonazepam and diazepam are long-acting ones. They can be used as sedatives for patients with sleep disturbances.

CONCLUSION

There is an urgent need for provision of comprehensive psychiatric care for people with Hansen's disease. As the mental health problems of this group of patients originate from social attitudes toward leprosy, an attitudinal change is the first goal to achieve. Health education is the most important measure in tackling this health problem. From every standpoint, any steps taken to reduce the emotional burden brought on by the disease are important.

FURTHER READINGS

1. Sengupta U. Elimination of leprosy in India: An analysis. Indian J Dermatol Venereol Leprol. 2018;84:131-6.
2. Singh GP. Psychosocial aspects of Hansen's disease (leprosy). Indian Dermatol Online J. 2012;3:166-70.
3. Bhatia MS, Chandra R, Bhattacharya SN, Imran M. Psychiatric morbidity and pattern of dysfunctions in patients with leprosy. Indian J Dermatol. 2006;51: 23-5.
4. Mahendra N, Yaduvanshi R, Sharma CS, Ali R, Rathore PK, Kuchhal A. Psychiatric co-morbidity in patients of Hansen's disease. Int J Contemp Med Res. 2018;5(1):1-5.
5. Govindasamy K, Jacob I, Solomon RM, Darlong J. Burden of depression and anxiety among leprosy affected and associated factors: A cross-sectional study from India. PLoS Negl Trop Dis. 2021;15(1):e0009030.
6. Erinfolami AR, Adeyemi JD. A case control study of psychiatric morbidities among subjects with leprosy in Lagos, Nigeria. Int J Psychiatry Med. 2009;39(1):89-99.
7. Govindharaj P, Srinivasan S, Darlong J. Quality of life of persons affected by leprosy in an endemic district, West Bengal, India. Indian J Dermatol. 2018;63:459-64.
8. Abdul Latheef EN, Riyaz N. Hypnotherapy: A useful adjunctive therapeutic modality in Hansen's disease. Indian J Dermatol. 2014;59:166-8.
9. Jindal KC, Singh GP, Mohan V, Mahajan BB. Psychiatric morbidity among inmates of leprosy homes. Indian J Psychol Med. 2013;35(4):335-40.
10. Somar P, Waltz MM, van Brakel WH. The impact of leprosy on the mental wellbeing of leprosy-affected persons and their family members: A systematic review. Glob Ment Health (Camb). 2020;7:e15.

CHAPTER 13

Psychodermatological Issues in Geriatric Population

Archana AG, Abdul Latheef EN

> **Key Messages**
> - Interaction between the skin and psyche is an established entity which often goes unnoticed by healthcare providers.
> - Generalized xerosis, asteatotic eczema, contact eczema, cutaneous infections, psoriasis, melasma, cutaneous ulcers, and various other dermatoses are common in elderly.
> - Growing age, age-related ailments, and neglect contribute to increased prevalence of depression, anxiety, and stress among the geriatric group.
> - Holistic healthcare in elderly requires management of both skin conditions and the mental health simultaneously.

INTRODUCTION

Old age is a special phase in human life where a person after enjoying the full youthhood and a very energetic phase of life goes to a relatively less active phase. That will produce immense health issues in the individual both physically and psychologically. The interaction between brain and skin is beyond a physiologic fact. Skin conditions can impose great effects on every aspect of the patient's life. Reciprocally, skin diseases may be evoked by psychological issues. The connection between mind and skin has been studied since the nineteenth century. The last 40 years have set the development of new research fields which helped to analyze how these two dimensions interact. Active researches are going on in the field of geriatrics also which brings forth the biopsychosocial issues in old age people. People aged 60 years and above are considered under the geriatric group as defined by the World Health Organization (WHO). India is an aging nation with 7.7% of the population above 60 years of age. Among Indians, culture, religion, and the belief in karma can all have a major impact on lifestyle, as well as the approach to managing various diseases, including dermatologic conditions. India is now the largest populated country in the world, with 149 million persons above 60 years of age as of 2022, and this number is likely to increase to 179 million in 2031 and further to 301 million in 2051. This constitutes 10.5% of the country's population.

This rapid demographic shift has created many challenges in the management of diseases in the geriatric population. The role of psychoneuroimmunology in the field of psychocutaneous disorders has gained momentum recently. The role of psychodermatology is increasing in geriatric population as they suffer from depression, anxiety, stress due to the disease, age-related ailments, and other hidden cofactors compared to general population. Geriatric population has their own peculiar mental and physical issues which are different from other age groups. In various dermatoses, prevalence of psychiatric morbidities like depression, anxiety, and somatoform disorders range from 25 to 43%. Epidemiological studies showed that the most frequent mental disorders in patients with skin diseases are depressive and anxiety disorders and body dysmorphic disorder.

As lifespan is rising, elderly constitute a significant population in dermatology clinics. Due to the growing knowledge regarding holistic health and well-being in the society, age-related changes have become a major concern to patients as well as dermatologists. Aging is a biological reality in which there is progressive structural and functional decline due to a series of physiological changes over time. Human skin undergoes chronological as well as photoaging and as a result various skin disorders develop due to the structural and physiological changes. This is termed intrinsic and extrinsic aging. Dermatologists need to be aware of these aging changes as well as equip themselves to treat these conditions. Psychiatric problems may play a role in the occurrence or relapse of dermatologic disorders. However, it is possible that psychiatric morbidity is secondary to dermatologic disorders because of their chronic course, effect on body image, and the associated stigma. Some of the principal reasons for the nonrecognition of mental disorders in elderly are high probability of these patients reporting only somatic symptoms and the lack of expertise of a doctor's in recognizing these symptoms as evidence of mental disorders. Besides these inherent aging changes, certain dermatoses are also more common in elderly and other age-related changes in health and lifestyle also reflect upon the mental well-being of elderly.

CHANGES IN AGING SKIN

Aging is a decrease in the ability of body in adapting to the extrinsic and intrinsic changes encountered in daily life. As skin is the largest organ in the body and acts as a barrier between the body and environment, the brunt of the aging process happens in skin. Skin protects the body from the environment, prevents excessive water loss from the body, and has an aesthetic effect. Aging is characterized by impaired ability of stem cells to regenerate tissues and restore the physiological integrity of the system. There are two types of aging processes: (1) chronological aging and (2) photoaging.

Chronological Aging

Xerosis, fine wrinkles, loss of elasticity, acrochordons, cherry angioma, sunken eyes, idiopathic guttate hypomelanosis, senile comedones, loss of luster of nails and hair, graying, and androgenetic alopecia (AGA) are examples of this group.

Photoaging

Deep wrinkles, cutis rhomboidalis nuchae, thick skin, dyschromias, citrine skin, colloid milium, melasma, pseudo stellate scars, Favre-Ricochet syndrome, etc., are few changes associated with photoaging. Constellation of all these sunlight-induced changes of aging is called dermatoheliosis.

DERMATOLOGICAL DISEASES WITH PSYCHIATRIC MORBIDITY IN ELDERLY

Even though any dermatological condition can affect the elderly, there are some conditions which are very commonly affecting the geriatric population. Some of them have profound psychiatric morbidity also.

Pruritus in Elderly

Pruritus is the most common skin disorder in elderly and is defined as unpleasant cutaneous sensation that provokes a desire to scratch. Pruritus in elderly is chronic and difficult to diagnose the underlying cause. Itching may be a protective mechanism but chronic itch, not responding to conventional therapies should be evaluated. This increased affliction may be attributed to three physiological aging changes:
1. Epidermal barrier defects—decreased lipid production and increased water loss
2. Activated immune system
3. Neurodegenerative disorders

Pruritus of an unknown cause is one of the dermatological manifestations of psychiatric morbidity, especially depression. The French Psychodermatology Group proposed a diagnostic criteria (**Box 1**).

Eczema

Asteatotic eczema is very common in old age because of decreased lipid production and increased water loss. Legs are common sites. Frequent application of moisturizers and protection from further

---

BOX 1: French psychodermatology group's diagnostic criteria for functional itch disorder.

3 compulsory criteria:
1. Localized or generalized pruritus sine materia (without primary skin lesion)
2. Chronic pruritus (>6 weeks)
3. No somatic cause

3 of 7 optional criteria:
1. A chronological relationship of pruritus with one or several life events that could have psychological repercussions
2. Variations in intensity associated with stress
3. Nocturnal variations
4. Predominance during rest or inaction
5. Associated psychological disorder
6. Pruritus that could be improved by psychotropic drugs
7. Pruritus that could be improved by psychotherapies

aggravating factors like frequent use of soaps and hot water should be avoided. Contact dermatitis is also common in legs, and most common allergens are fragrances, topical medications, steroids, and lanolin. Stasis eczema, atopy, and photodermatitis are also common.

Infections

Immunosenescence is not seen as an immune deficiency but rather as an immune dysregulation with certain immune activities exaggerated and certain others suppressed. Ultraviolet light, smoking, and several other extrinsic factors for many years along with intrinsic factors like degenerative and metabolic changes make the epidermis of elderly thin and fragile. Epidermis tears easily and the entry of infective organisms becomes easier. Comorbidities like diabetes mellitus, stasis dermatitis, and peripheral vascular disease make the skin even more fragile facilitating the entry of microorganisms.

Bacterial Infections

Cutaneous bacterial infections are very common in elderly persons owing to the waning immunity and reduced ability to stick on diligent hygiene practices due to other old age ailments. Cellulitis and infected ulcers are the most commonly encountered dermatological infections in the elderly. Intertrigo and erythrasma have a predilection for the flexures, especially axillae and groin. Secondary skin infections are often the result of persistent pruritus associated with increasing dryness of the aging skin.

Viral Infections

Herpes zoster is one of the most common viral infections in elderly which is very often severely painful and debilitating. It is caused by the reactivation of the varicella zoster virus that causes varicella zoster or chickenpox in childhood. Postherpetic neuralgia refers to pain lasting 2 months or more after an acute attack of herpes zoster. The pain may be constant or intermittent. It is usually lancinating and disturbs one's sleep and ability to do routine daily activities which may result in significant psychiatric morbidity. There is emergent resistance to acyclovir in these patients requiring higher antivirals like foscarnet or famciclovir which are expensive and demanding hospital stay. This can further result in the development of depression and anxiety. There is a strong but poorly understood bidirectional link between herpes zoster and functional decline. Herpes zoster is more common in elderly who are demented and those who have major difficulties in performing daily tasks. The disease itself further accentuates this functional decline. Elderly who are more depressed are to be affected more by herpes zoster. It has been noted that depression negatively affects immune function and leads to increased susceptibility to infection. Herpes simplex virus (HSV) most commonly affects the genitalia and perioral area. In the elderly, HSV infection is typically manifested at the vermilion border of the lip. The main concern of recurrent herpes labialis in the aged population is related to potential autoinoculation of the eye or genital area.

Fungal Infections

Cutaneous fungal infections are seen in a large proportion of aged population due to prolonged skin exposure and metabolic changes. *Candida albicans*, a normal commensal of skin, usually does not infect healthy young population, but causes candidiasis only when the normal immune balance is jeopardized. Oral candidiasis and chronic and recalcitrant fungal infections tend to be extensive and cause significant psychological issues in elderly.

Psoriasis

Psoriasis is a chronic, inflammatory papulosquamous disease with multiple remissions and exacerbations. The prevalence of patients of 60 years of age and older was about 0.1%. The most observed type of psoriasis is chronic plaque-type psoriasis. Several studies demonstrate a probable temporal association between psychological stress and onset, recurrence, and severity of psoriasis. In the light of this, they recommend that clinicians include "stress" as a trigger factor in psoriasis assessment and consider psychological interventions as adjuncts, particularly in those who identify as "stress responders". The relationship between psoriasis and psychological stress is like a vicious cycle because stress causes psoriasis to flare up and the flare-ups by themselves lead to increased stress, further exacerbating the disease. About 40–80% of psoriatic patients experience psychological stressors. Psoriasis can occur at any age, but two peaks in age onset have been documented: The first between 20 and 30 years and the second between 50 and 60 years. Disfigurement, social stigmatization, and dissatisfaction with prolonged and incomplete therapy could lead to depression and anxiety. When the patient has a lack of social support, which is more common in aged population, the anxiety is high because social support is considered a protective factor for psychosomatic diseases, like psoriasis. Stress disturbs the epidermal barrier. There is altered sympathetic nervous system activation with accelerated levels of epinephrine and norepinephrine and reduced levels of cortisol. This is due to dysregulation of both central and cutaneous hypothalamus–pituitary–adrenal (HPA) axis. This dysregulation of HPA axis upregulates proinflammatory cytokines, thus explaining the stress-induced exacerbation of psoriasis.

Lichen Planus

Lichen planus is a chronic, papulosquamous disorder of the skin, mucous membranes, nails, and hair. The typical clinical manifestations on the skin include the presence of pruritic, polygonal, flat-topped, violaceous papules and plaques with reticulated white lines, termed "Wickham's striae." Pruritus is a cardinal symptom of lichen planus which varies in intensity in each patient. It is the most unpleasant and worrisome symptom in most patients which greatly alter the well-being of patient and has significant impact on quality of life and results in depression and anxiety, stress, social phobia, obsessive thoughts, dysthymia, and panic symptoms in patients with lichen planus, especially in elderly.

Vascular Ulcers

Vascular ulcers mainly affect legs and foot, mainly due to their dependent nature. Leg and foot ulcers cause considerable physical and psychological burden to the patients as well as their families. Chronic wounds considerably affect the quality of life of sufferers due to the pain, functional disability, and physical deformity caused by them. Nevertheless, many patients suffering from leg ulcers do not get proper care and treatment, especially in developing countries like us, and hence they result in chronic disabilities

which finally make even palliative care difficult. Chronic wounds significantly reduce the quality of life due to impaired mobility and gait, pain, unpleasant odor, decreased appetite, insomnia, social isolation, frustration, and inability to perform day-to-day activities. Most common psychological reactions to chronic diseases, including chronic ulcers, are depression, anxiety, stress, aggression, and frustration. Psychological factors may not only be a result of delayed healing but may also have a negative impact on healing. Anxiety and depression have direct effects on endocrine and immune function which further delay the healing process. Several biobehavioral mechanisms are involved in the development of the psychological morbidity associated with chronic leg ulcers. The immune system has direct influence on the nervous system via secretion of several inflammatory cytokines. The level of cytokines has direct correlation with these symptoms. There are four categories of leg ulcers, mainly:
1. Venous leg ulcers
2. Arterial leg ulcers
3. Mixed venous and arterial ulcers
4. Hypertensive ischemic leg ulcers

Peripheral arterial disease can cause intermittent claudication, rest pain, necrosis, or gangrene of toes or forefoot which may lead to secondary infection, sepsis, infestation with maggots, and amputation. These may lead to marked impairment in the quality of life, depression, and anxiety. Patients suffering from these mental disorders are further prone to cardiovascular diseases, strokes as well as increased probability of worsening pain, and greater impairment in functional outcome. More than a quarter of patients with peripheral vascular disease suffer from depression and anxiety. Diabetic ulcer and diabetic foot are common complications of diabetes mellitus, especially in uncontrolled diabetics. Depression and anxiety are highly prevalent in patients with diabetic foot, and each of them perpetuates each other and diabetic foot complications. Depression is twice more associated with patients of type 2 diabetes who undergo amputation than those who do not. Diabetic ulcers and other vascular complications are associated with disturbed daily life including hypersomnia, lack of sleep, impaired mobility, loneliness, interference with sexual life, and lack of energy. Various studies demonstrate different causes of foot ulcers in diabetic patients like older age, rural residence, poor self-care practice, prolonged duration of disease, inadequate control of blood sugar values, high body mass index , type 2 diabetes, smoking, and peripheral neuropathy. The incidence of leg ulcers is very common in old age.

Urticaria/Angioedema

Chronic spontaneous urticaria is a common allergic skin disease that usually arises without any external stimuli. It is termed chronic when the disease lasts for more than 6 consecutive weeks. Various studies demonstrate increased prevalence of chronic urticaria among elderly compared to nonelderly. Intense pruritus of urticarial wheals, mild burning pain, and disfigurement of angioedema cause significant disturbance in a patient's quality of life and constitute other psychological morbidities. It accounts for stress, disturbed sleep, social disability, depression, negative self-image, anger, low mood, anxiety, and panic attacks in patients who develop frequent angioedema episodes. Psychiatric disorders are potential risk factors for chronic urticaria whereas the exact underlying pathomechanisms are not delineated. Stress has a vital role in activating T cells and has a role in creating abnormal tension in the autonomic nervous system, thereby elevating the levels of histamine in plasma and cells. A bidirectional relationship exists between brain and immune system. Neuropeptides from nerve endings may also provoke urticaria.

Melasma

Melasma is the most common pigmentary disorder in Indians. It is characterized by irregular, blotchy brown macules and patches, usually symmetrically distributed over face. It more commonly develops in women after the fourth decade of life and intensifies with age. Depressive disorder and adjustment disorder were significantly higher among melasma patients. Stress and depression are melanogenic due to skin stress response system by increasing adrenocorticotropic hormone (ACTH) and cortisol.

Acanthosis Nigricans

Acanthosis nigricans is a condition characterized by darkening and velvety thickening of skin into irregular folds. It is often related to endocrinological problems like obesity-associated insulin resistance and hyperandrogenism. It is more often seen in adolescents and aged obese persons. Depression, anxiety, and low self-esteem are commonly seen in acanthosis nigricans patients.

Androgenetic Alopecia

Androgenetic alopecia is the most common type of hair loss in Asian men. It is characterized by follicular miniaturization of terminal hair follicles into vellus hair follicles because of systemic androgen and genetic factors. Even though hair loss starts immediately after puberty and continues progressively, the age of onset is usually considered to be after the third or fourth decade. According to Hamilton study, the mean prevalence of AGA is 30% by 30 years and 50% by 50 years. Many of the treatments are expensive and do not offer much hair coverage resulting in considerable psychological morbidity. Even though elderly are more often not insecure about hair loss, a small proportion is associated with some psychological impact.

PSYCHOLOGICAL MORBIDITY

Depression

Depression is a growing concern in the current era. Depression in late life is more significant due to its increasing trend as well as its negative impact on the physical illness. It affects the person's global functional abilities like work, family, and interpersonal relationships and make the patients suffer.

Depression now affects 280 million people worldwide; still 76–85% of people in low- and middle-income countries receive no treatment for it. Social stigma associated with mental disorders, lack of resources, and lack of experienced professionals acts as barriers to effective treatment.

People who have gone through adverse life events are more prone to depression and considering this fact, elderly are more affected with depression. More than 5.7% of the people older than 60 years have depression. Physical ailments add to it and vice versa.

Anxiety

According to American Psychological Association, "Anxiety is an emotion characterized by feelings of tension, worried thoughts and physical changes like increased blood pressure." People with anxiety usually avoid certain situations that cause them to worry. They have recurrent intrusive thoughts or concerns and experience

physical symptoms like sweating, trembling, dizziness, or palpitation. Occasional anxiety is an unavoidable part of life, but anxiety disorders include more than transient worry or fear. The symptoms interfere with daily activities of life like school, work, and relationships. There are different types of anxiety disorders including generalized anxiety disorder, panic disorder, and various phobias.
- Feeling restless, wound-up, or on-edge
- Being easily fatigued
- Having difficulty concentrating; mind going blank
- Being irritable
- Having muscle tension
- Difficulty controlling feelings of worry
- Having sleep problems, such as difficulty falling asleep or staying asleep, or unsatisfying sleep

Social Anxiety Disorder or Social Phobia

It is the general intense anxiety toward social tasks or performances. They worry about the negative evaluation by others due to their actions or words and cause them embarrassment. This leads patients to avoid social situations and cause isolation. This is more common in elderly which make them isolate more and force them to confine to their rooms or houses.

Agoraphobia

Persons with agoraphobia have an intense fear of at least two or more of the following:
- Using public transportation
- Standing in line or being in a crowd
- Being outside of the home alone

Patients avoid these situations thinking that it could be impossible to leave or come out of that situation in case they develop panic attack or anxiety symptoms. In worst cases, the individual becomes housebound.

Separation Anxiety Disorder

Separation anxiety is usually seen in children, but adults, often elderly, are also prone to this. Patients experience fear of being parted from people to whom they are attached. They often think that some sort of harm or danger would happen to their attachment figures while they are apart. They have nightmares of being separated and develop anxiety symptoms when separation occurs or is anticipated.

Stress

Stress is an emergent process that involves the interaction between person and his environmental factors, past and current events, psychological and physiological activities. Stressors across life influence the reactivity and habitual responding of a person in his conscious and subconscious levels. Stress is a critical component in health throughout life span, especially in aging. Stressful events act as a precursor to many psychiatric disorders. Stress is also associated with a higher risk of physical ailments like hypertension, cardiovascular diseases, and infectious diseases. The term stress is used to describe the situations in life like separating from spouse or losing a job (stressors or stress exposures) and to the biological, emotional, and cognitive behaviors (stress responses) those situations evoke. So, stress can include antecedent stimulus or the response to it.

Chronic stress leads to activation of the HPA axis and this results in secretion of catecholamines and glucocorticoids.

Even though most of the dermatological diseases presenting in the outpatient department are of benign nature and many of them have only cosmetic outcome, dermatological illness constitutes a significant reason for declining quality of life. Increased number of hospital visits, cosmetic problems, prolonged and recurring nature of several diseases, lack of adequate response, and adverse effects of treatment make patients lead a difficult life. Skin appearance is negatively judged by people, especially in communities where physical appearance is very significant. The affected person experiences stigmatization, absence of acceptance due to their appearance and visible skin symptoms, distress, and anxiety. Patients are often glared at or avoided due to fear of infection and this leads to social isolation, low mood, poor body image, lack of self-care, loss of pleasure, low self-esteem, and high stress.

Adjustment Disorder

According to classifications in both the Diagnostic and Statistical Manual of Mental Disorders, 4th edition, text revision (DSM-IV-TR) and the International Classification of Diseases 10th Revision

(ICD-10), "Adjustment disorder is defined as subjective distress and emotional or behavioral disturbances that interfere significantly with social or personal functioning and that arise within 3 months after exposure to an identifiable psychosocial stressor, life change or stressful life event." Adjustment disorder is prevalent among older adults, particularly due to the effect of other mood disorders like depression and anxiety. The identification of adjustment disorder by a general practitioner in primary care remains to be very low.

CONCLUSION

Generalized xerosis and resulting asteatotic eczema are very common among elderly. Various other dermatological diseases like cutaneous infections, papulosquamous disorders, contact eczema, etc., are also common in elderly. The burden of dermatological diseases is substantially underestimated among geriatric population probably due to less care given to skin by patients themselves and care takers. Amidst systemic illness, skin seems to be unimportant to them, but patients may have a major impact in their quality of life and well-being due to dermatological disease. Here is the role of a physician who should probably expose the "hidden" but obvious skin problem and refer to a dermatologist whenever necessary. Then comes the role of a dermatologist who should recognize, diagnose, and treat the dermatological disease as well as the psychiatric comorbidity, if any, by either taking the help of a psychiatrist or by wearing the shoes of a psychodermatologist who can do a lot to improve the patient's overall well-being. It avoids the stigma of the patient being seen by a psychiatrist and develops more confidence and good rapport with the patient, thereby enhancing the response of medical management of both physical and psychiatric morbidity.

FURTHER READINGS

1. Ingle GK, Nath A. Geriatric health in India: concerns and solutions. Indian J Community Med. 2008;33(4):214-8.
2. Picardi A, Abeni D, Renzi C, Braga M, Melchi CF, Pasquini P. Treatment outcome and incidence of psychiatric disorders in dermatological out-patients. J Eur Acad Dermatol Venereol. 2003;17(2):155-9.
3. World Health Organization. (2020). Ageing. [online] Available from https://www.who.int/data/gho/whs-2020-visual-summary [Last accessed January, 2024].

4. Bhuvaneshkumar M, John KR, Logaraj MA. Study on prevalence of depression and associated risk factors among elderly in a rural block of Tamil Nadu. Indian J Public Health. 2018;62(2):89.
5. Greenberg SA. The geriatric depression scale (GDS). 2009;2(4):114-8.
6. Alshahwan MA. The prevalence of anxiety and depression in Arab dermatology patients. J Cutan Med Surg. 2015;19(3):297-303.
7. Kandwal M, Jindal R, Chauhan P, Roy S. Skin diseases in geriatrics and their effect on the quality of life: a hospital-based observational study. J Fam Med Prim Care. 2020;9(3):1453-8.
8. Liao YH, Chen KH, Tseng MP, Sun CC. Pattern of skin diseases in a geriatric patient group in Taiwan: a 7-year survey from the outpatient clinic of a university medical center. Dermatol Basel Switz. 2001;203(4):308-13.
9. Raveendra L. A clinical study of geriatric dermatoses. Our Dermatol Online. 2014;5:235-9.
10. Barua A, Ghosh MK, Kar N, Basilio MA. Prevalence of depressive disorders in the elderly. Ann Saudi Med. 2011;31(6):620-4.
11. Kim EK, Kim HO, Park YM, Park CJ, Yu DS, Lee JY. Prevalence and risk factors of depression in geriatric patients with dermatological diseases. Ann Dermatol. 2013;25(3):278-84.

CHAPTER 14

Sleep in Dermatology

Savitha Soman

> **Key Messages**
> - Human sleep occurs because of two processes: (1) Homeostatic sleep drive and (2) circadian rhythm.
> - There are two major phases of sleep: (1) Nonrapid eye movement (NREM) and (2) rapid eye movement (REM) sleep.
> - Skin plays a role in the physiology of sleep such as initiation of sleep.
> - Several sleep disorders like insomnia, rhythm disorders, sleep apnea, and sleep deprivation can have a possible effect on the skin.

INTRODUCTION

Sleep is an active process that arises from a complex interaction between several areas of the brain, multiple neurotransmitter pathways, and hormonal mechanisms. Human beings spend about one third of their lives sleeping. While sleep is very vulnerable to disruption, it is often ignored in the bigger challenge of treating the underlying condition. However, sleep disruption can lead to a myriad of health problems that affect several body systems.

Sleep disturbance is not uncommon for patients with dermatological problems, especially those with pruritus. There are relatively few studies that look at the association between skin diseases and sleep problems. This is especially ironical because melatonin, a key factor in maintaining the circadian rhythm, was in fact discovered by a dermatologist.

PHYSIOLOGY OF SLEEP

Human sleep occurs because of two processes: (1) Homeostatic sleep drive and (2) circadian rhythm.

There are two major phases of sleep: Nonrapid eye movement (NREM) and rapid eye movement (REM) sleep. During the NREM phase, the sympathetic tone reduces, and the parasympathetic activity is heightened, thus creating a state of reduced activity. It occurs in three stages: Stage 1 is a light sleep stage (10 minutes) and represents a shift from wakefulness to sleep, stage 2 (30 minutes) shows further slowing of breathing and brain activity, and person goes into deep sleep during stage 3 (20-40 minutes), followed by a transition to the REM phase where blood flow and metabolism are almost comparable to the wakeful state and most dreaming occurs. The end of the REM phase heralds a new sleep cycle. The initiation of sleep is regulated by the circadian and homeostatic signals from the diencephalon. The ultradian oscillator located in the mesopontine junction controls the shift between NREM and REM stages.

Wakefulness is "a state of arousal in which there is a conscious surveillance of the environment and the ability to respond to external stimuli", mediated by the posterior hypothalamus. Orexin and histamine neurons regulate sleep and wakefulness.

The daily sleep–wake cycle is dependent on the circadian clock located in the suprachiasmatic nucleus (SCN) which generates circadian rhythms within a period of approximately 24 hours and is regulated by several neurotransmitters and hormones. A key chemical agent is melatonin whose primary function is to carry information regarding this daily light and dark cycle to the different structures of the body, which is then utilized to harmonize various physiological activities. Other hormones implicated are growth hormone, corticotrophin-releasing hormone, galanin, neuropeptide Y, and somatostatin. A normal circadian rhythm ensures refreshing and consistent sleep, plays a role in thermoregulation, and mediates immune function.

As per the recommendations of the National Institutes of Health, preschool children must get an average of 10-12 hours of sleep, older children about 9 hours, and adults about 7-8 hours to maintain good health and functioning. Sleep deprivation is currently a well-recognized health problem, with a prevalence of 9-24%.

INTERFACE BETWEEN SKIN AND SLEEP

- Skin plays a role in the physiology of sleep such as initiation of sleep and thermoregulation.
- Skin symptoms are influenced by the body's circadian rhythms and peripheral circadian oscillators. For example, the physiological lowering of cortisol levels during the latter part of the day, which may contribute to the increased nocturnal pruritus in inflammatory dermatoses.
- Cutaneous symptoms like hyperhidrosis and itching can affect sleep and quality of life of patients and caregivers. Conditions like infantile eczema can prevent a parent from holding or hugging a child while trying to make him/her sleep.
- Reciprocally, several sleep disorders like insomnia, rhythm disorders, sleep apnea, and sleep deprivation can have a possible effect on the skin.
- Some dermatological disorders can be frequently comorbid with psychiatric disorders like depression and associated with sleep difficulties.
- Emotional stress can be associated with sleep difficulties and may often precede a worsening of an existing skin condition like acne.

DERMATOLOGICAL DISORDERS AND SLEEP PROBLEMS

The Diagnostic and Statistical Manual of Mental Disorders, 5th edition (DSM V) defines chronic insomnia as "loss of sleep three nights a week for at least 3 months" and includes difficulty in initiating sleep (initial insomnia), maintaining an unbroken sleep (middle insomnia), and waking up several hours earlier than the usual time (terminal insomnia) and/or having nonrestorative sleep, these being present in the context of the individual having adequate time and opportunity for sleep. Insomnia has been found to have a prevalence of approximately 10% in adults.

Amongst children, insomnia is reported by family members and encompasses resistance to go to bed, being unable to sleep independently or both. This can significantly affect sleep quality of the parents or caregivers. Insomnia due to medical condition is used to describe those situations where the patient has insomnia as well as a medical diagnosis that is known to disrupt sleep. Patients with diseases of the skin fit into this category. A cross-sectional study of 634 patients with dermatological conditions found that 27.92% of the participants had insomnia, of which 64.97% were reported to have subjective sleep disturbance. Skin-related causes accounted for the sleep problems in 55.65%, itch being the leading cause (64.49%), followed by pain (55.84%) and fearful thoughts about the skin (54.55%). Another study on 800 patients with varied dermatological diagnoses found that two thirds of their sample had poor sleep, which was associated with reduced quality of life, occupational dysfunction, and psychological distress. Poor sleep was independently related to the severity of the pruritis and nocturnal pruritis. A case-control study compared sleep quality in individuals with (2,871) and without cutaneous disorders (863). Patients had significantly higher levels of sleep disturbance (71.2% vs. 32.7%), itching, pain, and other subjective sensations being the predictors.

Pruritis

Pruritus/itch is a common symptom reported in the dermatology clinic. Several dermatological conditions like psoriasis, urticaria, eczema, prurigo nodularis, and atopic dermatitis (AD); infective conditions like scabies and mycoses fungoides; and other physical ailments like hematologic malignancies, hepatic disease, and cholestasis can present with pruritus. Nocturnal pruritis is present in almost 90% of patients with chronic pruritus, the severity of the sleep disturbance correlating with the severity of the nocturnal itch. Itching is more prevalent in NREM stage 1, stage 3 being rarely affected. Increased levels of C reactive protein have been found in patients with sleep difficulties; hence, a systemic inflammation theory has been postulated as a possible explanation for this association. Several itchy skin conditions can also have significant psychiatric morbidities, which can contribute to the degree of insomnia and cause a heightened itch perception.

Psoriasis

Psoriasis affects the thermoregulatory function of the skin, thus interfering with sleep initiation. The systemic inflammatory effects of psoriasis including arthritis cause fatigue and poor sleep. Insomnia prevalence in psoriasis ranges from 6 to 45%. A systematic review found that 93.7% of the studies assessed reported sleep disturbance in psoriasis patients. A recent cross-sectional study that compared sleep quality in 334 patients with psoriasis and 126 controls found that 59% of the patients had disturbed sleep as opposed to 34% of controls, the sleep duration being less by an hour. Anxiety and depression symptoms were found to be the strongest predictors of poor sleep, followed by nocturnal pruritis, age, being a woman, and the intensity of pruritus and gastroesophageal reflux disease. The circadian clock has also been postulated to play a role in psoriasis pathophysiology. The pruritus seems to worsen at night, indicating a circadian-rhythmic pathogenesis. Shift work, which plays havoc with the circadian rhythms, has been known to exacerbate or increase the risk for psoriasis. These features may be explained by the fact that the key elements in psoriasis like cell cycle, apoptosis, and inflammation lie under circadian control. Another possible link is the effect of sleep deprivation on the gut microbiome. A similar altered gut-bacteria ratio was found in psoriasis and in sleep dysfunction, indicating that sleep deprivation may have a role in psoriasis disease progression.

Atopic Dermatitis

Atopic dermatitis is associated with intense nocturnal pruritis, leading to disturbed sleep and impaired quality of life. Most of the literature on sleep in AD is based on studies in the pediatric population. About 60% of children with AD experience disturbed sleep, with a rise in frequency to 83% during flare-ups of the disease. In children < 6 years of age, 30% of the parents reported of co-sleeping due to AD; 66% found this bothersome. Children with eczema report more fatigue and reduced sleep efficiency; associations have been reported with short stature and attention deficits in children with AD who also have sleep problems. 33-87% of adults with AD experience difficulties in sleep, which include insomnia of all types, shorter sleep time, and higher sleep latency. Actigraphy studies have demonstrated a positive correlation between AD severity and degree of sleep disturbance. Studies on nocturnal scratching in AD have found that patients have a two times higher median number of sleep movements compared to control subjects.

Other Skin Conditions

Sleep has a role to play in wound healing as well as skin aging. Acute sleep deprivation is known to hamper the integrity of the skin. In one intriguing study from the military, sleep-deprived individuals took a day longer to heal blisters as compared to well-rested individuals. Oyetakin–White et al. compared healthy Caucasian women categorized as good- and poor-quality sleepers. Good sleepers were found to have lower intrinsic skin aging scores, 30% higher skin recovery 72 hours after tape stripping, and better recovery from erythema 24 hours after exposure to ultraviolet light and perceived themselves as physically attractive. Patients with chronic urticaria report pruritus and burning sensation of the skin, and more than 50% experience sleep disturbance. Histamine levels increase during dawn and dusk, causing terminal insomnia in these patients due to the pruritus. Skin infections like scabies can lead to nocturnal pruritus which can disturb sleep. In a study that evaluated sleep quality in patients with cutaneous warts, Karaali and Manav found that patients with warts had higher average Pittsburgh Sleep Quality Index (PSQI) scores than age- and gender-matched healthy controls. Those with genital warts had poorer sleep quality than patients with nongenital warts. Female patients with genital warts had the worst sleep quality. Autoimmune diseases of the skin like pemphigus vulgaris also have been known to impair sleep. These patients frequently have pain which can delay sleep onset as well as cause a disrupted sleep. This in turn leads to a greater sensibility to pain, thus sparking a vicious cycle. Schrom et al. assessed the relationship between sleep quality and acne severity in 40 adults using the Global Acne Grading Scale and PSQI. They found that the average subjective sleep scores were found to be reduced as the objectively rated severity of acne increased and vice versa. A systematic literature review (1979–2021) on the psychosocial aspects of vitiligo revealed that sleep disturbances ranged from 4.6 to 89%. Oztekin and Oztekin compared patients with vitiligo with an age- and sex-matched control group on measures for depression and sleep quality. They found higher median PSQI scores in the patient group, as well as scores for subjective sleep quality, sleep latency, and sleep disturbance. The chronic facial skin disease rosacea is also known to have an association with sleep. Wang et al. conducted a case–control survey on 608 rosacea patients and age- and sex-matched healthy controls using the PSQI and grading the rosacea severity by the guidelines of the National Rosacea Society. 52.3% of patients with rosacea had poor sleep quality as compared to controls (24%). The severity of the rosacea also affected the sleep quality. In a study that looked at sleep quality in patients with alopecia areata (AA), Shakoei et al. compared 51 AA patients with age- and gender-matched healthy controls and assessed them on PSQI, Epworth Sleepiness Scale (ESS), and Severity of Alopecia Tool (SALT). The mean PSQI score was higher in the AA group. More number of cases had higher ESS scores. The SALT scores did not show any association with the PSQI scores. Anxiety and depression were higher in the AA group, and these had worse PSQI scores. There is conflicting evidence regarding the association between sleep/circadian rhythms and skin malignancies.

OTHER SLEEP DISORDERS RELATED TO SKIN PROBLEMS

Obstructive Sleep Apnea

Obstructive sleep apnea (OSA) is a common breathing disorder where airway obstruction leads to impaired ventilation, during sleep. The frequent arousals from sleep can activate the sympathetic system which in turn alters the skin's neuroendocrine network homeostasis, thus precipitating inflammatory conditions like psoriasis. Rates of OSA are higher in psoriasis (36–56.3%). Children with AD can also have snoring and OSA, which indicates a comorbid allergic rhinitis and asthma. Vorona reported the case of an obese patient with severe OSA who developed hyperpigmentation and lichenification of the forehead skin after repeated rubbing of head against the wall, when trying to sleep.

Narcolepsy

Narcolepsy is a hypersomnia of central origin leading to sudden daytime sleep attacks. Daytime skin temperature is altered in narcolepsy. There have been case series and reports on the potential association between narcolepsy and AA, based on possible common autoimmune factors operating in both conditions as well as AD.

Parasomnias

Parasomnias are disorders of arousal from sleep that manifest as abnormal movements in sleep, dreams, behaviors like sleepwalking and autonomic arousal. An age-matched case–control study in AD showed that patients had more parasomnias, the frequency being related to AD severity, attributed to the "sensory hypersensitivity" in AD. A study that compared patients with vitiligo with other skin conditions revealed that the vitiligo patients reported more parasomnias in childhood and adolescence. A primary parasomnia may present as a sleep-related scratching behavior.

Restless Legs Syndrome

Restless legs syndrome (RLS) is a sensorimotor disorder in which the sufferer has an irresistible urge to move the legs, disrupting night sleep. There may be an unpleasant paresthesia in the leg, which may be misdiagnosed as a skin problem.

Problems related to treatment: Various drugs used to treat skin disorders can also contribute to problems with sleep. Corticosteroids reduce melatonin with a marked disturbance in the circadian rhythm and inhibit the brain uptake of tryptophan. The effect seems to be dose dependent; high doses of prednisolone have been known to reduce total REM sleep time. Isotretinoin, used for acne, can cause sleep apnea and insomnia. Antihistamines prescribed for pruritis can increase REM sleep latency, resulting in residual daytime sleepiness.

ASSESSMENT OF SLEEP

Questions regarding sleep needs to be a part of routine clinical evaluation of dermatology patients, especially those with chronic problems and nocturnal pruritus. Duration of sleep, type of insomnia, scratching behavior at night, daytime sleepiness, fatigue, comorbid emotional symptoms, stress, other medical conditions that can disturb sleep, and use of medications must be inquired into. In children, parents should be asked regarding the child's sleep pattern as well as co-sleeping. Using valid questionnaires [PSQI, Bergen Insomnia Scale (BIS), Insomnia Severity Index (ISI), ESS, etc.) can aid the process. Actigraphy and polysomnography are additional investigations that would help.

MANAGEMENT

Since one of the chief reasons for poor sleep is nocturnal itching and scratching, reducing the same is a key factor. Increased temperature can worsen pruritus; hence, reducing sweating, using clean and cool bed linen made of breathable fabric, and avoiding dust mites can help. Nails must be kept clean and short, as scratching with dirty nails can increase inflammation. Dry skin itches more; hence, using a moisturizer before going to bed is ideal. Maintaining the circadian rhythm by having a strict sleep-wake schedule can reduce inflammatory flares. The bed should be used only for sleeping; minimizing bright lights and loud noises in the sleeping area, trying relaxation methods (soft music and breathing exercises), avoiding screen use and stimulating activities an hour before bedtime, refraining from using caffeine and tobacco after evening hours, and having a cup of warm milk at bedtime aid in better sleep. Indiscriminate use of medications that can disrupt the sleep rhythm should be avoided; comorbid conditions need to be adequately treated. Adequate control of chronic skin condition is likely to improve sleep quality and duration; improving sleep may hasten disease control of the associated skin conditions (Mann et al. 2023, Anderson and Jeter 2023).

If these measures do not work adequately, a brief course of medications may be needed to improve sleep (Madari et al. 2021; Asnis et al. 2016). Various classes of drugs have been used to treat insomnia. Benzodiazepines which act as positive allosteric modulators on the $GABA_A$ binding site thereby enhancing the inhibitory effect of GABA are one of the commonly used class of drugs. Five benzodiazepines, namely, estazolam, flurazepam, quazepam, temazepam, and triazolam are FDA approved for insomnia treatment in adults. Since the other benzodiazepines also have sedative effects, they are also often used as off label hypnotics. The common adverse effects reported are drowsiness, dizziness, lethargy, ataxia, apnoea, and blurred vision.

A popularly used non benzodiazepine class is that of the Z drugs which act as benzodiazepine receptor agonists (BzRAs) and include Zolpidem, Eszopiclone and Zaleplon. Zolpidem which is the most prescribed is available in strengths of 5 and 10 mg as well as extended-release preparations of 6.25 and 12.5 mg. Abdominal symptoms, dizziness and somnolence are frequently reported adverse effects.

Certain antidepressants like Doxepin, trazodone and Amitriptyline have been used for treatment of insomnia due to their sedative effects. Headache and somnolence are common adverse effects. Only Doxepin is FDA approved for this particular use amongst the antidepressant class.

The naturally occurring hormone Melatonin secreted by the pineal gland is also used in the management if sleep problems. Melatonin is a full agonist at melatonin receptors 1 and 2. Though it chiefly targets circadian rhythm disorders, it is also a weak hypnotic agent. The dosing regime has varied between 0.1 to 5 mg. The Melatonin agonist Ramelteon is also an FDA approved drug useful for sleep onset difficulties.

Orexin receptor antagonists, Suvorexant and Lemborexant are also FDA approved hypnotic agents. Adverse effects include sleepiness, headaches, and abnormal dreams.

Off label hypnotics commonly prescribed by clinicians include antihistamines like Diphenhydramine and sedating atypical antipsychotics like Quetiapine.

CONCLUSION

Sleep is an important restorative process that is necessary for several physiological functions including maintaining the integrity of the skin. Skin and sleep are closely connected and affect each other in several ways. Most of the chronic skin conditions can lead to poor sleep, which in turn flares up the skin condition. Assessment of sleep must be an integral part of a clinical assessment in dermatology clinic and adequate steps must be taken to improve sleep in these patients.

FURTHER READINGS

1. Okechukwu CE. The neurophysiologic basis of the human sleep–wake cycle and the physiopathology of the circadian clock: a narrative review. Egypt J Neurol Psychiatr Neurosurg. 2022;58(34):1-7.
2. Liew SC, Aung T. Sleep deprivation and its association with diseases: a review. Sleep Med. 2021;77:192-204.
3. Gupta MA, Gupta AK. Sleep-wake disorders and dermatology. Clin Dermatol. 2013;31:118-26.
4. Morin MC, Jarrin DC. Epidemiology of Insomnia: Prevalence, Course, Risk Factors, and Public Health Burden. Sleep Med Clin. 2022;17(2):173-91.
5. Tamschick R, Navarini A, Strobel W, Muller S. Insomnia, and other sleep disorders in dermatology patients: A questionnaire-based study with 634 patients. Clin Dermatol. 2021;39:996-1004.

6. Spindler M, Przybyowicz K, Hawro M, Weller K, Reidel U, Metz M, et al. Sleep disturbance in adult dermatologic patients: A cross-sectional study on prevalence, burden, and associated factors. J Am Acad Dermatol. 2021;85(4):910-22.
7. Halioua B, Misery L, Seite S, Delvigne V, Chelli C, Taieb J, et al. Influence of Skin Subjective Symptoms on Sleep Quality in Patients with Cutaneous Disorders: A Study of 2871 Subjects. Clin Cosmet Investig Dermatol. 2021;14:143-52.
8. Lavery MJ, Stull C, Nattkemperi LA, Sanders KM, Lee H, Sahu S, et al. Nocturnal Pruritus: Prevalence, Characteristics, and Impact on Itchy QoL in a Chronic Itch Population. Acta Derm Venereol. 2017;97:513-5.
9. Podder I, Mondal H, Kroumpouzos G. Nocturnal pruritus and sleep disturbance associated with dermatologic disorders in adult patients. Int J Women's Dermatol. 2021;7:403-10.
10. Patel SP, Khanna R, Choi J, Williams KA, Roh YS, Hong MS, et al. Sleep disturbance in adults with chronic pruritic dermatoses is associated with increased C Reactive Protein levels. J Am Acad Dermatol. 2021;84(2):265-72.
11. Gupta MA, Gupta AK. Psychodermatology: an update. J Am Acad Dermatol. 1996;34:1030-46.
12. Gupta MA, Gupta AK, Schork NJ, Ellis CN. Depression modulates pruritus perception: a study of pruritus in psoriasis, atopic dermatitis, and chronic idiopathic urticaria. Psychosom Med. 1994;56:36-40.
13. Gupta MA, Simpson FC, Gupta AK. Psoriasis and sleep disorders: A systematic review. Sleep Med Rev. 2016;29:63-75.
14. Henry A, Kyle SD, Bhandari S, Chisholm A, Griffiths CEM, Bundy C. Measurement, Classification and Evaluation of Sleep Disturbance in Psoriasis: A Systematic Review. PLoS ONE. 2016;11(6):1-18.
15. Sahin E, Hawro M, Weller K, Sabat R, Philipp S, Kokolakis G, et al. Prevalence and factors associated with sleep disturbance in adult patients with psoriasis. J Am Acad Dermatol Venereol. 2022;36:688-97.
16. Li WQ, Qureshi AA, Schernhammer ES, et al. Rotating night-shift work and risk of psoriasis in US women. J Invest Dermatol. 2013;133:565-7.
17. Luengas-Martinez A, Paus R, Iqbal M, Bailey L, Ray DW, Young HS. Circadian rhythms in psoriasis and the potential of chronotherapy in psoriasis management. Exp Dermatol. 2022;31:1800-9.
18. Myers B, Vidhatha R, Nicholas B, Stephanie C, Quinn T, Chang HW, et al. Sleep and the gut microbiome in psoriasis: clinical implications for disease progression and the development of cardiometabolic comorbidities. J Psoriasis Psoriatic Arthritis. 2021;6:27-37.
19. Camfferman D, Kennedy JD, Gold M, Martin AJ, Lushington K. Eczema and sleep and its relationship to daytime functioning in children. Sleep Med Rev. 2010;14:359-69.
20. Chamlin SL, Mattson CL, Frieden IJ, Williams ML, Mancini AJ, Cella D, et al. The price of pruritus: sleep disturbance and co-sleeping in atopic dermatitis. Arch Pediatr Adolesc Med. 2005;159:745-50.
21. Fishbein AB, Vitaterna O, Haugh IM, Bavishi AA, Zee PC, Turek FW, et al. Nocturnal eczema: Review of sleep and circadian rhythms in children with atopic dermatitis and future research directions. J Allergy Clin Immunol. 2015;136(5):1170-7.

22. Jeon C, Yan D, Nakamura M, Sekhon S. Frequency and Management of Sleep Disturbance in Adults with Atopic Dermatitis: A Systematic Review. Dermatol Ther. 2017;7:349-64.
23. Yu SH, Attarian H, Zee P, Silverberg JI. Burden of sleep and fatigue in US adults with atopic dermatitis. Dermatitis. 2016;27(2):50-8.
24. Jernelov S, Höglund CO, Axelsson J, Axén J, Grönneberg R, Grunewald J. Effects of examination stress on psychological responses, sleep, and allergic symptoms in atopic and non-atopic students. Int J Behav Med. 2009;16(4):305-10.
25. Bender BG, Leung SB, Leung DY. Actigraphy assessment of sleep disturbance in patients with atopic dermatitis: an objective life quality measure. J Allergy Clin Immunol. 2003;111(3):598-602.
26. Bringhurst C, Waterston K, Schofield O, Benjamin K, Rees JL. Measurement of itch using actigraphy in pediatric and adult populations. J Am Acad Dermatol. 2004;51(6):893-8.
27. Smith TJ, Wilson MA, Karl JP, Orr J, Smith CD, Cooper AD, et al. Impact of sleep restriction on local immune response and skin barrier restoration with and without "multinutrient" nutrition intervention. J Appl Physiol (1985). 2018;124:190-200.
28. Oyetakin-White P, Suggs A, Koo B, Matsui MS, Yarosh D, Cooper KD, Baron ED. Does poor sleep quality affect skin ageing? Clin Exp Dermatol. 2015;40(1):17-22.
29. Mann C, Gorai S, Staubach-Renz P, Goldust M. Sleep disorders in dermatology: a comprehensive review. J Dtsch Dermatol Ges. 2023;21:577-84.
30. Karaali MG, Manav V. Evaluation of Sleep Quality in Patients with Genital and Non-genital Cutaneous Warts: a Prospective Controlled Study. Dermatol Pract Concept. 2022;12(4):e2022167.
31. Pedroni MN, Hirotsu C, Porro AM, Tufik S, Anderson ML. The role of sleep-in pemphigus: a review of mechanisms and perspectives. Arch Dermatol Res. 2017;309(8):659-64.
32. Schrom KP, Ahsanuddin S, Baechtold M, Tripathi R, Ramser A, Baron E. Acne severity and sleep quality in adults. Clocks Sleep. 2019;1:510-6.
33. Ezzedine K, Eleftheriadou V, Jones H, Bibeau K, Kuo FI, Sturm D, et al. Psychosocial Effects of Vitiligo: A Systematic Literature Review. Am J Clin Dermatol. 2021;22:757-74.
34. Oztekin A, Oztekin C. Sleep quality and depression in vitiligo patients. Eurasian J Fam Med. 2020;9(1):35-42.
35. Wang Z, Xie H, Gong Y, Ouyang Y, Deng F, Tang Y, Li J. Relationship between rosacea and sleep. J Dermatol. 2020;47(6):592-600.
36. Shakoei S, Torabimirzaee A, Saffarian Z, Abedini R. Sleep disturbance in alopecia areata: A cross-sectional study. Health Sci Rep. 2022;1(53):e576.
37. Anderson EJ, Jeter JP. Dermatologic implications of sleep deprivation in the US military. Cutis. 2023;111(3):146-9.
38. Chng SY, Goh DYT, Wang XS, Tan TN, Ong NBH. Snoring and atopic disease: a strong association. Pediatric Pulmonol. 2004;38:210-6.
39. Vorona RD. Skin pigmentation changes in a patient with a sleep disorder. J Clin Sleep Med. 2007;3:535-6.

40. King Jr LE, Eastham AW, Curcio NM, Schmidt AN. A potential association between alopecia areata and narcolepsy. Arch Dermatol. 2010;146:677-9.
41. Nigam G, Pathak C, Riaz M. Alopecia areata and narcolepsy: A tale of obscure autoimmunity. BMJ Case Rep. 2016:bcr2015211523.
42. Chin J, Bearison C, Silverberg N, Lee Wong M. Concomitant atopic dermatitis and narcolepsy type 1: psychiatric implications and challenges in management. Gen Psychiatry. 2019;32(5):e100094.
43. Shani-Adir A, Rozenman D, Kessel A, Engel-Yeger B. The relationship between sensory hypersensitivity and sleep quality of children with atopic dermatitis. Pediatric Dermatol. 2009;26:143-9.
44. Mouzas O, Angelopoulos N, Papaliagka M, Tsogas P. Increased frequency of self-reported parasomnias in patients suffering from vitiligo. Eur J Dermatol. 2008;18:165-8.
45. Nigam G, Riaz M, Hershner SD, Goldstein CA, Chervin RD. Sleep related scratching: a distinct parasomnia? J Clin Sleep Med. 2016;12(1):139-42.
46. Walters AS, Hickey K, Maltzman J, Verrico T, Joseph D, Hening W, et al. A questionnaire study of 138 patients with restless legs syndrome: the "Night-Walkers" survey. Neurology. 1996;46:92-5.
47. Gillin JC, Jacobs LS, Fram DH, Snyder F. Acute effect of a glucocorticoid on normal human sleep. Nature. 1972;237:398-9.
48. Gupta MA, Vujcic B, Gupta AK. 1031 Isotretinoin (13-cis retinoic acid) is associated with a higher frequency of sleep apnea syndrome: results from the US FDA adverse event reporting system (FAERS). Sleep. 2017;40(1):A3834.
49. Assiri SH, Alosiami AK, Adler JR. Severe Insomnia Induced by Isotretinoin Use for the Management of Acne Vulgaris: A Rare Side Effect. Cureus. 2023;15(1):e33658.
50. Ozdemir PG, Karadag AS, Selvi Y, Boysan M, Bilgili SG, Aydin A, et al. Assessment of the effects of antihistamine drugs on mood, sleep quality, sleepiness, and dream anxiety. Int J Psychiatry Clin Pract. 2014;18(3):161-8.
51. Suilmann T, Zeidler C, Osada N, Riepe C, Stander S. Usability of Validated Sleep-assessment Questionnaires in Patients with Chronic Pruritus: An Interview-based Study. Acta Dermatol Venereol. 2018;98(8):722-7.

CHAPTER 15

Suicide Prevention in Patients with Dermatological Conditions

Shubh Mohan Singh, Eepsita Mishra

> **Key Messages**
> - Dermatological conditions show significant psychological burden and can lead to suicidality.
> - Certain skin conditions such as psoriasis, atopic dermatitis, and severe acne have relatively high risk.
> - Suicidality is an indicator of psychiatric illness and is a preventable cause of death.
> - If the primary treating doctor is able to recognize and interfere timely with the help of a psychiatrist, a valuable life can be saved.

INTRODUCTION

Chronic medical illnesses have long been known to have adverse impacts on the mental and emotional well-being of the person suffering from them. However, when one thinks of such chronic debilitating illnesses, dermatological conditions often fall lower on the rung of considerations. This may be in part due to the fact that they are viewed as largely benign conditions and do not bear the tag of "terminal illnesses". In fact, for a long time, dermatologists were considered to be the "physicians treating patients who never die". In recent times, scientific research and anecdotal reports show that dermatological conditions impose a significant psychological burden, and associated depression, anxiety, and suicidality are common. These studies are briefly reviewed below.

A significant proportion of people with dermatological illnesses experience adverse psychological outcomes stemming from multiple and varied causes. The foremost, and perhaps most obvious, is the disfigurement that many of these diseases are associated with. This toll on physical appearance is often associated with social isolation by adversely impacting family and community perceptions, employment, and marital prospects—all of which are well-established independent risk factors for depression. Another important cause is the chronic nature of the disease itself and the consequent sense of the sufferer always feeling "unhealthy", which may at times yield to hopelessness. Chronic illnesses are often accompanied by the need for long-term medication which, in addition to posing a financial burden on the patient, may at times carry the risk of inducing depressive symptoms or suicidality as an adverse reaction. It has been reported that around a fourth of patients afflicted by dermatological illnesses have some form of psychiatric morbidity, mostly in the form of depression or anxiety disorders. Psoriasis, acne, and atopic dermatitis are among the dermatological conditions with the highest association of psychiatric comorbidity.

Suicidality is a phenomenon that exists on a spectrum and therefore presents as such. It may range from feelings of life weariness and death wishes to thoughts and plans of committing suicide and ultimately to a suicidal attempt, which may be aborted or completed. On the one hand, it may be possible that a person with a primary psychiatric illness also has a dermatological condition; suicidality in such a case would likely be due to the compound effect of these two conditions. However, the main focus of this chapter is the second situation, that is, the psychological toll that dermatological illnesses take on a person leading to suicidality due to factors that are unique to these conditions. Suicidal ideation varies anywhere between 6 and 18% depending on the underlying skin condition as is reviewed below.

The importance of identifying suicidality as early as possible on the aforementioned spectrum is obvious. As in general psychiatric practice, it may not always be possible to prevent a suicidal attempt, but it is feasible and desirable to screen patients with dermatological diseases, especially those known to be associated with a higher risk of suicidality—such as psoriasis, acne, eczema, and atopic dermatitis—for psychiatric morbidity (mainly depression and anxiety) as well as suicidality.

This chapter attempts to provide an overview of the literature with regards to suicide and suicidality in the context of dermatoses and the management and prevention of the same.

SUICIDE AND SUICIDALITY IN DERMATOSES

As presented in **Table 1**, studies show that certain skin diseases present a higher risk of suicide. Some important ones are given in the following text.
- *Psoriasis*: Two large-scale studies have shown that patients with psoriasis express a higher degree of suicidality compared with healthy controls as well as other skin diseases such as alopecia areata and vitiligo. Depending on the instrument used, suicidality in psoriasis ranges from 7 to 21%. It is higher in women and inpatients, the former mostly attributable to more importance given to physical appearance by and in women. Rating of disease severity by dermatologists was found to correlate poorly with patient ratings, which goes on to highlight the severity of the psychological impact of the disease.
- *Acne*: As it primarily affects the face, acne can lead to great stigma and low self-esteem. A large-scale study found patients with mild-to-moderate acne to report suicidal ideations and death wishes. Indeed, some studies have found that the risk of suicide in acne at times corelates with its severity. Moreover, isotretinoin, one of the commonly used drugs to treat severe acne, has been reported to independently cause suicidal thoughts; however, the data on this is as yet inconsistent. Patients with moderate-to-severe acne are at a higher risk of completed suicide, especially those affected postadolescence.
- *Atopic dermatitis*: It is a debilitating condition affecting all age groups and is associated with significant suicide risk, especially in the more severe forms of the disease.

Other diseases found (inconsistently) to have an elevated risk of suicidality include eczema, alopecia areata, and vitiligo.

UNDERSTANDING THE PSYCHOLOGICAL IMPACT OF DERMATOLOGICAL CONDITIONS IN RELATION TO SUICIDE

Of all the organ systems in the human body, the skin is the largest and most exposed to the external environment. Its visibility, compounded by sociocultural overemphasis on physical perfection, gives rise to unrealistic standards of beauty and physical appearance

Table 1: Review of studies assessing suicidality in persons with dermatological illnesses.

Year	Authors	Sample size	Outcome measures	Skin conditions	Results
1998	Gupta et al.	480	Carroll Rating Scale for Depression (CRSD) including one item for assessing suicidality ("I have been thinking about trying to kill myself")	Noncystic facial acne, alopecia areata, AD, and psoriasis	• In-patients with severe psoriasis scored higher on CRSD as compared to others • Prevalence of suicidal ideation was 7.2% in psoriasis inpatients, 2.5% in psoriasis outpatients, and 2.1% in AD • Mild-to-moderate facial acne—suicidal ideation (5.6%) and death wishes (8.3%) • Suicidal ideation had association with greater severity of depressive symptoms
2001	Khan et al.	50		Acne	• Suicidal ideations in 8% of patients with acne
2004	Zachariae et al.	798 (333 outpatients, 172 inpatients, and 293 healthy controls)	Beck's Depression Inventory (BDI), Dermatology Life Quality Index, Brief Symptom Inventory	Psoriasis, acne, AD, urticaria, and eczema	• Greater percentage of patients with psoriasis (21.2% of 113) and AD (18.9% of 95) had thoughts about suicide compared with healthy controls • Inpatient status was associated with suicidal ideation

Continued

Continued

Year	Authors	Sample size	Outcome measures	Skin conditions	Results
2005	Arima et al.	51	BDI, Self-Anxiety Scale (SAS)	AD	BDI scores were significantly higher in patients with severe AD
2006	Picardi et al.	466 (294 outpatients and 172 inpatients)	Patient Health Questionnaire (PHQ), General Health Questionnaire (GHQ-12), and Skindex-29	Acne, psoriasis	• Overall prevalence of suicidal ideation—8.6%, with highest proportionate prevalence in psoriasis • Suicidal ideation in acne—7.1% • Suicidal ideation associated with depression
2006	Kimata et al.	10,323 (6,748 patients and 3,575 healthy controls)	Questionnaire enquiring about suicidal ideation	AD	Lifetime prevalence of suicidal ideation—19.6% in severe AD, 6% in moderate AD, and 8.1% in healthy controls
2006	Purvis et al.	9,567	Reynolds Adolescent Depression Scale, Multidimensional Anxiety Scale for Children, self-reported acne and suicide attempts	Acne	Association present between acne and suicide attempts after controlling for depressive symptoms and anxiety (OR 1.5; 95% CI 1.21–1.86)
2008	Rehn at al.	315 (165 patients and 150 controls)		Acne	No relationship between acne and self-reported depressive symptoms

Continued

Continued

Year	Authors	Sample size	Outcome measures	Skin conditions	Results
2009	Dieris-Hirche et al.	124 (62 patients and 62 healthy controls)	Hospital Anxiety and Depression Scale (HADS), Poldinger's scale	AD	• Higher prevalence of suicidal ideation and greater HADS scores in patients with AD as compared to healthy controls • Strong correlation between patient-rated severity of dermatological disease, psychological burden, and suicidal ideation
2011	Halvorsen et al.	3,775	GHQ-12, BDI, Alcohol Use Disorders Identification Test and Rosenberg Self-Esteem Scale	Acne	• 1 in 4 adolescents with severe acne reported suicidal ideation • Prevalence of suicidal ideation in severe acne as compared with no or little acne was twice as high in girls and thrice as high in boys • Significant association between substantial acne and suicidal ideation in both genders after controlling for other factors, including depression

(AD: atopic dermatitis; CI: confidence interval; OD: odds ratio) which are impossible to meet for a "normal" person, let alone someone afflicted by skin disease. Understandably, a person having scarring or outwardly visible skin lesions is more often than not subject to stigma—both self and external. Such persons may be unduly critical of their physical appearance which translates to low self-esteem and feelings of worthlessness. They may also be excluded from social and religious gatherings, lose out on marital prospects, and face discrimination at the workplace, which leads to social isolation. Moreover, the chronicity of the conditions leads to a sense of hopelessness, which is one of the most important predictors of suicide.

Vulnerable Subpopulations

A recent review article found that children and adolescents with dermatological conditions were at a higher risk of suicide compared to adults with similar illnesses. This may be attributed to several factors such as the psychological need to "fit in" with their peer group, higher levels of concern and preoccupation with physical appearance, emotional immaturity, and impulsivity. Moreover, individuals with pre-existing mental health conditions who then go on to develop dermatological illnesses (e.g., a patient of bipolar disorder on lithium contracting drug-induced acne) are at a higher risk of death by suicide due to the compounding effect of the two illnesses and interwoven complex psychosocial factors.

Impact of Stigma and Social Support

As discussed previously, skin conditions are associated with greater self, public as well as institutional stigma, which lead to not only loneliness and social isolation but also reduced help seeking and consequent increased risk of suicide.

Strong social support networks, in the form of familial and community ties, support groups, online forums, etc., may aid in the reduction of stigma and contribute to a sense of being included. It also offers the opportunity to seek out help when in distress and acknowledge one's fears and insecurities without the risk of "othering".

RECOGNIZING SUICIDE WARNING SIGNS

In nonpsychiatric settings, consultations can often feel rushed and overly focused on symptoms and laboratory values; in such a situation, a patient may find it difficult to discuss any ongoing mental health issues or bring up experience of suicidal thoughts. Hence, the importance of an unhurried, compassionate clinical interview cannot be overstressed. Contrary to the widely held view, patient inquiry into mental health status does not prolong the length of the consultation and proves to be an invaluable tool for assessing mental health issues and planning appropriate interventions.

While it is nearly impossible to "predict" suicide, there are often several warning signs to look out for. Early identification of such signs and a subsequent prompt response can significantly reduce the risk of suicide attempts.

Some common warning signs may include the following:
- Expressing a feeling of shame or guilt
- Expressing feeling like a burden on others
- Talking about wanting to die
- Increased substance abuse or risk-taking behavior
- Gestures of finality such as saying goodbye to friends, making a will
- Making a plan or researching ways to die

COLLABORATIVE CARE APPROACH

Effective care and suicide prevention can be possible by the use of a multidisciplinary approach involving dermatologists, mental health professionals, and support groups. It is important that there is efficient communication and collaboration among healthcare providers to address both the physical and the psychological aspects of care.

The first step is to routinely screen all patients with chronic dermatological illnesses for depression and suicidality. This can be done using screening instruments, such as Patient Health Questionnaire-9 (PHQ-9) and General Health Questionnaire-12 (GHQ-12), and/or as a part of interview during clinical consultation. The dermatologist must not hesitate to ask about feelings of sadness or thoughts of dying for the unfounded fear that such questions may in fact precipitate suicidality. Rather, patients are more likely to communicate openly about any such issues when they feel that their physician is understanding and nonjudgmental.

If the dermatologist feels that the patient's responses extend beyond a normal psychological reaction to the illness, a prompt referral to a mental health professional is warranted, in addition to proper management of the primary skin disease to the best extent possible.

PSYCHOLOGICAL INTERVENTIONS

Evidence-based psychological interventions to help patients cope with the emotional toll of their skin condition include cognitive behavioral therapy (CBT) and acceptance and commitment therapy (ACT), among others.

Cognitive behavioral therapy is correlated with improved outcomes in quality of life, mental health, and skin status for patients suffering from conditions like psoriasis, atopic dermatitis, acne, vitiligo, and alopecia areata. In addition to positive psychological impact of CBT, the stress hypothesis postulates that stress reduction through CBT positively modulates the immune system which in turn leads to reduction in flare-ups of the skin condition.

Acceptance and commitment therapy aims to weaken the rumination cycle and "fused thoughts" related to skin conditions with body-image concern, shame, and self-criticism for extending kindness and understanding to oneself; to build self-perspective, that is, perceiving one's experience as part of the larger human experience; to inculcate a sense of self-kindness with acceptance of one's experience; and to take steps to act on values while practicing kindness and compassion.

Peer counseling groups offer a good alternative to such structured therapies which require the skills of a qualified professional as well as significant time and monetary investment. In addition to education about the illness, discussion about positive coping strategies, and providing the opportunity to share one's experience with the illness, such groups also act as social and community support networks.

PHARMACOLOGICAL CONSIDERATIONS

Patients identified to have comorbid depression must be offered pharmacological treatment without delay. Literature is scarce on specific pharmacological agents to be used for the treatment of depression in persons with dermatological illnesses, and the current standards of practice mostly adhere to existing guidelines for treating depression. Selective serotonin reuptake inhibitor (SSRI) drugs are usually the first line of treatment and may be combined with benzodiazepines or other anxiolytics.

Interestingly, recent studies have found use for certain antidepressants in the treatment of dermatological conditions. Mirtazapine, and less commonly, fluoxetine and sertraline, have been found to have antipruritic effects in eczema, with mirtazapine being especially advantageous owing to its sedative property, as eczema is often associated with severe night time itching, sleep disturbance, and reduced quality of life. Other studies have found paroxetine and fluvoxamine to be effective antipruritic agents in atopic dermatitis. While the exact mechanism for this action continues to elude us, anti-inflammatory properties of anti-depressants are generally considered to be responsible for the same.

Certain antidepressants, such as fluoxetine and fluvoxamine, inhibit cytochrome P450 (CYP) enzymes, which may lead to increased blood levels of certain drugs metabolized by the same isoenzyme. However, commonly used drugs in dermatological practice, such as prednisone and isotretinoin, are generally not known to have significant pharmacokinetic interactions with antidepressants.

Electroconvulsive therapy (ECT) may be useful in patients where suicidality is severe and there is an imminent danger of a suicide attempt.

Suffice to say, suicidality should always be taken seriously and an expression of the same should usually necessitate a detailed evaluation and referral to specialist psychiatrist services.

PATIENT EDUCATION AND EMPOWERMENT

While it is relatively easy to formulate standard operating protocols for dermatologists for dealing with suspected psychiatric morbidity in their patients, a referral to a mental health professional can be deeply stigmatizing in and of itself for patients. Fears related to "losing one's mind" or "being called crazy" are common. The role of the dermatologist as well as peer support groups in dispelling such notions and encouraging help seeking is fundamental to patient empowerment and improvement in the quality of their lives. Where resources permit, it may be easier for the patient to access mental healthcare services if a mental health professional is available within the confines of the dermatological establishment itself. This would circumvent the stigma of visiting a psychiatrist's office and thus improve service utilization and help-seeking behavior.

CREATING A SUPPORTIVE ENVIRONMENT

The road to health for patients with comorbid dermatological and psychiatric illnesses does not extend only from the physician's office to the psychiatrist's couch; rather it involves a much broader policy-level commitment to proposing and implementing strategies to promote a supportive and compassionate environment within healthcare settings for patients with skin disorders. Information and education activities must be conducted for healthcare providers to enhance their understanding of mental health issues related to dermatological conditions.

CRISIS INTERVENTION AND REFERRAL PROCEDURES

If a patient expresses suicidal thoughts during the course of the consultation, the clinician should attempt to engage them in productive conversation about the same, with a general attitude of empathy and nonjudgement, expressed by both verbal and nonverbal cues on part of the clinician. Contrary to popularly held belief, asking or talking about suicide in a person with suicidality does not increase their risk of harming themselves. Rather, it is a sound approach to cultivating empathic curiosity when dealing with a suicidal patient, which includes expressing support and empathy and gently enquiring about the details of their suicidal thoughts, such as planning, means that they intend to use and whether they have a time frame in mind.

If a person expresses having suicidal thoughts but no imminent planning or means for the same and/or is able to exert reasonable control over such thoughts, it may be helpful for the primary treating doctor to initially discuss safety strategies such as designating safe places to be, safe people to call, and self-soothing strategies. The patient should then be encouraged to seek psychiatric help and referred to a psychiatrist for further evaluation. Even if the person is unwilling for consulting a psychiatrist at the time, it is of utmost importance that the conversation with the primary doctor regarding suicidality should be ongoing and the doctor should continue supportive listening and encourage the patient to see a psychiatrist at the earliest if these thoughts are persistent or worsen in any way.

On the other hand, if a patient expresses a perceived lack of control over their suicidal thoughts, imminent plans for a serious attempt, have access to lethal means of self-harm, or have a past history of a suicide attempt, emergency services must be contacted immediately so that patient safety can be ensured. In such cases, a separate referral to a psychiatrist is usually not necessary as psychiatric intervention is more often than not part of emergency care for such patients. A close liaison with the psychiatrist should be established for holistic management of the patient's skin disease as well as mental health condition.

It would be naive to assume that patients neatly fit into such a cookie-cutter view of suicidality. As discussed previously, suicidality exists on a spectrum and presents as such. Many a time, the clinician may feel unsure and find it difficult to accurately ascertain a person's degree of suicidality. In case of doubt, it is always prudent to involve mental health professionals at the earliest.

PUBLIC HEALTH INITIATIVES AND POLICY RECOMMENDATIONS

As discussed earlier, improving the mental health of persons with dermatological conditions requires concerted efforts from multiple stakeholders including policy makers and public health officials. Regular organization of public health initiatives aimed at raising awareness of mental health issues in patients with dermatological conditions, such as television and radio broadcasts, skits and street plays, etc., are examples of low-investment strategies promising to bear high returns in terms of education.

Policy changes to improve mental health screening and access to mental health resources for this patient population may include (but are not limited to) proper training of dermatologists and physicians in identifying warning signs of suicide, using screening instruments for suicide risk, discussing mental health concerns with their patients, mandatory mental health screening of patients visiting dermatology clinics, free availability of pamphlets and flyers on depression and suicide risk in dermatology clinics, focused resource allocation to ensure availability of an "on-site" mental health professional for ready referrals, and addressing the psychological problems of patients.

CONCLUSION

Suicidal thoughts, ideation, behavior, and attempts are more prevalent in persons suffering from dermatological conditions than previously thought. It is more common in certain skin conditions such as psoriasis, atopic dermatitis, and severe acne, compared to others. Suicidality is an indicator of psychiatric illness, has significant adverse bearing for the patient, their loved ones, and society at large, and is a preventable cause of death and morbidity. It is thus incumbent upon the primary treating doctor to be sensitive to the occurrence of such phenomena, properly assess the same during their consultation, employ crisis intervention strategies, ensure timely referral to mental health professionals, and work in close collaboration with them to ensure well-being of the patient.

FURTHER READINGS

1. Harris EC, Barraclough BM. Suicide as an outcome for medical disorders. Medicine (Baltimore). 1994;73(6):281-96.
2. Goodwin RD, Marusic A, Hoven CW. Suicide attempts in the United States: the role of physical illness. Soc Sci Med. 1982. 2003;56(8):1783-8.
3. Humphreys F, Humphreys MS. Psychiatric morbidity and skin disease: what dermatologists think they see. Br J Dermatol. 1998;139(4):679-81.
4. Picardi A, Lega I, Tarolla E. Suicide risk in skin disorders. Clin Dermatol. 2013;31(1):47-56.
5. O'Carroll PW, Berman AL, Maris RW, Moscicki EK, Tanney BL, Silverman MM. Beyond the Tower of Babel: a nomenclature for suicidology. Suicide Life Threat Behav. 1996;26(3):237-52.
6. Gupta MA, Gupta AK. Depression and suicidal ideation in dermatology patients with acne, alopecia areata, atopic dermatitis and psoriasis. Br J Dermatol. 1998;139(5):846-50.
7. Khan MZ, Naeem A, Mufti KA. Prevalence of mental health problems in acne patients. J Ayub Med Coll Abbottabad. 2001;13(4):7-8.
8. Zachariae R, Zachariae C, Ibsen HHW, Mortensen JT, Wulf HC. Psychological symptoms and quality of life of dermatology outpatients and hospitalized dermatology patients. Acta Derm Venereol. 2004;84(3):205-12.
9. Arima M, Shimizu Y, Sowa J, Narita T, Nishi I, Iwata N, et al. Psychosomatic analysis of atopic dermatitis using a psychological test. J Dermatol. 2005;32(3):160-8.

10. Picardi A, Mazzotti E, Pasquini P. Prevalence and correlates of suicidal ideation among patients with skin disease. J Am Acad Dermatol. 2006;54(3):420-6.
11. Kimata H. Prevalence of suicidal ideation in patients with atopic dermatitis. Suicide Life Threat Behav. 2006;36(1):120-4.
12. Purvis D, Robinson E, Merry S, Watson P. Acne, anxiety, depression and suicide in teenagers: a cross-sectional survey of New Zealand secondary school students. J Paediatr Child Health. 2006;42(12):793-6.
13. Rehn LMH, Meririnne E, Höök-Nikanne J, Isometsä E, Henriksson M. Depressive symptoms, suicidal ideation and acne: a study of male Finnish conscripts. J Eur Acad Dermatol Venereol. 200822(5):561-7.
14. Dieris-Hirche J, Gieler U, Kupfer J, Milch W. Suicidal ideation, anxiety and depression in adult patients with atopic dermatitis. Hautarzt Z Für Dermatol Venerol Verwandte Geb. 2009;60:641-6.
15. Halvorsen JA, Stern RS, Dalgard F, Thoresen M, Bjertness E, Lien L. Suicidal ideation, mental health problems, and social impairment are increased in adolescents with acne: a population-based study. J Invest Dermatol. 2011;131(2):363-70.
16. Germain N, Augustin M, François C, Legau K, Bogoeva N, Desroches M, et al. Stigma in visible skin diseases - a literature review and development of a conceptual model. J Eur Acad Dermatol Venereol. 2021;35(7):1493-504.
17. Beck AT, Weissman A, Lester D, Trexler L. The measurement of pessimism: the hopelessness scale. J Consult Clin Psychol. 1974;42(6):861-5.
18. Prabhakar D, Peterson EL, Hu Y, Rossom RC, Lynch FL, Lu CY, et al. Dermatologic Conditions and Risk of Suicide: A Case Control Study. Psychosomatics. 2018;59(1):58-61.
19. Brådvik L. Suicide Risk and Mental Disorders. Int J Environ Res Public Health. 2018;15(9):2028.
20. Janowski K, Steuden S, Pietrzak A, Krasowska D, Kaczmarek Ł, Gradus I, et al. Social support and adaptation to the disease in men and women with psoriasis. Arch Dermatol Res. 2012;304(6):421-32.
21. Grover S, Mehra A, Dogra S, Hazari N, Malhora N, Narang T, et al. Internalized Stigma and Psychiatric Morbidity among Patients with Psoriasis: A Study from North India. Indian Dermatol Online J. 2020;12(1):97-104.
22. Hardavella G, Aamli-Gaagnat A, Frille A, Saad N, Niculescu A, Powell P. Top tips to deal with challenging situations: doctor–patient interactions. Breathe. 2017;13(2):129-35.
23. Detmar SB, Muller MJ, Wever LD, Schornagel JH, Aaronson NK. The patient-physician relationship. Patient-physician communication during outpatient palliative treatment visits: an observational study. JAMA. 2001;285(10):1351-7.
24. Hawton K, van Heeringen K. Suicide. Lancet Lond Engl. 2009;373(9672):1372-81.
25. Kessler RC, Borges G, Walters EE. Prevalence of and risk factors for lifetime suicide attempts in the National Comorbidity Survey. Arch Gen Psychiatry. 1999;56(7):617-26.
26. Moutier C, Mortali MG. Suicide Warning Signs and What to Do. Vet Clin North Am Small Anim Pract. 2021;51(5):1053-60.
27. Kromer C, Mohr J, Celis D, Poortinga S, Gerdes S, Mössner R. Screening for depression in psoriasis patients during a dermatological consultation: A first step towards treatment. JDDG. 2021;19(10):1451-61.

28. Revankar RR, Revankar NR, Balogh EA, Patel HA, Kaplan SG, Feldman SR. Cognitive behavior therapy as dermatological treatment: a narrative review. Int J Womens Dermatol. 2022;8(4):e068.
29. Chong YY. Embodying a Compassionate Self Through Acceptance and Commitment Therapy for Parents and Children With Eczema: A Family Based Eczema Management Programme. [online] Available from https://clinicaltrials.gov/study/NCT04919330 [Last accessed January, 2024].
30. Kanji A. Perspective on Living With a Skin Condition and its Psychological Impact: A Survey. J Patient Exp. 2019;6(1):68-71.
31. Thorneloe RJ. The use of online peer support communities in dermatology. Br J Dermatol. 2019;181(5):888-9.
32. Yadav S, Narang T, Sendhil Kumaran M. Psychodermatology: A comprehensive review. Indian J Dermatol Venereol Leprol. 2013:79:2;176-92.
33. Fried RG, Gupta MA, Gupta AK. Depression and skin disease. Dermatol Clin. 2005;23(4):657-64.
34. Patel P, Patel K, Pandher K, Tareen RS. The Role of Psychiatric, Analgesic, and Antiepileptic Medications in Chronic Pruritus. Cureus. 13(8):e17260.
35. Kiecka A, Szczepanik M. The potential action of SSRIs in the treatment of skin diseases including atopic dermatitis and slow-healing wounds. Pharmacol Rep. 2022;74(5):947-55.
36. Hakkola J, Hukkanen J, Turpeinen M, Pelkonen O. Inhibition and induction of CYP enzymes in humans: an update. Arch Toxicol. 2020;94(11):3671-722.
37. Hoffelt C, Gross T. A review of significant pharmacokinetic drug interactions with antidepressants and their management. Ment Health Clin. 2016;6(1): 35-41.
38. Medscape Drug Reference Database. Drug Interactions Checker. [online] Available from https://reference.medscape.com/drug-interactionchecker [Last accessed January, 2024].
39. Ahmedani BK. Mental Health Stigma: Society, Individuals, and the Profession. J Soc Work Values Ethics. 2011;8(2):4-1-4-16.
40. Dazzi T, Gribble R, Wessely S, Fear NT. Does asking about suicide and related behaviours induce suicidal ideation? What is the evidence? Psychol Med. 2014;44(16):3361-3.
41. Practice Guideline for the Assessment and Treatment of Patients With Suicidal Behaviors. In: APA Practice Guidelines for the Treatment of Psychiatric Disorders: Comprehensive Guidelines and Guideline Watches, 1st edition. Arlington, VA: American Psychiatric Association; 2006.
42. Gupta MA, Gupta AK. Psychiatric and psychological co-morbidity in patients with dermatologic disorders: epidemiology and management. Am J Clin Dermatol. 2003;4(12):833-42.
43. Hawton K, Fagg J. Suicide, and other causes of death, following attempted suicide. Br J Psychiatry J Ment Sci. 1988;152:359-66.
44. Pandya A, Shah K, Chauhan A, Saha S. Innovative mental health initiatives in India: A scope for strengthening primary healthcare services. J Fam Med Prim Care. 2020;9(2):502-7.
45. Dhyani A, Gaidhane A, Choudhari SG, Dave S, Choudhary S. Strengthening Response Toward Promoting Mental Health in India: A Narrative Review. Cureus. 2022;14(10):e30435.

CHAPTER 16

Assessment Tools and Questionnaires in Psychodermatology

Sreejayan Kongasseri

> **Key Messages**
> - Scales can supplement clinical assessment in a psychodermatology clinic.
> - Choosing an appropriate scale is important for meticulous assessment.
> - While choosing a scale, the clinician or researcher should consider "what, where, who, and how" of the assessment.

INTRODUCTION

Clinical interviewing of patients with psychological symptoms can often be complemented with use of rating scales. It should be emphasized here that use of rating scales and questionnaires should not replace the clinical evaluation. Assessment tools can be used to screen, diagnose, quantify, and document the psychological status. They can be used over different time periods to assess changes in the symptoms.

Scales can be self-rated or clinician rated. In the first type, the subject themselves go through the items and decide the appropriate response. The subjects may be the patient (e.g., in rating depression or anxiety) or the caregiver (rating themselves). Sometimes, a caregiver may rate the patient (e.g., teachers or parents rating of child's behavioral problems). In the clinician-rated scales, trained professional rates the subject based on interview and observation.

Depending on the purpose of the scale, it may be categorized as mentioned in the following text.

DIAGNOSTIC SCALES

Diagnostic scales identify specific mental disorders. These take long time to administer and the clinician has to be trained in their administration, e.g., present-state examination (PSE), diagnostic interview schedule (DIS), and mini-international neuropsychiatric interview (MINI). These are used for research and are not appropriate for clinical use.

Symptom-based Scales

Symptom-based scales assess particular symptoms or set of symptoms and not the specific diagnosis itself, e.g., child behavioral checklist (CBCL) detects emotional and behavioral problems in children and adolescents.

Diagnosis-specific Scales

Diagnosis-specific scales are used to rate the symptoms in a specific diagnosis, e.g., the Hamilton rating scale for depression (HRSD).

SCREENING TOOLS

These scales screen for symptoms or disorder. They have high rate of false positives but have good sensitivity. These are appropriate to administer to a large number of subjects in a short time, e.g., to screen all the patients coming to a busy dermatology clinic using the Self-Reporting Questionnaire (SRQ).

Most of the scales used in psychiatric research are ordinal scales. They categorize the symptoms, e.g., sleep disturbance can be: not present, mild, moderate, or severe. Here the difference between the groups may not be the same. In the interval scales, the unit changes are constant and of the same value.

For a good outcome, the interviewer should be trained in administering and scoring the scale. Before starting the interview, the rater should have all the information available, ask all items, and do it in a calm environment. For self-rating scales, the clinician should be well-versed with the scales so that they can clarify if subject has any queries.

Screening Scales

Screening scales are screening tools that can be administered on large number of subjects.
- *Self-reporting questionnaire* (SRQ): This scale has been developed by the *World Health Organization* to screen for psychiatric disorders. It can be either self-administered or interviewer administered and consists of 20 questions with yes or no answers. The 20 questions are related to neurotic disorders. Four additional questions can be added to rule out psychotic disorders and one for convulsions. SRQ at the cut-off point of 10 shows a sensitivity of 83% and specificity of about 93%. This can be used in the waiting rooms of busy dermatology clinics.
- *General health questionnaire* (GHQ): This is a measure of psychological well-being in community. There are short versions: GHQ 12 and GHQ 5 consisting of 12 and 5 questions, respectively.

Rating Scales

Rating scales are used to rate the severity of an illness. Once treatment is started, scales may be repeated to assess improvement. There are different scales for each psychiatric disorder.

Depression

There are many scales that rate the severity of depression. These scales can be administered at two points of time to assess the change with treatment.
- *Hamilton Depression Rating Scale* (HAM-D) and *Montgomery–Åsberg Depression Rating Scale* (MADRS) are interviewer-administered scales that are commonly used. However, the interviewer needs to be trained in the administration of these scales.
- *Geriatric Depression Scale* (GDS) is a 30-item self-administered scale to assess depression in elderly. A shorter version with 15 items is also available. The responses are marked as yes or no. Due to its simple structure, GDS can be administered on medically ill and in elderly with mild cognitive dysfunction. *Zung Depression Scale* (ZDS) is another self-administered scale consisting of 20 items. The questionnaire takes about 10 minutes to complete. The scores provide indicative ranges for depression severity that can be useful for clinical purpose. ZDS also provides a simple tool for monitoring changes in depression severity over time.

CHAPTER 16: Assessment Tools and Questionnaires in Psychodermatology

Anxiety

Hamilton Anxiety Scale is a clinician rated scale with 14 items. The individual scores are used to compute an overarching score that indicates a severity of severity. *Zung Anxiety Scale* is a self-reported with 20-items to measure anxiety. The anxiety can be grouped into four symptom groups: (1) cognitive, (2) autonomic, (3) motor, and (4) central nervous system symptoms. The individual items are added up to obtain a raw score that can be converted into anxiety index using a chart. The "Anxiety Index" score can then be used to clinically interpret level of anxiety.

Some of the symptoms of depression and anxiety overlap with that of medical illness and this could result in over estimating the severity of psychological symptoms in medically ill. The *hospital anxiety depression scale* (HADS) avoids these mutually common symptoms and is an appropriate scale to use in medically ill.

The *depression anxiety stress scale* (DASS) is a 42-item self-reported scale that has been validated in psychodermatology population. In addition to depression and anxiety, it also measures stress through its items on tension and irritability.

The *Yale–Brown Obsessive-Compulsive Scale* measures the severity of obsessions and compulsions. This scale has been modified for neurotic excoriation. *Skin Picking Impact Scale* (SPIS) measures the psychosocial impact of skin picking.

SUBSTANCE USE

Patients may use substances to cope with stress and also to manage the physical symptoms of skin diseases. Substance use disorder can present additional challenges in management of both skin diseases and psychological disorders. Asking four questions from the CAGE (Cut down, Annoyed, Guilty, Eye-opener) questionnaire helps to determine if substance abuse exists:

1. Have you ever felt you should cut down on your drinking?
2. Have people annoyed you by criticizing your drinking?
3. Have you ever felt bad or guilty about your drinking?
4. Have you ever had a drink first thing in the morning to steady your nerves or to get rid of a hangover (eye-opener)?

A yes answer to two or more of these questions identify people with substance use disorders.

QUALITY OF LIFE

The term "quality of life (QoL)" refers to the physical, psychological, and social domains of health and is influenced by a person's experiences, beliefs, expectations, and perception. The clinician's goal is not just to treat the symptoms but to improve the overall quality of life of the patient.

Short form (36) health survey (SF-36), which has been used in dermatological research, is a self-report questionnaire to measure general health-related QoL. It takes 5–10 minutes to complete. The scale assesses physical and mental domains.

Dermatology-specific QoL questionnaires have been developed to accurately capture the impact of skin diseases. *The Dermatology Life Quality Index* (DLQI) is a dermatology-specific quality of life instrument with 10 simple questions. It has been used in over 40 different skin conditions. DLQI can be used for routine clinical work without charge and without seeking permission, but for other purposes, please contact dermqol@cf.ac.uk.

SKindex, which was originally developed as a 61-item scale (SKindex 61), was later redeveloped into briefer versions, SKindex 29 and SKindex 16. SKindex 29, assesses QoL in three domains: symptoms, emotions, and functioning. The shortest version, *SKindex-16* unlike other instruments, measures the "bother" rather than frequency of the experiences. The authors can be contacted at ude.fscu.mred@mnerhc for permission to use. SKindex 29 can be used in research when to understand and investigate the effect of the disease on QoL or to compare with other diseases. SKindex 16 may be better suited when the burden on the subject is being investigated. SKindex is also sensitive to detect change in QoL.

STIGMA

Stigma is the mark of disgrace or dishonor that sets a person part from others. When a person receives a label of an illness, they are seen as part of a certain group and provoke negative attitudes, which create prejudice leading to negative actions and discrimination. There are various scales to assess stigma in patient with skin diseases. These scales can be for general dermatology or for specific skin diseases. The *6-item stigmatization* scale scores anticipation of rejection, feelings of being flawed, sensitivity to the opinions of others, guilt and shame, negative attitudes, and secretiveness on three-point scale. Higher scores indicate worse experience of stigmatization. *Short version of the Questionnaire on Experience with Skin Complaints (QES)* and Perceived Stigmatization Questionnaire (PSQ) are longer scales with 38 and 23 items, respectively. *Explanatory model interview catalog* (EMIC) is relevant for cross-cultural research because it is not a fixed scale but a catalog of explanatory model interviews based on an adaptable operational framework. It addresses illness experience (patterns of distress), perceived causes, general illness beliefs, preferences for help seeking, and lastly, the stigma caused by the illness.

DISABILITY

Disability is a term that covers impairments, activity limitations, and participation restrictions. It is not just a health problem but the result of complex between person's body and the society.

WHO disability assessment schedule 2.0 (WHODAS 2.0): It is an instrument for the assessment of health and disability which can be used in all diseases including dermatological disorders and it is applicable over all cultures. This covers six domains of functioning, which includes cognition, mobility, self-care, getting along, life activities, and participation. *Participation scale* (P scale) scale is a reliable instrument to assess client perceived participation in social activities which can be an indicator of disability. Initially used in patients with leprosy, it can be used in other dermatological disorders as well. Patients rate their participation in comparison with a "peer," defined as "someone similar to the respondent in all respects except for the disease or disability." It is based on the participation domains of international classification of functioning disability and health (ICF).

There are scales that measure disease-specific disability such as *Psoriasis Disability Index, Cardiff Acne Disability Index,* and *Eczema Disability Index.*

SUICIDAL RISK

Patients attending the psychodermatology clinic may have suicidal ideations and it is important to identify these thoughts to manage risk and avoid an adverse health outcome. The *suicide behaviors questionnaire-revised* (SBQ-R) is a brief four-item self-rated questionnaire that measures different dimensions of suicidality.

Though not a comprehensive scale, its brevity and that it is self-rated makes it an ideal instrument to use in dermatology clinics. *Suicide affecting behavior cognition scale* (SABCS) is a six-item self-rating questionnaire. There are not cut off values but, by using the answers provided by the patient the clinician can predict the risk from a "Risk Barometer" given along with the scale. *Suicide intent scale* is a more comprehensive clinician administered scale.

CHILDREN

Pediatric symptom checklist is a psychosocial screen designed to facilitate the recognition of cognitive, emotional, and behavioral problems in children. There are two versions; the parent-completed version (PSC) and the Youth self-report (Y-PSC), which can be administered to adolescents 11 years and above. Children who score more than the cut off values need to be evaluated further. *Child behavior checklist* is completed by parents and it helps to identify emotional and behavioral problems in children and adolescents. There are two versions—the preschool checklist (CBCL/11/2-5) to be used with children aged 18 months to 5 years and the school-age version (CBCL/6-18) is for children aged 6-18 years. Similar questions are grouped into a number of syndromes. This tool is appropriate for research purpose since it takes a long time to complete. *Children's Dermatology Life Quality Index* (CDLQI) can be used to measure QoL among children.

DISEASE-SPECIFIC SCALES

Individual dermatological disorders have different presentations. While the dermatological scales measure the overall impact of the disease, there are disease-specific scales that can measure the influence of that particular presentation on the psychological functioning of the individual. *Vitiligo impact scale 22 (VIS22), Vitiligo Quality of Life (VitiQoL), VLQI (Vitiligo Life Quality Index), and Vitiligo Impact Patient scale (VIPs)* measure impact on vitiligo in the QoL. *Cardiff Acne Disability Index*, a short 5-item questionnaire derived from *Acne Disability Index* can be used in routine practice to assess the impact of acne on patients' life. *Acne-QoL* measures four domains of self-perception, emotional role, social role, and symptoms of acne. *Acne Quality of Life (AQoL)* scale evaluates the two dimensions of social impact and vocational impact of acne. The 15-item AQoL scale also evaluates for depression and anxiety; however, it does not have any published validating studies. *Psoriasis Index of Quality of Life (PSORIQoL)* is reliable and valid method of measuring QoL in psoriasis. *Psoriasis arthritis quality of life scale (PsAQoL)* can be used specifically in those patients who have developed arthritic complications and the *Nail Psoriasis Quality of Life Scale (NPQ10)* among patients who have nail involvement. Psoriasis Family Index (PFI-15) measures the QoL among families of patients with psoriasis. *Adolescent Psoriasis Quality of Life instrument (APso-QoL)* is a developmentally appropriate disease-specific instrument for 12-17 years old.

CONCLUSION

Psychodermatologists use rating scales to support their clinical assessments. Screening scales can be used to identify patients with psychological issues. Self rating screening tools can be made available in the waiting area, whereas clinician rated scales are administered by the psychodermatologist during their assessment. In addition to identifying clinical conditions such as depression, anxiety and substance use, scales can also be used to rate psychosocial concepts such as stigma, disability and quality of life. They are used in psychodermatology research to understand the impact of the dermatological condition on the psychological and social aspects of the patient. The research scales are constantly refined through research and clinicians should ensure they use scales with good validity and reliability in their practice.

FURTHER READINGS

1. Brenaut E, Halvorsen JA, Dalgard FJ, Lien L, Balieva F, Sampogna F. The self-assessed psychological comorbidities of prurigo in European patients: a multicentre study in 13 countries. J Eur Acad Dermatol Venereol. 2019;33(1):157-62.
2. Brown GE, Malakouti M, Sorenson E, Gupta R, Koo JY. Psychodermatology. Clinical Challenges in the Biopsychosocial Interface. 2015:34:123-34.
3. Dréno B. Assessing quality of life in patients with acne vulgaris: implications for treatment. Am J Clin Dermatol. 2006;7:99-106.
4. Jafferany M, Ferreira BR, Patel A. The essentials of psychodermatology. Springer International Publishing; 2020.
5. Land B, Blais MA. Handbook of Clinical Rating Scales and Assessment in Psychiatry and Mental Health. New York: Humana Press; 2010.
6. Sajatovic M, Ramirez LF. Rating Scales in Mental Health, 3rd edition. Baltimore, MD: Johns Hopkins University Press; 2012.

CHAPTER 17

Psychodermatology Counseling: A Holistic Approach to Skin and Mind

Sudipta Roy

> **Key Messages**
> - There is bidirectional connection between skin and mind.
> - Stress plays an important role in manifestation of skin conditions.
> - Skin conditions impact body image, self-esteem, social anxiety and isolation, generalized anxiety and depression.
> - Skin conditions require a holistic approach to intervention.
> - Dermatologists, Psychiatrists, Psychologists and Counselors can work together to manage skin conditions.
> - Different skin conditions have varying psychological ramifications that are discussed here.
> - Assessments can provide useful insights into the nature and severity of psychological problems.
> - Counseling approaches that can be used includes, cognitive behavior therapies, mindfulness, relaxation techniques, supportive counseling, resilience training, training for coping strategies and ways to promote self-esteem are emphasized.
> - Role of family and social support are discussed.

INTRODUCTION TO PSYCHODERMATOLOGY: UNDERSTANDING THE SKIN–MIND CONNECTION

Psychodermatology is at a relatively nascent stage, yet it is fair to say that it is a rapidly evolving field, which sits at the intersection of dermatology and psychology. It delves into the intricate relationship between the skin and the mind. From the stand point of a psychologist, our role is to address the emotional, cognitive, and behavioral facets, which can accompany skin conditions while complementing more traditional biological treatments. In this chapter, we embark on an exploration of the role of counseling in the realm of psychodermatology, beginning with the mechanisms underlying the skin-mind connection. We will look at differences between traditional dermatology and psychodermatology while emphasizing a collaborative approach. We will also examine the psychological impact of common skin conditions and illuminate the role of counseling in ameliorating these challenges. As we navigate this evolving landscape, it becomes evident that psychodermatology not only enhances our understanding of health but also highlights the importance of treating individuals holistically and allows for an acknowledgment of the intricate interplay between their external appearance and internal emotional experiences.

The relationship between skin health and psychological well-being is far from unidimensional. A complex interplay, where changes in one domain can significantly influence the other and vice versa, is evident to practitioners and researchers today. This bidirectional connection makes evident that there is a profound impact of our emotional state on our skin's health and appearance, as well as that the condition of our skin can shape our mental and emotional states. Psychodermatology acknowledges that skin health is intricately linked to psychological well-being. Stress, for instance, can trigger or worsen conditions like psoriasis and eczema through the release of inflammatory molecules. Additionally, the visible nature of skin disorders can adversely affect self-esteem and body image, leading to psychological distress. Psychodermatological interventions recognize this synergy and aim to improve both skin health and mental well-being, thus helping us to get out of this vicious cycle.

Psychological Impact on Skin Health

- *Stress and inflammation*: The skin has long been confirmed to be both an immediate stress perceiver and a target of stress responses. Psychological stress can trigger a cascade of hormonal and neurochemical changes that lead to inflammation in the body. Skin and its appendages are not only targets of key stress mediators but also a local source for these factors which induce various immune and inflammation responses. Inflammatory skin conditions like psoriasis, eczema, and acne can flare up or worsen due to increased stress levels.

- *Itch and scratching*: Emotional distress and anxiety can intensify sensations of itchiness, leading individuals to scratch excessively. Scratching can aggravate skin conditions and result in a vicious cycle of worsening symptoms. In some cases, individuals with psychological disorders like excoriation may compulsively pick at their skin, resulting in scarring and injuries that further fuel anxiety.
- *Impaired immune function*: Acute stress is linked to elevated levels of proinflammatory cytokines, leading to chronic systemic inflammation, which subsequently suppresses both cellular and humoral immunity. This compromised immune response can hinder the body's ability to effectively combat infections, impeding the healing process of skin wounds and infections.
- *Skin barrier function*: Mental stress and poor sleep have been found to be harmful to the skin barrier. The production of sebum by the skin, which is an oily substance produced to keep the skin moisturized, is also positively correlated with the severity of anxiety. A compromised skin barrier increases susceptibility to irritants, allergens, and pollutants therefore contributing to the development or aggravation of skin conditions such as acne.

Skin's Impact on Psychological Well-being

- *Body image and self-esteem:* Physical appearance wields significant influence over our self-perception and our interactions with society. Cutaneous body image (CBI) is a construct that encompasses how individuals perceive their hair, skin, and nails. Recent research has shown how CBI acts as a mediator of the relationships between having a skin condition and anxiety and depression. Negative perceptions of one's appearance can result in social withdrawal, heightened anxiety, and even depression.
- *Social stigma and isolation*: Visible skin diseases (VSDs) such as psoriasis, acne, and atopic dermatitis have immense self and social stigma attached to them, impacting the mental health of patients. Isolation often becomes a coping mechanism for those living with VSDs. The fear of rejection and humiliation can lead to self-imposed isolation, limiting social interactions and experiences. This can result in loneliness, depression, and anxiety, further compounding the burden of the skin condition itself.

- *Psychosocial distress*: Chronic skin conditions exhibit remarkable unpredictability, perpetually influenced by factors such as an individual's dietary choices, stress levels, sleep patterns, and various uncontrollable environmental elements. This capricious nature often leads to feelings of frustration, anger, and a pervasive sense of helplessness. When coupled with the existing stigma associated with these conditions, this unpredictability can intensify psychological distress, exerting a profound impact on an individual's overall quality of life.
- *Anxiety and depression*: Research indicates that individuals with visible skin conditions are more susceptible to experiencing anxiety and depression. In most cases, chronic skin disease patients who have comorbid depression also have suicidal ideation. The magnitude of depression among patients with chronic skin conditions ranges from 9 to 70%. The emotional burden of living with chronic skin issues can contribute to the onset or exacerbation of these mental health disorders.

The mind-body connection has long been ignored in medical care; therefore, understanding the bidirectionality of this relationship is pivotal in psychodermatology. Addressing skin conditions purely from a medical standpoint might not yield complete resolution if the emotional aspects are left unattended. Likewise, solely focusing on the psychological impact neglects the potential physiological factors that can perpetuate skin issues. A comprehensive approach involves treating both the skin and the mind and recognizing that improvement in one domain can positively influence the other. By offering interventions that target both the visible and invisible aspects of skin-mind health, clinicians can provide more holistic and effective care, enhancing the overall well-being of individuals facing these challenges.

Differences between Traditional Dermatology and Psychodermatology Counseling

Traditional dermatology primarily focuses on diagnosing and treating the physical manifestations of skin conditions. Dermatologists prescribe medications, offer medical procedures, and advise on skincare routines to manage symptoms. While these interventions are essential, they may not comprehensively address the core issues, which are the psychological and emotional aspects of skin disorders.

Psychodermatology counseling, on the other hand, goes beyond the surface to recognize that skin health is intertwined with mental well-being. Acting as a virtuous circle for skin health, counselors work collaboratively with individuals to address the emotional repercussions of skin conditions, such as body image concerns, self-esteem issues, anxiety, and depression. They also focus on skin problems that are exemplified by stress or other turbulent emotional states. This approach acknowledges that effective treatment extends beyond creams and medications to encompass strategies that enhance emotional resilience and coping skills.

Psychodermatology is most effective when practiced as a collaborative effort involving dermatologists, psychologists, and counselors. Psychocutaneous diseases, which are essentially psychiatric disorders with visible skin manifestations, exemplify a critical intersection where the collaboration between dermatologists and psychologists is imperative. Individuals are often reluctant to seek psychiatric assistance, yet they may be more receptive to doing so when presented with dermatological concerns as a motivating factor.

This multidisciplinary approach acknowledges the multifaceted nature of skin-mind health and leverages the expertise of each discipline to provide holistic care.

- *Dermatologists*: Medical expertise is essential in diagnosing and treating skin conditions. Dermatologists prescribe medications, recommend treatments, and monitor the physical aspects of skin health.
- *Psychologists*: They delve into the cognitive and emotional dimensions of mental health. They assess and treat psychological disorders, applying therapeutic techniques to address issues like anxiety, depression, and body dysmorphia.
- *Counselors*: They bridge the gap between dermatology and psychology by focusing on the emotional impact of skin conditions. They offer counseling interventions that empower individuals to manage the psychological distress caused by skin disorders and improve their overall well-being.

This collaborative approach ensures that individuals receive comprehensive care tailored to their unique needs. By working together, dermatologists, psychologists, and counselors can create treatment plans that integrate medical management, psychological support, and emotional coping strategies. This synergy acknowledges that the path to healing involves addressing both the visible and unseen aspects of skin–mind health, ultimately promoting a higher quality of life for individuals facing these challenges.

Role of Counseling in Psychodermatology

The importance of counseling in dermatology might be unclear to many clients, medical practitioners, and even counselors. However, we can conceptualize the role of counselors as two-pronged: Firstly, directing the patients with chronic skin conditions on the use of stress management. Instead of assuming the underlying cause of the condition, counselors can guide patients to adopt a more holistic approach in handling acceptance, understanding avoidance behaviors, and building self-esteem. Secondly, psychologists can help to deal with deeper psychopathology that may maintain or aggravate skin conditions using different psychotherapies such as dealing with social phobias using cognitive behavioral therapy (CBT) or working with trichotillomania using habit reversal training, etc. Let us explore these two possibilities.

Exploring the Role of Counselors in the Context of Psychodermatology

Counselors play a pivotal and multifaceted role in the emerging field of psychodermatology, where the focus extends beyond the physical aspects of the skin to encompass individuals' psychological and emotional well-being. They are uniquely positioned to address the emotional toll of skin conditions, providing support, guidance, and interventions to enhance the overall quality of life for individuals grappling with both visible and concealed challenges.

In an increasingly appearance-focused world, individuals may harbor fears and anxieties related to their skin conditions. It falls upon counselors to provide a safe and empathetic space for them to explore their emotions without any underlying judgment. This channel of communication can help individuals manage distressing emotions and develop coping strategies to navigate the psychosocial impact of their skin disorders.

Dealing with Deeper Psychopathology

Dermatologic disorders go beyond simply being cosmetic disfigurements, as they are associated with a variety of psychopathologic problems that can affect the patients and their families. It is a common misconception that the objective severity of a dermatological condition should correlate with the psychological impact it has on the patient. On the contrary, Rick Fried, a US-based clinician who specialized in psychodermatology stated that he has found people with nodulocystic acne who albeit unhappy are not psychologically distraught and also seen patients with one zit on their chin who have attempted suicide. It is clear that a deeper psychopathology exists affecting the patients' abilities to manage skin conditions.

Even self-inflicted skin disfigurements, such as body-focused repetitive behavior which encompasses a cluster of behavior in which individuals repeatedly engage in body-focused acts such as hair pulling (trichotillomania) or skin picking (dermatillomania), can be worked upon by a psychologist through therapeutic interventions. Research evidence shows multitudes of nonpharmacological interventions in the management of psychodermatological conditions, such as hypnosis, support groups, biofeedback, meditation, guided imagery, progressive muscle relaxation, CBT, and other forms of psychotherapy. The purpose of these interventions is to give the patients a sense of control over their conditions by regulating how they react to them.

Common Psychodermatological Conditions and their Psychological Impact

Skin conditions such as psoriasis, eczema, acne, and dermatitis not only are physical ailments but also carry profound psychological implications. These conditions can significantly impact an individual's mental and emotional well-being, triggering a range of psychosocial challenges that often remain hidden beneath the surface.

Psoriasis

This chronic autoimmune condition is characterized by red, scaly patches on the skin. Beyond its physical discomfort, psoriasis can lead to intense self-consciousness and embarrassment due to its visible nature. Individuals with psoriasis often experience lowered self-esteem, body image issues, and anxiety related to social interactions. The persistent nature of the condition and the unpredictable flare-ups can contribute to feelings of frustration and helplessness.

Eczema

Eczema, or atopic dermatitis, manifests as itchy, inflamed skin. The constant itchiness and discomfort can lead to sleep disturbances, further impacting emotional well-being. Individuals with eczema may struggle with feelings of irritation, embarrassment about visible skin changes, and a sense of isolation due to their condition. The relentless itching and the sometimes visible lesions can evoke feelings of self-consciousness and social withdrawal.

Acne

Acne is a common skin condition that affects people of various ages. Its appearance on the face, chest, and back can result in significant emotional distress. Adolescents and adults alike often experience lowered self-esteem, anxiety, and depression due to concerns about their appearance. Acne's visibility can lead to self-imposed isolation, avoidance of social activities, and even bullying, all of which contribute to psychological challenges. A study conducted by Tasoula and colleagues (2012) revealed that among young students with severe acne, there was a pronounced psychosocial and emotional impairment, significantly impacting their self-esteem, body image, and interpersonal relationships.

Dermatitis

Dermatitis encompasses a range of skin inflammations, including different types of dermatitis. These conditions can cause redness, itching, and discomfort. Constant itching and visible symptoms can lead to feelings of frustration and embarrassment. Additionally, the discomfort and the appearance of the affected skin can impact an individual's self-confidence and overall emotional well-being.

Vitiligo

Vitiligo is a condition in which patches of the skin lose their pigment, resulting in white or depigmented areas. The visible nature of vitiligo can lead to emotional distress, self-consciousness, and reduced self-esteem. In countries where colorism is prevalent, this can cause further distress in the form of loss of identity. In a sample of 200 people, the proportion of vitiligo patients with depression and anxiety disorders as compared to healthy controls was found to be 62% versus 25%.

Psychological Impact

The psychological impact of these conditions extends beyond the physical discomfort and compromises well-being. Individuals often experience negative emotions such as anxiety, depression, shame, and frustration. The visibility of skin conditions can evoke a sense of self-consciousness and social isolation, leading to decreased self-esteem and impaired quality of life. The uncertainty of flare-ups, the chronic nature of these conditions, and the societal pressure to conform to beauty standards further contribute to emotional distress.

ASSESSMENT AND EVALUATION IN PSYCHODERMATOLOGY COUNSELING

Using psychological tools with psychodermatology clients can have many explicit benefits. Firstly, they can help a dermatologist identify potential areas of distress in the client beyond the skin condition. Secondly, using an objective measuring tool can help with identifying primary, secondary, or comorbid psychiatric conditions that may sometimes miss the clinician's eye. Thirdly, they provide a stepwise entry into enrolling the client's consent to seeking help for psychological concomitants to skin conditions.

Koo and Lee have provided a widely utilized classification system for psychodermatological conditions, which serves as a framework for assessments and is listed below:

- *Psychophysiological disorders*: These conditions exhibit a clear and chronological connection between stress and the onset or exacerbation of a skin ailment, as seen in cases like psoriasis and acne.
- *Primary psychiatric disorders with dermatological symptoms*: In these instances, there is no underlying skin disease; instead, the symptoms arise due to a psychiatric disorder, as observed in conditions like delusional infestation, body dysmorphic disorder, and trichotillomania.

- *Secondary psychiatric disorders*: These conditions involve psychological issues that develop as a consequence of a skin disease and are often more severe than the underlying dermatological disorder, as exemplified in cases such as alopecia areata and acne excoriee.

Assessment Tools

Various assessment tools can be employed for evaluating psychodermatological disorders. Some common ones include:
- Dermatology Life Quality Index (DLQI) or Children's Dermatology Life Quality Index (CDLQI)
- Person-Centered Dermatology Self-Care Index (PeDeSI)
- Psoriasis Disability Index (PDI)
- Dermatitis Family Impact (DFI) questionnaire

Details of these can be referred to elsewhere, e.g., Shreejayan (2016). Assessments need to be supplemented with interviews and observations as well.

Interview Assessment and Evaluation

The psychologist needs to have keen powers of observation and the ability to provide an empathetic therapeutic atmosphere, to conduct an effective psychiatric assessment of the patient with dermatological conditions. A preinterview study of the available medical records might help in making a diagnosis. A structured interview can be helpful in outlining the chronology of the symptoms, including the problems associated with it.

Thereafter each symptom should be explored qualitatively, such as anxiety, depression, and suicidal ideation. An assessment of the stressors in the patient's life needs to be made along with the exploration of the patient's attitude toward the illness. In some cases, the patients may also have discovered secondary gains through the skin conditions (intentional self-injuries to get social advantages) that should be addressed.

Presence of psychological distress adds significantly to the morbidity associated with the dermatological condition. Hence, a combined biopsychosocial approach is essential in understanding and managing psychodermatological conditions.

THERAPEUTIC APPROACHES IN PSYCHO-DERMATOLOGY COUNSELING

Psychodermatology counseling employs a range of therapeutic techniques to address the intricate interplay between skin health and psychological well-being. These approaches aim to empower individuals to manage the emotional challenges associated with skin conditions, enhance coping strategies, and improve overall quality of life. Common ingredients of therapy with psychodermatology clients necessitate that the counselors or psychologists consistently convey unconditional positive regard to patients, given the multiple self-esteem challenges they often grapple with. Beyond this, many different psychotherapies have the potential to address the psychological issues that accompany skin conditions. These include the well-known approaches of CBT, mindfulness approaches, supportive psychotherapy, integrated approaches, biofeedback, hypnotherapy, habit reversal training, and the like.

Cognitive-behavioral Interventions

Cognitive restructuring for negative thought patterns: Cognitive restructuring involves identifying and challenging negative thought patterns related to appearance. Individuals with skin conditions often develop distorted beliefs about their appearance, contributing to low self-esteem and social withdrawal. Counselors work with clients to recognize these negative self-perceptions, reframe them with more balanced perspectives, and replace them with constructive thoughts that promote self-acceptance.

Behavioral techniques for habit reversal: Skin-picking disorders, like dermatillomania, can worsen skin conditions and impact psychological well-being. Behavioral techniques such as habit reversal involve identifying triggers for skin-picking behaviors, developing alternative responses, and implementing strategies to redirect the impulse. Counselors guide individuals in building awareness, self-control, and healthier coping mechanisms.

Mindfulness and Relaxation Techniques

Mindfulness-based stress reduction (MBSR): Mindfulness practices help individuals stay present and nonjudgmentally aware of their thoughts, emotions, and bodily sensations. MBSR, specifically tailored for psychodermatology, can reduce stress-induced flare-ups by mitigating the physiological responses triggered by stress. By practicing mindfulness, individuals develop a greater capacity to manage distress and minimize the impact of stress on their skin.

Relaxation strategies for self-care: Relaxation techniques, such as deep breathing exercises, progressive muscle relaxation, and guided imagery, can alleviate symptoms of skin conditions and promote overall well-being. These techniques are effective in reducing stress, minimizing itchiness, and improving sleep quality, which in turn positively impacts skin health.

Supportive Counseling

Creating a safe emotional space: Supportive counseling provides individuals with a nonjudgmental and empathetic environment to express their emotions. This space allows clients to discuss their fears, anxieties, and frustrations openly, which can alleviate emotional distress and promote a sense of relief.

Addressing body image and self-esteem: Counselors play a pivotal role in helping individuals with skin conditions address body image concerns and build self-esteem. Through guided conversations, individuals learn to recognize and challenge unrealistic beauty standards, embrace their uniqueness, and develop a positive self-image irrespective of their skin appearance.

Integration and Holistic Care

Therapeutic approaches in psychodermatology counseling are not mutually exclusive; they can be integrated to create a comprehensive treatment plan tailored to individual needs. This holistic approach acknowledges the interconnectedness of physical and emotional well-being. By combining cognitive-behavioral interventions, mindfulness techniques, relaxation strategies, and supportive counseling, clinicians can empower individuals to manage the psychological impact of skin conditions effectively.

Ultimately, these therapeutic strategies offer individuals a toolbox of skills to manage their emotions, improve their self-perception, and enhance their ability to cope with the challenges of living with skin conditions. The integration of these approaches fosters resilience, empowers individuals to reclaim control over their emotional well-being, and cultivates a positive relationship between their skin and mind.

BUILDING RESILIENCE AND COPING SKILLS

Skin conditions can place a substantial emotional burden on individuals, affecting their overall well-being and quality of life. Building resilience and cultivating effective coping skills are essential components of psychodermatology counseling. By empowering individuals to navigate the emotional challenges associated with skin disorders, counselors play a pivotal role in enhancing their psychological well-being.

Identifying and Enhancing Resilience Factors

Resilience refers to an individual's ability to adapt and thrive in the face of adversity. Psychodermatology counseling focuses on identifying and enhancing resilience factors in individuals with skin conditions. These factors can include social support systems, problem-solving skills, optimism, and the capacity to manage stress. By recognizing and bolstering these strengths, individuals are better equipped to cope with the emotional impact of their conditions.

Teaching Adaptive Coping Strategies

Counselors collaborate with clients to develop adaptive coping strategies that effectively address the emotional toll of skin disorders. These strategies help individuals manage distress, reduce anxiety, and navigate the challenges posed by their conditions. Some techniques commonly employed include:
- *Problem-solving*: Teaching clients how to identify specific challenges related to their skin condition and develop practical solutions in a stepwise manner to address them
- *Emotion regulation:* Providing tools for managing intense emotions, such as anxiety and frustration, through techniques like deep breathing, mindfulness, and grounding exercises
- *Social support:* Encouraging individuals to reach out to their support networks, share their experiences, and seek comfort from friends, family, or support groups

- *Distraction techniques:* Guiding clients in finding healthy distractions or engaging in activities they enjoy to redirect their focus away from negative thoughts and emotions
- *Positive self-talk:* Helping individuals replace self-critical thoughts with more compassionate and self-affirming statements
- *Behavioral activation:* Encouraging engagement in positive and fulfilling activities to counteract the tendency to withdraw due to emotional distress.

Emphasizing Self-compassion and Self-acceptance

Skin disorders can lead to feelings of shame, embarrassment, and self-criticism. Psychodermatology counseling emphasizes the importance of self-compassion and self-acceptance as integral components of emotional healing. Counselors guide individuals to treat themselves with kindness and understanding, just as they would offer support to a friend facing similar challenges. Practicing self-compassion allows individuals to develop a healthier relationship with themselves and their skin condition.

Self-acceptance involves acknowledging one's condition without judgment and reframing it as just one aspect of who they are. Counselors help individuals recognize their intrinsic worth beyond their appearance and skin health. By cultivating self-acceptance, individuals can reduce the negative impact of societal beauty standards and external judgments on their self-esteem.

ADDRESSING BODY IMAGE AND SELF-ESTEEM

Body image and self-esteem are intricately linked to skin health, and psychodermatology counseling plays a vital role in helping individuals navigate these complex connections.

Exploring the Link between Body Image, Self-esteem, and Skin Health

Skin conditions can significantly impact how individuals perceive their bodies and themselves. Visible skin issues can lead to negative body image and lowered self-esteem. The way individuals feel about their appearance can influence their overall sense of self-worth and confidence. This relationship is particularly pertinent in a society where societal beauty standards often prioritize flawless skin.

Strategies to Promote a Positive Body Image and Improve Self-esteem

Psychodermatology counseling offers tailored strategies to promote a positive body image and enhance self-esteem for individuals with skin conditions:

- *Self-appreciation:* Counselors help individuals shift their focus from perceived flaws to acknowledging their strengths and attributes beyond physical appearance.
- *Self-compassion:* Encouraging self-compassion involves treating oneself with kindness and understanding. This approach helps individuals develop a more forgiving and gentle attitude toward themselves and their skin conditions.
- *Positive self-talk:* Counselors assist individuals in recognizing negative self-talk patterns and replacing them with affirming and realistic thoughts. This process supports the development of a healthier self-image.
- *Gratitude and mindfulness:* Practicing gratitude for the body's functionality and being present through mindfulness can foster acceptance and appreciation for one's physical self.

FAMILY AND SOCIAL SUPPORT IN PSYCHODERMATOLOGY

Social support stands as one of the most intricate factors contributing to the enhancement of the quality of life for individuals grappling with psychodermatological issues. Several studies have consistently demonstrated how the perception of social support can impact the psychopathological levels of patients. Specifically, when a dermatological patient perceives lower levels of social support and exhibits reduced overall appearance satisfaction before undergoing dermatological treatment, their predicted psychopathology levels tend to be higher.

Receiving familial and social support in the form of acceptance is crucial, as it directly influences the patient's self-esteem. Furthermore, patients who reported higher levels of social support experienced a significantly better quality of life, lower levels of depression, and greater acceptance of life despite their condition. Among the various types of social support, tangible support emerged as the most effective predictor for all adaptation indices.

ETHICAL CONSIDERATIONS IN PSYCHODERMATOLOGY COUNSELING

Psychologists and therapists are bound by fundamental principles that guide their practice, including beneficence and nonmaleficence, fidelity and responsibility, integrity, justice, and respect for people's rights and dignity. Within the realm of psychotherapy, specific ethical considerations must also be upheld, such as ensuring informed consent in therapy, safeguarding privacy and confidentiality, preventing harm, avoiding unfair discrimination, and addressing issues related to sexual harassment.

CASE STUDIES AND PRACTICAL APPLICATIONS

Case Studies

Case Study 1: Jayati's Psoriasis Journey

Jayati, a 32-year-old professional, struggled with severe psoriasis since her early twenties. The visible plaques on her arms and legs made her feel constantly exposed, leading her to avoid social gatherings and even workplace interactions. Her self-esteem plummeted, causing her to withdraw from relationships. Psychodermatology counseling helped Jayati to develop coping strategies, challenge negative self-perceptions, and regain her confidence. Gradually, with integrated care from her dermatologist and counselor, her physical and emotional well-being improved.

Case Study 2: Manu's Battle with Acne

Manu, a 16-year-old high school student, faced severe acne that resulted in relentless bullying from his peers. His acne impacted his self-esteem, making him avoid school and extracurricular activities. Manu's psychologist helped him develop resilience and self-acceptance strategies, while his dermatologist prescribed a tailored treatment plan. Through counseling and medical intervention, Manu's skin improved, and he learned to navigate the emotional challenges of acne with greater confidence.

These case studies exemplify the intricate interplay between skin health and mental well-being. The emotional distress experienced by individuals with these common skin conditions underscores the significance of psychodermatology in addressing both the physical and psychological aspects of their lives. By offering tailored interventions that encompass medical management, psychological support, and coping strategies, clinicians can empower individuals to lead fulfilling lives while managing their skin conditions and the associated emotional burdens.

FUTURE DIRECTIONS IN PSYCHO-DERMATOLOGY COUNSELING

Given the relatively new status of this field, much work lies ahead to serve clients of psychodermatology. There is a need for professionals form the different fields of dermatology, clinical psychology, and psychiatry to come together and develop a collaborative communication channel along with a set of disease-wise common operative procedures that can be used for different skin conditions. Another area to take forward is to develop psychological assessment tools for psychodermatological concerns such as body image, self-esteem, quality of life, etc., specific to the different cultural contexts.

Role of Counseling in Redefining Beauty Standards

An area that complicates and impacts skin conditions, as well as guides, the client's reactions to them are the standards of beauty in any society. Thus, another potential area for intervention in the coming decades would be to help develop new standards for beauty in a society. Media can, in fact, play an enormous role to bring about macrolevel change in this regard. Counseling, on the other hand, can play a crucial, mediatory role at a microlevel in helping individuals redefine beauty standards and challenging societal norms that equate skin perfection with self-worth. Counselors create a safe space to explore and challenge these harmful ideals, enabling individuals to recognize the diversity of beauty and their inherent value beyond appearance.

By empowering individuals to cultivate self-acceptance and redefine beauty in a broader sense, psychodermatology counseling assists in reshaping the narrative around skin health and self-esteem. This shift ultimately promotes a more positive body image, bolsters self-esteem, and improves overall emotional well-being.

CONCLUSION

The role of counselors and psychologists in psychodermatology is one of great importance. Building resilience and coping skills is a cornerstone of psychodermatology counseling and enables individuals to manage the emotional and psychological toll of skin conditions. Through identifying resilience factors, teaching adaptive coping strategies, and emphasizing self-compassion and self-acceptance, counselors empower individuals to lead fulfilling lives despite the challenges they face. The benefits of counseling for individuals having dermatological conditions can encompass: Improved overall well-being, increased self-esteem, and enhanced quality of life, which are worthy goals for every treating clinician and their suffering client.

FURTHER READINGS

1. American Psychiatric Association. (2022). Diagnostic and statistical manual of mental disorders (5th ed., text rev.). [online] Available from https://doi.org/10.1176/appi.books.9780890425787 [Last accessed January, 2024].
2. Chen Y, Lyga J. Brain-skin connection: Stress, inflammation and skin aging. Inflamm Allergy Drug Targets. 2014;13(3):177-90.
3. Costeris C, Petridou M, Ioannou Y. Social Support and Appearance Satisfaction Can Predict Changes in the Psychopathology Levels of Patients with Acne, Psoriasis, and Eczema, before Dermatological Treatment and in a Six-Month Follow-up Phase. Psych. 2021;3(3):259-68.
4. Dalgard FJ, Gieler U, Tomas-Aragones L, Lien L, Poot F, Jemec GB, et al. The psychological burden of skin diseases: A cross-sectional multicenter study among dermatological out-patients in 13 European countries. J Invest Dermatol. 2015;135(4):984-91.
5. Hinkley SB, Holub SC, Menter A. The Validity of Cutaneous Body Image as a Construct and as a Mediator of the Relationship Between Cutaneous Disease and Mental Health. Dermatol Ther. 2020;10:203-11.
6. Janowski K, Steuden S, Pietrzak A, et al. Social support and adaptation to the disease in men and women with psoriasis. Arch Dermatol Res. 2012;304(6):421-32.
7. Kieć-Swierczyńska M, Dudek B, Krecisz B, et al. The role of psychological factors and psychiatric disorders in skin diseases. Medycyna Pracy. 2006;57(6):551-5.
8. Koo JY, Lee CS. (Eds). General approach to evaluating psycho-dermatological disorders. In: Psychocutaneous Medicine. New York: Marcel Dekker; 2003. pp. 1-29.
9. Latheef AEN Skin and psyche. In: Latheef A, Prabhu S, Shenoi S (Eds), Handbook of Psychodermatology. New Delhi: Jaypee Brothers Medical Publishers; 2016. pp. 1-8.

10. Layegh P, Arshadi HR, Shahriari S, Pezeshkpour F, Nahidi Y. A Comparative Study on the Prevalence of Depression and Suicidal Ideation in Dermatology Patients Suffering from Psoriasis, Acne, Alopecia Areata and Vitiligo. Iran J Dermatol. 2010;13(4):106-11.
11. Lyu F, Wu T, Bian Y, Zhu K, Xu J, Li F. Stress and its impairment of skin barrier function. Int J Dermatol. 2023;62:621-30.
12. Mhatre M, Mysore V. Skin, mind and beauty. In: Latheef S, Prabhu S, Shenoi S (Eds), Handbook of Psychodermatology. New Delhi: Jaypee Brothers Medical Publishers; 2016. pp. 9-15.
13. Mitchell AE. Bidirectional relationships between psychological health and dermatological conditions in children. Psychol Res Behav Manag. 2018;11: 289-98.
14. Shreejayan K. Asssessment tools and questionnaires in psychodermatology. In: Latheef A, Prabhu S, Shenoi S (Eds), Handbook of Psychodermatology. New Delhi: Jaypee Brothers Medical Publishers; 2016. pp. 21-28.
15. Tasoula E, Gregoriou S, Chalikias J, Lazarou D, Danopoulou I, Katsambas A. The impact of acne vulgaris on quality of life and psychic health in young adolescents in Greece: results of a population survey. An Bras Dermatol. 2012;87(6):862-9.
16. Vernwal D. A study of anxiety and depression in vitiligo patients: new challenges to treat. Eur Psychiatry. 2017;41(S1):S321-1.

CHAPTER 18

Psychological Intervention in Psychodermatological Conditions: Part 1

Shweta Rai

> **Key Messages**
> - Stress can worsen many skin conditions.
> - Hence, dealing with stress is a way to improve skin conditions.
> - Psychotherapies like habit reversal, supportive therapy, relaxation procedures, and cognitive behavior therapy are highly useful in stress-related dermatology cases.

INTRODUCTION

The aim of psychotherapy is to recognize the emotional issues that may affect the way skin problems respond to medical treatment. As there is well-established connection between skin and mind, there is no doubt that many of the dermatological conditions are a result of stress. Therefore, intervention needs to target stress, anxiety, and worry which may be secondary to skin condition or may lead to aggravation of illness.

Before starting the psychological intervention, it is very important to know which psychodermatological conditions will be targeted. In primary psychiatric illness (delusion of parasitosis, obsessive compulsive disorder, dysmorphophobia, etc.), the target is to modify or remove the symptoms of illness with specific models and approaches.

If stress is playing an active role in etiology and course of skin conditions (psoriasis, atopic dermatitis, urticarial, etc.), or it is delaying the improvement, then the aim should be to apply the psychological intervention which reduces the stress and worries.

In some skin conditions (pemphigus vulgaris, Hansen's disease, etc.), where stress has not much role in aggravation, the aim of the intervention should be to strengthen the defenses and teaching new and better mechanisms to maintain the control.

The following psychological interventions will be discussed:
- Habit reversal
- Supportive therapy (ST)
- Relaxation procedures
- Cognitive behavior therapy (CBT)

HABIT REVERSAL

Habit reversal is used successfully in the treatment of trichotillomania (TTM) and body focused repetitive behavior (e.g., skin picking). It has four important components:
1. Awareness training (AT)
2. Competing response (CR)
3. Habit control motivation
4. Generalization

Awareness Training

Awareness training is the most important step and aims at the patient being aware of the whole behavior chain. For example, in TTM, the patient needs to identify how he starts to pull the hair with the help of therapist. For example, he may start with touching the hair, then holding one or four to five hair in index and thumb finger, then strokes over it, and finally pulls it from the root.

Identifying a high-risk situation is another important part, e.g., reading, watching TV, sleeping, sitting free, or thinking. In case of children, parents should also be involved. Patients apply CR after immediately noticing the very first warning signs of pulling hair.

Competing Response

The patient is trained in performing movements which are incompatible with pulling hair or skin picking, etc. The patient has to perform it for 1–3 minutes each time the problematic behavior occurs. CR has to be applied before the problematic behavior (when

the urge to pull the hair) begins. In case of unfocused pulling, if the patient has already started pulling the hair, then they can immediately stop it and apply CR. Sometimes, children find it difficult to practice CR for a minute; in such cases, they can start with 30 seconds and gradually increase the time to a maximum of 3 minutes. The therapist should decide a CR which is easy for patients. The following CR can be suggested to the patients to perform:
- Grasping object firmly
- Making fist and squeezing
- Sitting on one's hands
- While reading, holding the book firmly or holding cushion while watching TV
- Squeeze rubber balls kept at strategical positions

Some of the warning signs can be used to enhance AT and as a reminder of CR, for example, putting "NO pulling" signs or red dot in bedroom or in the middle of the mirror and in other high-risk situations.

Motivation and Social Support

This is the most important and challenging aspect of the technique. The therapist needs to regularly review the record sheet of the behavior either in the session or telephonically. Regular feedback and positive reinforcement should be given. Support of family members, close friends, and class teacher, in case of children, should be ensured.

Record Sheet

Date and time	Location (where were you?)	Activity (what were you doing?)	Strength of urges (0–10)	Thoughts	Notable sensation	Site	No. of pulled

RELAXATION PROCEDURES

When the patient reports of excessive fear, anxiety, and stress which include autonomic arousal, then in such conditions relaxation procedures can be applied, which help to calm down. These include muscular relaxation training, autogenic training (AT), biofeedback (BF), meditation, imagery, and paced breathing. Here, four techniques will be discussed in detail: Jacobson progressive muscular relaxation (JPMR), imagery, BF, and AT.

These techniques basically help the patients to reduce the arousal. Deep state of relaxation could reduce arousal in both central nervous system (CNS) and autonomic nervous system (ANS), and as a result it could resort or promote psychological and physical well-being. This view is consonant with theory that there is close and interactive relation between bodily state and emotional state.

Jacobson Progressive Muscular Relation

Before starting the procedure, the patient should be explained about how anxiety plays a role in aggravation of his skin condition and how relaxation can help. This procedure will take 30–40 minutes. There are two important components in relaxation exercise, one is relaxing the muscles and second is tensing the muscles. Before initiating the procedure, the therapist should demonstrate how to tense and relax the muscles in each group of muscles. The therapist must inquire as to any injury or disabilities that might cause pain or discomfort when certain groups of muscles are tensed. In such conditions, such groups of muscles can be skipped or only focusing relaxation without prior tension.

A calm dim light room can be used. Tight clothing can be avoided and tight rubber bands and wristwatch can be removed; legs should not be crossed while lying down and sitting on a recliner chair. All parts of the body should be supported by the bed or chair.

In JPMR, the therapist starts from the head muscles and moves to toe muscles. Like this, he completes all groups of muscles in a progressive manner. To start with, first the patient is asked to tense the muscles for 15 seconds and lose them gently and feel the difference in muscles for 30 seconds. These same instructions are given for all groups of muscles from head to toe. The rationale for this is that tensing the muscles before attempting to relax allows the patient to become more aware of muscle tension so as to be able to identify it when it occurs. The contrast between the tense and relaxed states may also help the patient to achieve a deeper state of relaxation than would be possible when beginning from resting state. While tensing the muscles, the therapist may give the instructions "feel the tension of your muscles" and while relaxing the therapist may direct the patient's attention to the feeling of relaxation. During the initial session, the tension-release cycle, typically, is performed twice on each muscle group to ensure complete relaxation. The patient needs to practice it every day for at least 2 months to maintain the improvement.

The steps of a modified version of Jacobson's progressive relaxation procedure are as follows:

Take a comfortable position on the bed...lie down on the bed as comfortably as you can on your back, with all the parts of your body loose...light...and free. Be calm and comfortable keep your eyes closed tightly. Now let us start the practice...as you go on doing it concentrate on the feelings from within. Avoid stray thought as best as you can, be calm, quiet and still, on the bed. Avoid extra movement of the body.

1. *Clench your right fist... As tightly as you can...tighter and tighter... good. Now observe the tightness or tension within your palm muscles, hold it for some time, slowly release it, make it completely loose and light...let your fingers be completely loose and light... now observe the soothing sensation within...feel the lightness in your palm good...keep the entire body loose and light, be calm and relaxed. Repeat it again...clench it as hard as you can... now observe the tension within...slowly release it...make it free and light...feel the soothing lightness, within and be relaxed... still more calm and relaxed. Breathe freely and gently. The same instructions of tightening and loosening the muscles as mentioned in the first step in detail, have to be followed for the rest of the steps.*
2. *Clench your left fist...*
3. *Clench both fists at a time*
4. *Clench your fist and bend your arms...tighten your arms muscles...*
5. *Now straighten your hands as tightly as you can make them stiff and press them by the body...*
6. *Wrinkle your forehead...*
7. *Twitch eyebrows as if you are frowning on someone*
8. *Now press your tongue to the roof (palate) of your mouth in a flat manner...do not coil your tongue...*
9. *Bite your teeth tightly (pressing of jaws...*
10. *Press your lips against each other (do not bite)*

11. *Bend your head forward and let your chin touch the chest...turn your face to right as tightly as possible and observe the tension in your neck muscles and now turn it to the left...again bring it to the middle...touch the chin to the chest...and slowly keep it back on the bed...make it loose and free...*
12. *Bend the head backwards and turn it left and right, observe the tension and slowly release it.*
13. *Bend your shoulders upwards in an arc-like manner...as tightly as you can...*
14. *Bend your shoulders backwards...press them against your back...*
15. *Take a deep breath and expand your chest......as best as you can...*
16. *Swell your belly with air (abdomen...*
17. *Shrink your belly in...*
18. *Tighten your thigh muscles as tightly as possible...*
19. *Bend your heels down and tighten your calf muscles...*
20. *Bend your toes upwards*
21. *Bend the toes downwards*
22. *Now slowly draw in a deep breath and slowly release it. Keep the entire body loose and light and free. Concentrate on the growing lightness in your hands, face, neck, shoulder, chest and abdomen back,...relax more and more...further...deeper and deeper.*
23. *Termination: Now you are calm, comfortable relaxed. I will be counting from 1-10 and you prepare yourself to open your eyes (1, 2, 3,... 9, 10). Now slowly open your eyes, slowly get up sit for a while, now you are completely relaxed, fresh comfortable.*

Guided Imagery

Guided imagery can be applied in skin conditions when the patient expresses excessive distress due to illness or due to any life event. It makes the patient calm and relaxed. The therapist should use a scenery which is soothing to the patient. For example, if the therapist is describing a scene of beach and the patient has the fear of the same, it would lead to panic and then relaxation. The scenes should be embellished with as much minute details as possible, sensory details to make the imagery scene more real and to make the patient completely involved in the experience.

Guided imagery can also be used as a distractor while the patient is anxious, stressed, and in physical pain. The success of guided imagery depends on the patient's ability to imagine vividly, which can be assessed by asking a patient to imagine an object or a pleasurable event which has happened in the past. Then the therapist can ask many details of that event and object. Guided imagery may not be effective for patients who are unable to imagine. An example of guided imagery is as follows:

Close your eyes, take a comfortable position, take a deep breath, and try to imagine as I say. Imagine that this is morning time, you are in the garden and you are sitting on the bench. The cold breeze is blowing on...you can feel the coldness of the breeze on your body, on your face, arms, feet, etc. You can see the beautiful colorful flowers... you can smell the fragrance of the flowers. You are enjoying all this and now you get up from the bench and start walking on the grass. You are walking bare feet and could feel the coldness of grass on your feet. You can hear the bird's sound. You are feeling relaxed...more and more relaxed. You are enjoying every moment of the morning. Continue enjoying and be calm and relaxed.

Biofeedback

Biofeedback techniques can be applied in many medical conditions (hypertension, chronic pain, migraine headache, etc.), and in psychiatric conditions. In psychodermatology, it can be implicated when a patient reports of anxiety, stress, autonomic arousal, and pain. It has been effectively used in hyperhidrosis. BF would be more effective with patients who report of various physiological changes as result of anxiety.

The basic mechanism of BF is that it gives feedback about involuntary physiological changes, e.g., alpha and beta brain waves, heart rates, body temperature. This feedback is given to the patient in either visual or auditory mode. There are also computerized video game-based BF which gives feedback in the form of gaining and losing the points while the patient plays. This is usually used in child cases.

Before starting the session, the patient can be explained how physiological changes are related to anxiety. It can be done through a small experiment: The electrodes can be fixed on the patient's body (based on the type of BF) and then the patient can be asked to imagine a most pleasant moment of his life and immediate physiological changes can be shown to the patient in a BF machine. After this, the patient can be given a cognitively demanding task so that he feels the pressure to perform. For example, he can be asked to solve a puzzle or given a task of problem solving and planning can be given. And while he is performing on this task, the immediate physiological changes can be brought to the patient's notice through the BF machine. Now it will be very clear to the patient that involuntary physiological changes are in his control which cause so much distress to him. And this control can be gained through BF training procedures. There are different types of BF: Electromyography, temperature BF, sweat gland activity, and electroencephalogram. Here, temperature BF will be discussed in detail.

Temperature Biofeedback

In the first session, the therapist should explain the rationale of temperature biofeedback (TBF). It gives feedback about the body temperature. The electrodes are placed on the patient's finger (index or little) with the help of paper tape. The therapist should be careful that the flow of blood should not be cut off while fixing the electrodes on the finger. The patient will be assured that it will not give any electric current. After fixing electrodes, TBF's monitor starts reflecting temperature either in Fahrenheit or in Celsius as set by the therapist. Now the patient can be given instructions as, "you need to increase the temperature of your body as it is indicator of your ANS functions. That means when your body temperature increases your sympathetic nervous system calms down and parasympathetic nervous system gets activated, which eventually indicates that you are going in to relaxed state. And to do this you can imagine a pleasant scene or a moment from your experience". When the patient imagines, he starts feeling relaxed gradually and his temperature starts increasing. Now, the feedback for increase and decrease in the temperature can be given in auditory or visual mode. For example, the patient can read the temperature in monitor or BF machine will give beep sound whenever temperature increases or decreases from a threshold of temperature set by the therapist. Some patients would like to close their eyes and want the therapist to give verbal feedback. Every time there is an increase in temperature, verbal positive reinforcement can be given. Sessions have to be given on a daily basis and after 10–12 sessions, the patient can practice it at home. Booster sessions can be given.

Autogenic Training

Autogenic training was developed by German physician Johannes Schultz (1932) to help client switch from stress to relaxation. It induces an optimal level of arousal, which may involve an increase or decrease in one's current level of physiological arousal depending upon the circumstances. It is an autosuggestion technique which a client can self-produce after a minimal amount of training. It has a set of six psychophysiological exercises that use short auto suggestion. These exercises emphasize on heaviness and warmth in extremities, regulation of cardiac activities and respiration, abdominal warmth, and cooling of the forehead. The exercise is learnt in a specific sequence and the client needs to learn each state before initiating the next exercise. An example of the training procedure is as follows:

The client needs to sit on a chair in a relaxed posture. Basic rules of relaxation need to be followed before starting exercise, which have already been mentioned in detail while explaining JPMR. Once the client is settled in to relaxed position with eyes closed, the therapist begins in calm voice (first formula), "I am at piece…my right arm is heavy". The client has to repeat this silently for about 20 seconds. After a week's interval, the heaviness formula is modified to include other parts of the body. Then, the second formula of warmth in limb can be introduced. The therapist can say, "my right arm is very warm". Then, the third formula of heart regulation will be introduced. The therapist says, "my heart is beating calmly and strongly". Fourth is breathing regulation—many times the client brings voluntary changes in breathing pattern out of anxiety which is undesirable. The therapist uses passive phrase here as "it breaths me". Fifth is regulation of visceral organs. The therapist says, "warmth radiates over my stomach". Sixth is regulation of the temperature of the head. The therapist says, "my forehead is cool".

COGNITIVE BEHAVIOR THERAPY

The basic assumption of CBT is that thinking influences our emotions and emotions influence our thinking. So, the aim of the therapy is to modify thinking so that it would bring positive changes in emotions. There are well-established cognitive models for depression, anxiety, personality, psychosis. Many times, patients suffering from debilitating skin illness express excessive negative automatic thoughts (NAT),

worries, and appraise events negatively due to present skin conditions. Before starting CBT, the therapist should check the amenability of the patient for the technique. For example:
- Capacity to access and identify NAT
- Awareness and differentiation of emotions
- Acceptance of responsibility to change
- Understanding and acceptance of cognitive rationale for the therapy

For the success of the therapy, it is important that the therapist should have good therapeutic alliance with the patient so that they both can work collaboratively for the problem. In CBT, unlike other therapies, the patient has to take an active role for the desirable changes. In initial sessions, the therapist tries to elicit NAT of the patients. There are many ways to assess NAT but the most commonly used is thought diary.

Date	Situation	Emotion	Automatic thought	Outcome
3/11/15	Friend called for get together	Anxious	Everyone will notice my scars on face. I am not pretty. I look stupid	Did not go for the party

The cognitive techniques are used to restructure NAT, beliefs, assumptions, and schemes. The techniques which would be discussed here are embedded in Socratic dialogue.

Defining and Operationalizing Terms

Many times, the meaning of a patient's NAT is not clear. It is important to understand the meaning of appraisal a patient makes because it is difficult to challenge a thought if it is meaning is obscure. For example, a patient with vitiligo says, "I cannot cope with this illness". Now the therapist needs to know what requires coping with—facing society, low confidence, financial load, physical pain. Once the actual nature of fear is clear, verbal reattribution can be specifically targeted at the concept. Some useful questions for operationalizing terms are:
- When you say that you cannot cope, what do you mean?
- If you could not cope, what is the worse that could happen?
- What would not being able to cope look like to you?
- If that was true, what would it mean to you?
- If that was true, what would be bad about that?
- If you could cope well, how would things be different from the way they are now?

Questioning the Evidence

Questioning the evidence in support of NAT, beliefs, and assumptions helps a patient to understand the irrationality of the thought. However, the thoughts may not be always irrational in patients with skin conditions. For example, a patient with psoriasis expresses the thought that people avoid him looking at his skin condition. Now in this case, the patient might be right; however, this may not be happening always. But in view of NAT, he might become socially withdrawn. Now the patient and therapist have to work collaboratively to explore the quality of evidence in support of NAT. The following questions can be asked:
- What is the evidence that all do not like you and reject you?
- What makes you think that?
- How do you know that will happen?
- What is your reason for believing that this will happen?

Many times, the evidence might be available but the quality of evidence has to be reinterpreted. This can be done through reviewing alternative explanation of evidence and counter evidence. So, the therapist may ask:
- What is the evidence that people will not reject you?
- What other way you can look at your problem?
- What is the evidence to support an alternative way of looking at it?
- Have all people rejected you? Why not?

Worst, Best, Most Likely

Here, the therapist may first ask what best could happen in the situation and then what worst could happen. Finally, the therapist would discuss what could be the most likely things to happen out of the best and worst possibilities. This kind of questioning helps a patient to reduce catastrophize thinking.

Use of Rationale Response

This is the ultimate of cognitive restructuring that converts NAT into rationale response or alternative thoughts. Once rationale responses are generated, the patient can write them on flashcards and keep those flashcards always with him so that he can use them whenever a situation arises. For example, a 25-year-old female suffering from acne vulgaris might have thoughts about that she will not get a good marriage proposal. A rationale response to this may be, "physical appearance plays important role in getting a good match but there are other important attributes which are more important for a relationship." The patient can also be reminded that she does have good close friends or other people who accept her in spite of this skin condition.

An example of cognitive restructuring, using techniques mentioned above, is as follows:

A 32-year-old male suffering from psoriasis.

Therapist (T): When you say that you are not a fit in social gathering, what do you mean by that?

Patient (P): People stare at me.

T: What happens if they stare at you?

P: I feel embarrassed.

T: What do you do at that time?

P: I feel like running away, do not give eye contact, and when someone talks to me, I do not know what to say and my heart starts beating fast. I start feeling that I am ugly looking, do not even know how to talk, that's why people think I am dumb.

T: So, your NATs are—you are ugly looking; you do not know how to talk; people think you are dumb.

P: Yes I guess so.

T: Do you have any evidence people actually think so?

P: It has happened earlier when I was anxious in a similar situation. I do not know what to say and my mind goes blank.

T: It is true that you do not get words to communicate and you go blank but what makes you think that people find you dumb.

P: I am not sure but may be my looks.

T: Well how physical appearance is related to being dumb. (Here, the therapist may also probe further what does it mean when a patient says that people see him dumb). On the other hand, how would people react to you if they think you were dumb and ugly looking?

P: They will not talk to me and will not call me for social gathering.

T: Is there any evidence people do that to you?

P: No, some people might but not all and not always.

This is how a therapist goes on eliciting NAT and challenging them.

SUPPORTIVE THERAPY

There are some dermatological conditions in which the damage is irreversible or chronic. The patients lose self-confidence and become dysfunctional and hopeless. Here, ST can be applied, which aims to bring about equilibrium by promoting psychological and social adaptation, by restoring and reinforcing abilities to cope with challenges of life which are caused by the illness. ST has the following components.

Catharsis

Empathy and warmth in a patient–therapist relationship bring trust in therapy so that the patient ventilates his feelings of sorrow, frustration, and fear to the therapist, no matter however, painful and embarrassing they may be, leading to a sense of relief.

Reassurance

A 30-year-old woman with chronic pemphigus vulgaris could not complete her education and did not marry in view of the skin condition. At present, facing a financial constrain due to never-ending treatment, she believes that life has been unfair to her. She was rejected in college, did not have friends, and had not done well in her personal and professional life as well. In such a condition, the therapist can reassure the patient by removing doubts and misconceptions and by pointing to their assets. The patient should be reassured that fear of being unwanted and having not done well is irrational and help in regaining her confidence, albeit realistically. To promote hope unreasonably that is groundless may be effective in short term but is bound to backfire later.

Suggestions and Guidance

In some skin conditions when patients lose their looks, they become socially withdrawn, leave their jobs, or become irregular, consequently facing financial crises and family conflicts. In such cases, the patient can be advised for personal care, job (e.g., changing a job, getting a job), family (marital conflict, how to deal with problematic children), and social life (how to reconnect to people, enhancing social circle, joining social club). The therapist's main aim is to teach the patient requisite skills for coping with the problem as well as assist him in doing the same.

Encouragement

A patient with long-standing illness needs regular doses of encouragement whenever required. Encouragement helps the patient to combat feelings of inferiority and promote self-esteem. The therapist can give verbal reinforcement, e.g., "I am fully confident you can do it". It can also be expressed nonverbally through a display of eagerness and optimism. Again, past achievements can be pointed out. Caution is necessary while extending encouragement. To encourage a patient unrealistically toward a goal hopelessly out of his reach may well have contrary results.

CONCLUSION

Psychotherapeutic techniques discussed here are efficacious treatment in various psychodermatological conditions. However, one needs to select a right approach depending upon the condition and the patient's suitability for approach.

FURTHER READINGS

1. Bloch S. An Introduction to the Psychotherapies, 3rd edition. Oxford: Oxford University Press; 1979.
2. Franklin M, Tolin D. Treating Trichotillomania Cognitive-Behavioral Therapy for Hairpulling and Related Problems. New York: Springer; 2007.
3. Rimm D, Masters J, Thomas GB, Steven DH. Behavior Therapy: Techniques and Empirical Findings, 3rd edition. New York: Academic Press; 1974.
4. Sanders D, Wills F. Cognitive Therapy: An Introduction, 2nd edition. London: Sage Publications; 2005.
5. Wells A. Cognitive Therapy of Anxiety Disorders: A Practice Manual and Conceptual Guide. Chichester: Wiley; 1997.
6. Harth W, Gieler U, Kusnir D, Tausk FA (Eds). Clinical Management in Psychodermatology. Germany: Springer; 2009.

CHAPTER 19

Psychological Interventions in Psychodermatological Conditions: Part 2

Abdul Latheef EN, Julaila Thasneem

> **Key Messages**
> - Many dermatological conditions are stress-related, which leads to psychiatric comorbidity.
> - Unless we manage the underlying psychosocial issues, response to therapy will be less.
> - Psychotherapies like psychoeducation, hypnotherapy, group therapy, family therapy, behavior therapy, and neurolinguistic programming are equally effective to pharmacotherapy.

INTRODUCTION

Psychological interventions are essential part of psychodermatology management.

Psychoeducation, Hypnotherapy, Behavior therapy, Group therapy and Family therapy are very useful psychological techniques. Familiarizing few techniques will be highly useful in patient management.

PSYCHOEDUCATION

Psychoeducation is very important in the management of psychocutaneous disorders. It implies teaching of psychosomatic concepts by providing information and knowledge about the problem, thereby teaching a biopsychosocial model of the disease. Patients with dermatitis artefacta syndrome, body dysmorphic disorder, or delusional disorders are frequently not open to biopsychosocial concepts and are not willing for psychotherapy. These patients usually have a purely somatic concept and a desire for somatic therapy only. There are so many myths, misconceptions, and anxieties regarding many diseases. The educator should be able to give them a comprehensive picture of the disease, to help alleviate the anxieties and to cope up with the disease. Thus, "soothing assurances" can contribute to the reduction of anxiety and gaining knowledge for self-management, even in unmotivated patients. The following points are highly relevant in giving psychoeducation.

Etiology

Most of the time, the patient will have their own concept of etiology. For example, in prurigo nodularis, spider bite is attributed as the cause by many and they approach a quack handling poison (*visha vydya - malayalam language*) for treatment. The doctor should teach them that scratching is the main culprit in the progression of the disease. Once they stop scratching, the skin problem will subside rapidly.

- The genesis of the disease is known (psychosomatic). The doctor should convince the patient that the cause and progression of the disease are well known and common and that we are familiar with such conditions.
- The patient's problem is not a rare case. Usually, the patient thinks that his problem is a rare one and that is why there is no response to treatment. If we tell them that others too suffer from the same disease, their anxiety will be alleviated.
- The nonserious nature of the disease. Some patients think that their disease is very serious and incurable.
- *Precipitating factors*: The intelligent patient can be given an idea regarding precipitating factors, to avoid recurrences or delay in treatment.
- *Role of stress*: The importance of stress in the disease causation or precipitation should be discussed. Many patients will not be ready to admit stress as the precipitating factor, and a denial response is very common. If the doctor succeeds in convincing stress as a precipitating factor, only then stress-reduction therapies and coping strategies can be implemented. A little bit of expertise is needed for a successful communication.
- *Noncontagious nature*: Many patients are afraid of spreading the disease to the family members and others even though the condition is purely noncontagious. Family members too think so and behave accordingly, increasing the stress burden of the patient.

- *Treatment options*: The doctor should share the various treatment options, both pharmacological and nonpharmacological, for a better result and should emphasize the need for strict adherence to therapy.
- *Consequences*: Many patients are afraid of malignancy and other serious conditions. It is better to ask the patient what do you think it is? And what are your fears regarding the disease? Then convince him that the disease is unpleasant but not dangerous.
- *Prognosis*: It is better to inform the prognosis in a palatable way. Good prognosis can be openly told, but if it is bad, disclose only step by step. Deteriorations will be dealt with in therapy.
- Need of new emotional experiences and modification of behavior
- *Relate patient successes*: Better to share the history of successfully treated cases, their attitude toward treatment, their adherence to therapy, and belief in treating doctor
- Refer to your earlier experiences (life experiences, therapy experiences). It is better to share the success story of your treatment in similar cases that will increase their hope and belief in your treatment and help for a better outcome.
- Simple psychoeducation (even though time consuming) alone will bring dramatic changes in patient's attitude, coping skills, and treatment responses.

HYPNOTHERAPY

Introduction

Hypnotherapy is a psychotherapeutic procedure used since antiquity. The word hypnos is derived from the "Greek God of Sleep" **(Fig. 1)**. All individuals enter the spontaneous mild trances daily

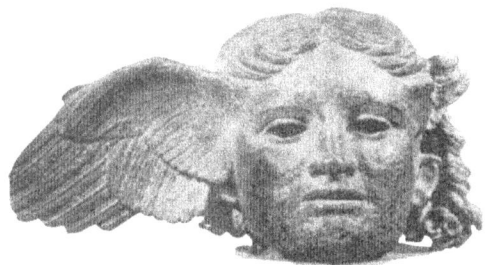

Fig. 1: Hypnos: The Greek God of Sleep.

during watching television or movies, reading book or magazine, meditation, self-hypnosis, or just before sleeping. Hypnosis is the intentional induction, deepening, maintenance, and termination of the natural trance-like state for a specific purpose. Hypnotherapy is used in varied conditions like pain disorders, phobias/fears, panic attacks, irritable bowel syndrome, atopic dermatitis, alopecia areata, and Hansen's disease but less utilized in the field of dermatology. Only limited data exist on its role in various skin diseases.

History

Franz Anton Mesmer (1733-1815), an Austrian physician, was the pioneer and the term Mesmerism is used as a synonym for hypnotherapy. He proposed the cosmic fluid theory (a curative force could be stored in lifeless objects like magnets and transferred to patients to cure the disease) and animal magnetism (he considered himself as a magnet with fluid-like force and transferred to others). Thousands rushed to his clinic in Austria and treated diseases like blindness, paralysis, headache, and joint pains.

Dr James Braid (1795-1860), a Scottish physician, gave mesmerism a scientific perspective and coined the term hypnosis. It is his early evaluation of hypnotherapy that forms the basis for the use of therapeutic suggestions to help patients deal with physiologic ailments. Milton H Erickson (1901-1980), a psychiatrist in the mid-1900s, popularized hypnotherapy. Sigmund Freud (1856-1939) further propagated hypnotherapy and it was accepted as a valid medical procedure by the American Medical Association and Psychological Association in 1958 and British Medical Association in 1953.

Stages of Hypnosis

Induction Phase

Various techniques are used for induction of hypnosis—relaxation techniques, music, colored lights, eye fixation method, meditation, deep breathing, and drugs like ketamine. By utilizing any one or a combination of different methods, hypnosis can be induced.

Suggestion Phase (Trance)

Trance is a state of deep relaxation with altered consciousness, narrowed awareness, restricted and focused attentiveness, selective

Table 1: Comparison of normal sleep and hypnotic trance.	
Normal sleep	**Hypnotic trance**
• No response to stimuli/suggestions	• Responds to suggestions
• Reflexes like knee-jerk/absent	• Reflexes present
• Muscle tone-limbs flaccid	• Tonic rigidity of arms and legs
• No reasoning capacity	• Capable of reasoning
• Not induced by another person	• Could be induced by another person
	• EEG waves of hypnotics and waking state almost similar

wakefulness, and heightened suggestibility **(Table 1)**. In this phase, we can give suggestions, use guided imageries, or even do systematic desensitization. Hypnoanalysis can also be done during this phase. The various levels include the following:

- *Light trance (lethargic state)*:
  - Closed eyes
  - Loss of awareness of the surroundings
  - Increased awareness of internal functions, e.g., heartbeat, breathing
  - Increased receptivity of senses
  - Intensified imagery
- *Medium trance (hallucinatory state)*:
  - Further reduction of activity and energy output
  - Stiffness of limbs
  - Narrowing of attention
  - Increased suggestibility
  - Able to visualize suggested scenes
  - Decreased auditory receptivity and environment awareness
  - Heightened function of creative process
- *Deep trance (somnambulistic state)*:
  - Suspension of voluntary exercise
  - Severe reduction or absence of conscious thought
  - Can open eyes, talk, obey instructions, still in hypnosis

Medical hypnotherapy aims to decrease sufferings, promote healing, and help the person alter a destructive behavior.

How Does it Work?

- Past events are stored in our brain as memories, which will produce a particular physical and emotional response (healthy/unhealthy).

- During hypnotic trance, unhealthy responses can be substituted by healthy responses by giving positive suggestions, guided imageries, or neurolinguistic programming (NLP) techniques.

Suggestions: Key Points
- Give positive suggestions.
- Use unambiguous and clear phrases based on the level of intelligence.
- Repeat the suggestions.
- Reinforcement
- Give time for response to take place.
- Avoid unpleasant suggestions.
- Remove extraneous suggestions before awakening.

Benefits of Hypnotherapy
- Calming the mind and body
- Normalization of sleep
- Decreases pain
- Decreases itching and breaks itch scratch cycle
- Decreases anxiety and depression
- Rapid clearance of diseases
- Enhances self-esteem and enables a positive attitude to physical, mental, and spiritual life
- Helps to strengthen the coping mechanisms
- Increases concentration and memory
- Breaks bad habits

Ideal Age
Children aged 5–15 years are excellent subjects, though the age group of 16–65 years is most practical.

There is no difference in genders and only a minimal level of intelligence is needed, motivation and ability to concentrate being more important.

Usually, 4–10 sittings are advised depending upon the response.

Risks and Complications
These are minimal and patients are safe in experienced hands, but a thorough clinical examination is needed before labeling as a

Table 2: Hypnosis—myths and realities.

Myths and misconceptions	Reality
• Hypnosis is an unnatural phenomenon • Under hypnosis, the subject loses consciousness • Hypnosis is dangerous and will reveal innermost secrets • Hypnosis will weaken one's mind and will power • Hypnosis is addictive • Under hypnosis, the subject will not awaken	• Hypnosis is a normal psychophysiological phenomenon • No loss of consciousness • In trained hands, no danger arises • Even in the deepest trance the subject is in contact with reality, will not disclose anything against his will • It is spontaneous in nature • It is a pleasurable experience • Heterohypnosis is a close interpersonal relationship • Hypnosis is a mean to heighten and direct the suggestibility, inherent characteristic of all human beings

BOX 1: Dermatological conditions where hypnotherapy can be tried.

- Atopic dermatitis
- Acne excoriee
- Alopecia areata
- Dyshidrotic dermatitis
- Erythromelalgia
- Vitiligo
- Trichotillomania
- Urticaria
- Neurodermatitis
- Nummular eczema
- Glossodynia
- Phallodynia
- Herpes simplex
- Hyperhidrosis
- Lichen planus
- Verruca vulgaris
- Postherpetic neuralgia
- Psoriasis
- Rosacea
- Pruritus

psychological disease. Various myths and realities related to hypnosis are given in **Table 2**.

Dermatological Conditions

There are anecdotal reports of usefulness of hypnotherapy in various dermatological conditions. Only limited literature is available in this area. Some of the conditions where hypnotherapy is useful are given in **Box 1**.

> **BOX 2: Conditions where hypnotherapy was tried by the author.**
> - Hansen's disease (neuralgia, ENL)
> - Trichotillomania
> - Chronic urticaria
> - Prurigo nodularis
> - Pemphigus
> - Psoriasis
> - Exfoliative dermatitis
> - Vitiligo
> - Atopic dermatitis
> - Neurodermatitis
> - Nummular eczema
> - Pruritus
> - Venereo phobia
> - Impotence (psychogenic)
> - Factitious dermatitis
> - Factitious cheilitis
>
> (ENL: erythema nodosum leprosum)

Author's Experience

The author tried hypnotherapy in the following conditions either as a sole therapy or along with standard dermatological treatment with varying success rates **(Box 2)**.

Conclusion

- Hypnotherapy is not a panacea for all diseases.
- Healthy body exists only where there is a healthy mind.
- Hypnotherapy can be used alone or as an adjunctive therapeutic procedure along with standard treatment to promote rapid healing and alleviate the sufferings of humanity.

Limited studies are there mentioning the usefulness of hypnotherapy in alopecia areata and Hansen's disease. It is hypothesized that hypnotherapy could provide benefit for various psychodermatological conditions like trichotillomania, factitious dermatitis, body dysmorphophobia, and other diseases like Hansen's disease neuralgia and recurrent reactions, atopic dermatitis and alopecia areata, psoriasis, etc. There are only very few studies in the world literature regarding usefulness of hypnotherapy in dermatology practice.

> **Case Vignette 1**
>
> A 35-year-old female presented with Hansen's disease—lepromatous leprosy with recurrent erythema nodosum leprosum (ENL) lesions. The patient was on multidrug therapy (MDT) for 8 months, systemic corticosteroids and thalidomide. The course of the reaction was characterized by repeated remissions and exacerbations necessitating

five admissions to the hospital during a span of 3 months. On psychological evaluation, she was observed to be depressed [Hospital Anxiety and Depression (HAD) scale-19, Dermatology Life Quality Index (DLQI)-29]. After obtaining informed consent, we subjected her for hypnoanalysis and could realize that the fear of spreading the disease to her family members was the reason for her stress. We asked her to visualize that her body was infected with the lepra bacilli and after taking the MDT, all the bacteria were killed completely and not even a single bacterium was left behind to infect her family members. After the first session, her fear was markedly decreased (HAD scale-11, DLQI-18). The ENL lesions started subsiding. We repeated two more sessions at 3 day intervals. Psychologically, she became stable (HAD scale-5, DLQI-6) and the ENL lesions subsided completely by 3 weeks. We could reduce the dose of corticosteroids and thalidomide quickly. We continued the MDT for up to 1 year and followed up with the patient for 2 years. She had no more ENL recurrences and admissions thereafter.

Case Vignette 2

A 10-year-old girl presented with generalized burning pain and itching mainly at around 7 PM. She was unable to read and sleep. Routine history taking and physical examination did not reveal any clue to the diagnosis. She was given antihistamines and analgesics, but there was no response. Due to the unusual presentation and no clue in history and physical examination, the patient was subjected to hypnoanalysis. Under hypnosis, the patient disclosed that she got the symptoms after watching a circus—the scene of a death well. That was at about 7 PM. She became afraid and got generalized burning and after that everyday at the same time, she got the same symptoms. Under hypnosis, she was asked to visualize the scene repeatedly and to relax by breathing when she feels difficulty. The procedure continued for 30 minutes. She became all right after a single sitting.

BEHAVIOR THERAPY

Behavior therapy comprises applications derived from learning theory (classical and operant conditioning) and utilizing them to the treatment of persistent, maladaptive, learned habits. The various techniques that come under this include relaxation training (e.g., autogenic and progressive muscle relaxation, biofeedback), habit-reversal training, imagery (already discussed in detail in previous chapter), systematic desensitization, assertiveness, and social skills training. The aim of these techniques is to progressively diminish maladaptive behavioral responses by repeatedly inhibiting the anxiety by means of competing responses. The clinician conducts a detailed behavior analysis to collect information about the relationship between stimuli and behavioral responses in order to understand the role of anxiety. Different behavioral therapeutic strategies have been applied, either separately or in combination with other psychological techniques, to dermatological conditions.

Systematic Desensitization

Systematic desensitization is a highly useful technique for the treatment of skin conditions with features of anticipatory anxiety. The fear and apprehension of the patients with skin disease may be challenged by this technique. This is useful in conditions like psoriasis, atopic dermatitis, and vitiligo and in infectious conditions like leprosy and sexually transmitted disease (STD) with features of anxiety. It is also useful in phobias with cutaneous symptoms. Through graded exposure, the patient enters situations that they may fear and avoid. A physiological state inhibitory of anxiety is induced in the patient by means of muscle relaxation and he is then exposed to a weak anxiety arousing stimulus for a few seconds. If the exposure is repeated several times, the stimulus progressively loses its ability to evoke anxiety. Then successively stronger stimuli are introduced and a similar procedure is repeated. This procedure enables us to overcome many neurotic habits in a short span of time.

Case Vignette

A 60-year-old man presented with generalized burning and itching, especially at night. He had lack of sleep and when he falls asleep he dreams of snakes and is very much afraid of them. Then his skin symptoms increase and he continue the rest of the night without sleep. He was on many drugs without much improvement. His snake phobia was treated with systematic desensitization. He was asked to close the eyes and relax by taking deep breath. Then he was asked to visualize a small snake for a few moments. That induced his anxiety, and he was then suggested to relax by breathing. Then he was suggested to visualize a big snake and after that multiple snakes in a graded manner and to relax by breathing when he feels anxious. This procedure was continued for 20–30 minutes. Three sessions at 3 day interval were given under guidance and he was advised to repeat it himself at home. By this procedure, his fear disappeared and skin symptoms subsided. All the drugs were stopped.

GROUP THERAPY

Group therapy is a mode of intervention that helps individuals with a common problem to enhance their social functioning through group exercises. Topic-centered group therapy is a highly effective approach in group therapy. The participants should be informed and agreed on a common topic, e.g., in psoriasis and vitiligo, "What are the problems faced in the society?" Group members are given the opportunity to share their experiences, feelings, and difficulties in a safe atmosphere. Using a combination of instruction, modeling, feedback, role play, and open discussion, members of the group are encouraged to discover more about the interaction process. This procedure may lead to embarrassment or silence initially; the facilitator of the group can take the initiative and moderate the session. The treating doctor can act in this role and he can invite at least three or more patients to this discussion. A weekly session of at least 2 hours is ideal. After the initial silence, they will slowly participate and share their difficulties faced in the society and the method of their management. The adage tells that "a problem shared is a problem halved". In my personal experience, it is a highly useful simple method for sharing their experiences in the family and society, as they come to trust and value one another and develop group cohesiveness. It will facilitate acquiring new coping skills, enhance self-esteem, manage anxieties, and prevent from social withdrawal; moreover, group members can bolster one another's self-confidence and self-acceptance. This method can be adopted in any chronic dermatological condition. It is highly useful in incurable conditions, where they will understand the coping skills from their group.

FAMILY THERAPY

Family therapy is another useful psychotherapeutic method in chronic diseases, especially dermatological conditions where skin diseases produce so many misconceptions that will affect their normal relationship, care, and support. In family therapy parents, spouses, children, siblings, and other strong support givers can be included even though not belonging to the family. There will be interpersonal problems like fear of spreading infection to family members and a feeling of lack of hygiene which will negatively affect their interpersonal relationship; for example, shaking hand, eating together, sharing utensils, sleeping together and caressing, using same toilets, and mingling with children in the family and among spouses even can affect sexual relationships. If the above problems can be solved by giving a good counseling and psychoeducation, the patient will get a good support from family. This will boost up the morale of the patient and help in sharing the problem and in turn reduce the anxiety, social withdrawal, depression, and other psychiatric comorbidities.

NEUROLINGUISTIC PROGRAMMING

Neurolinguistic programming is a simple, skillful method developed by Richard Bandler and John Grinder for studying how the brain works, people think, feel, learn, motivate themselves, interact with others, make choices, and achieve realistic goals, used by many thousands of people around the world. NLP is the process of creating models of excellence using our own nervous system (neuro-brain hardware) and our language (linguistic software) to program ourselves and others to achieve the results we want. The main objective of NLP is to increase the behavioral choices available to us and it helps us to study what goes on inside a person (the processes people use to build their unique distinctive maps or models of the world) by identifying the language and the nonverbal cues. NLP classifies individuals into visual, auditory, and kinesthetic depending upon the mode of perception. Each group of individuals has their common mode of perception and accordingly the behavior. A presupposition in NLP is that the more choices and possibilities we become aware of and make available to ourselves, the more we will become aware of and be able to fulfill our desire. The founders developed models of tools and techniques that enable anyone to change from a troubling behavior to a useful one. Various tools used in NLP for generating new behavior, communication skills, rapport establishment, visual kinesthetic dissociation (useful for phobia management), reframing (useful for cognitive therapy and cognitive behavior therapy), and NLP Swish (useful for behavior modification) are useful in the management of dermatological disorders.

CONCLUSION

Psychodermatology deals with the diseases of skin and mind. So dermatological management along with psychological intervention is essential in treatment. Familiarizing few psychological techniques will be highly useful for Dermatologists.

FURTHER READINGS

1. Harth W, Gieler U, Kusnir D, Tausk FA (Eds). Clinical management in Psychodermatology. Germany: Springer; 2009.
2. Pattabhi Ram BV. Hypnotism for Beginners. New Delhi: Pustaka Mahal; 2001.
3. Richard P, McHugh SJ (Eds). Mind with a Heart: Creative Pattern of a Personal Change. Gujarat: Sahithya Prakash Publisher; 2005.
4. Walker C, Papadopoulos L (Eds). Psychodermatology: Psychological Impact of Skin Disorders. New York: Cambridge University Press; 2005.
5. Abdul Latheef EN, Riyaz N. Hypnotherapy: A useful adjunctive therapeutic modality in Hansen's disease. Indian J Dermatol. 2014;59:166-8.
6. Wolpe J. Behaviour therapy for psychosomatic disorders. Psychosomatics. 1980;21:379-85.

CHAPTER 20

Meditation: An Experience beyond Words

Sreekanth Sukumarakurup

> **Key Messages**
> - Meditation, even if its greater dimensions are not explored, can be a useful stress reduction and relaxation technique.
> - In many scientific studies, meditation has been shown to be providing wide-ranging medical benefits.
> - Meditation systems use various techniques like contemplation, passive noticing and nonjudgmental perception, concentration, and activities that can lead to a meditative state.

INTRODUCTION

Since meditation is an experience beyond words, there is a multiplicity of definitions, sometimes conflicting and confusing to the beginners. Even though the word meditation initially meant contemplation or thinking, many meditation systems talk about a state of reduced or no thoughts and going beyond the mind. Such differences might have been due to the differences in techniques used to attain the final goal and the fact that there is some kind of thought process taught in most of the techniques initially, and in advanced stages, thoughts become lesser and lesser. Definitions vary with the method one follows, the level of advancement reached, and hence the state one has experienced. There are umpteen methods for meditation, all slowly progressing to the advanced state where only an indefinable peaceful bliss prevails. Until one is able to see things in its totality,

CHAPTER 20: Meditation: An Experience beyond Words

there may be arguments regarding definitions and the direction in which each method goes.

Since none of the available definitions of meditation is comprehensive and compatible with the various stages and diverse techniques of meditation, the author would suggest to define it as follows: Meditation is a trained or sometimes untrained thought process or contemplation (deep reflective thinking) or some specific mental or physical activities, leading initially to an inner state of peaceful and pleasant calmness, which may progress in advanced stages to a thoughtless, yet blissful state, which is sometimes referred to as pure awareness, the constant practice of which may lead a person to a realized and contented life.

If you find this difficult to understand, imagine a state where you are thoughtless, calm, and peaceful as in a deep sleep without dreams and still you are aware and experiencing it. Then you are somewhere near meditation. Meditation is actually thoughts leading to thoughtlessness, i.e., specific types of thoughts that calm down your mind, leading finally to a peaceful state of reduced or absent thoughts. It is the way of thinking that can consume all thoughts. Many of us may not digest the idea of "absence of thoughts" which occurs only in the peak levels of a true meditation and may argue that it is thought that makes us know that state. Experts in the field of meditation call it as awareness, rather than thought. The same domains within you, which experienced and knew the thoughts (which may be called the witness within you), experience in advanced stages of meditation just a plain peaceful bliss without any form or content as in a thought. The awareness of that blissful peace with nothing else may or may not be a form of thought, but the quality of it is far different from the usual thoughts we know. Far from being definite or indefinite, it gives a feeling of something infinite, where you are not thinking, but just experiencing a state where you just exist and is aware of the experience.

The advanced states of meditation described here are attainable only after years and years of practice for many, but achieving even the initial steps is helpful to most, for calming of mind and for a peaceful living. While practicing meditation, rather than expecting a jump into the final states, one should peacefully accept what one gets, as the result for the moment. "Does meditation have something beyond the material world seen or known" is beyond the scope of this book.

MEDITATION AS MEDICATION: EXPLORING THE MEDICAL BENEFITS OF MEDITATION

Scientific studies have shown benefits by meditation in many conditions like:
- Hypertension
- Post-traumatic stress disorder
- Anxiety
- Depression
- Migraine
- Cardiovascular diseases
- Pain
- Sleep disturbance in cancer survivors
- Prevention of Alzheimer's disease
- Slowing the rate of cellular aging, which has a relation to human longevity

Studies have shown that meditation can lead to decrease in muscle sympathetic nerve activity, systolic blood pressure (BP), diastolic BP, and mean arterial pressure. It has been shown that experienced meditators exhibit higher parietal-occipital electroencephalography (EEG) gamma activity during nonrapid eye movement (NREM) sleep. It is also found that meditation practitioners exhibit greater gray matter volume and fewer reported cognitive failures. Meditation has also been reported to enhance attention, memory, mood, and emotional regulation.

The dermatological relevance for meditation comes from the fact that many dermatological diseases are known to be associated with anxiety, depression, and stress. Meditation has been shown to increase the rate of improvement in psoriasis when it is done along with other modalities of treatment.

Although certain mental and physical side effects are also reported for meditation, it is an area where no definite and undisputable knowledge is available.

CLASSIFICATION

Classifications available are few and incomplete. Here, an attempt is made for devising a comprehensive classification. This classification is based on the predominant technique used in a type of meditation, although there may also be elements of other techniques in it:

- *Meditations using either (1) contemplation or (2) passive noticing and non-judgmental perception of multiple things around and inside you:* Although (1) and (2) are seemingly nonsimilar, both are attributes of thinking and many techniques use a combination of these and hence grouped together here. Examples of some age-old practices in this group are the ancient Indian "*Vedanta*"-based philosophical meditation (predominantly a contemplation about what we really are) and the medically well-explored mindfulness meditation (predominantly a passive noticing and nonjudgmental perception of multiple things happening not only outside you, but also inside your body and mind). Other known examples are meditations using a stream of philosophical or other peaceful thoughts or imagination of peaceful situations and meditations using specific feelings like love and kindness. If the contemplation is about the true nature of our self, like in *Vedanta*-based meditation, then it can be associative type or dissociative type. In associative type, the thoughts are directed toward what we really are (like thinking that I am limitless, beyond time and space), while in dissociative type, thoughts are directed toward excluding things which we are really not (like thinking that I am not anything which I see, I am not my body, etc.).
- *Concentration techniques*: Concentrating on a single thing, i.e., a picture, substance, scene, mental image, meditative music, voice or imagined voice, is used in these techniques. Concentration on something is used here as a technique to divert the mind from thoughts. Meditation by concentrating on objects like diamond, transcendental meditation by concentrating on sound, etc., are examples. The concentration need not be intense or strenuous as popularly thought; it can be just keeping the mind in a thing without distractions.
- *Meditation based on activities*: Even though you are doing nothing in the advanced states of meditation, either mentally or physically, like the way you use specific thought processes in the initial part of meditation to reach that final serene, tranquil, and almost thoughtless state, activities can also be used to reach that goal. Various "*kriya* yogas", i.e., meditation using "*kriya*" (meaning performance of an activity in Indian languages), comes under this category. Various "*pranayamas*" (regulation of the rhythm of breath), like the "*Sudarshan kriya*" are examples for this. There are occult and less-known forms of meditation, where a realized

master uses his touch or even gaze to induce the state of meditation in the student, known as "initiation". Whether such forms utilizes only the psychological effect of the situation, or is there anything more, is not known.

All the above-mentioned techniques can be practiced as either a (1) *guided meditation*, where the practitioner is following the step-by-step instructions of an experienced teacher through either recorded or real-time voice command or following steps described in a book; or a (2) *partially guided self-practiced meditation*, using accumulated knowledge already gained through hearing or reading or any other source; or a (3) *self-practiced meditation*, based on his own intuitions. Some schedules of meditation may use a mixture of techniques classified above. All of these are done either as a group meditation or as an individual meditation.

Some well-established and known systems of meditation are discussed in the following text: (Mindfulness meditation, which is an important type of meditation, is not discussed under this heading, as it is included as a separate chapter, with detailed description.)

Transcendental meditation: Even though all meditations have a state transcending the known areas of mind in the advanced stages, the name transcendental meditation is usually used for a system derived from the ancient Indian knowledge and presented to the modern world by Maharishi Mahesh Yogi. It is a sound-based meditation using "mantra". Studies have shown health benefits in conditions like cardiovascular disease, hypertension, psychological distress, and post-traumatic stress disorder.

Yoga: The practices described by the ancient Indian sage Patanjali is popular by the name Yoga. The word Yoga means *union* in Sanskrit language. It implies a union with our inner self or the higher consciousness, and the term may be applicable to other types of meditation also. But by usage it has become synonymous with the Indian system by Patanjali, even though some other Indian systems also use the term. In addition to training various physical activities, breathing techniques, and postures, and advising a philosophical and peaceful way of life, it teaches meditation. Even though the activity component of Yoga is more well known, in advanced learning, it also utilizes all techniques of meditation, including *pranayama*, contemplation, and, to some extent, the passive noticing and nonjudgmental perception. Since yoga has a physical activity component and a meditation component, it is difficult to assess whether the proven health benefits are due to the physical component or meditation component. It has been found that Yoga has considerable health benefits, including improved cognition, reduced cardiovascular risk, body mass index, BP, and diabetes. It has also been shown to influence immunity and to ameliorate joint disorders. Prenatal Yoga has also been shown to be well suited for depressed and anxious pregnant women, especially in the view of preference for nonpharmacological treatments in pregnancy. Yoga has also been shown to reduce trauma-related distress and emotional and behavioral difficulties among children.

"Vedanta"-based philosophical meditation: It is the earliest known and one of the most advanced forms of meditation which has its roots in ancient Indian civilization. Even though it has elements of other techniques also, it predominantly uses contemplation in the early stages of meditation, reaching a thoughtless and absolutely blissful pure awareness in the advanced stages. It has a wide range of techniques for going beyond the mind or in other words going beyond the known areas of mind. The inner search for the answer of the basic question, "Who am I?" is one of its components. It teaches to experience the witness inside us, i.e., the witness of every sense experience, emotion, or thought. The understanding that the real "I" is not the experience, thoughts, or emotions, but is really the "experiencer" of these, gives great insight into our real nature, which has infinite dimensions. Detached from the waves of unruly emotions, it helps to develop a personality that is stable, peaceful, and blissful. It also teaches to see things in a universal point of view, rather than in an individualistic point of view, which instantly takes off many of our worries. Vedantic philosophy is an ocean, beyond the scope of discussion here, with a variety of techniques to explore the mind and transcend.

Pranayama: It is based on regulation of breathing rhythm. *Pranayama* is used in many meditations including "*Sudarshan kriya*" and other "*kriya* yogas" that are followed by many lineages, and it is also considered a component in the traditional Yoga by Patanjali. Fast respiration without much bodily activity is sometimes one of the steps. It may induce a state of carbon dioxide washout, and this state of hypocarbia which is known to produce a dizzy mental state can probably aid in spiritual feelings or meditation. *Pranayama* should not be practiced without proper training and guidance of an experienced teacher.

Suggesting one simple and generalized method: A simplified method using elements of many techniques mentioned above is suggested here for further scientific studies. Those having psychiatric illnesses or those who are not psychologically stable enough to try new practices should avoid doing it. It is to be practised only after understanding the risk of possible physical and mental side effects, since it is an area which is not definitely understood or adequately researched. But the author has not faced any side effects on doing this, either for himself or for persons trained by him, so far.

PREMEDITATION STEPS

- Sleep adequately on the day of meditation and the days before.
- Take moderate food, not too heavy, not too light. Especially, avoid a heavy food immediately before meditation. Both a heavy meal just before meditation and a hungry abdomen can act as a hindrance.
- Physical tiredness can also be a hindrance.
- Immediately after waking up from a good sleep in the morning is the most ideal time for meditation, although any other time of the day can also be used.
- Use loose and comfortable clothing.
- Find a place, as silent and lonely as possible.
- Detach yourselves from the connection through mobile phones, as situation allows.

Posture

Comfortable sitting posture is ideal. Indian traditions advocate sitting posture with an erect spine. A too uncomfortable posture may disturb the mind in meditation and a too relaxed posture like lying down may invite sleep, the greatest enemy of meditation. But in the early days of meditation practice, where a mild relaxation may be the only benefit that can be expected, even a sleep may be considered as acceptable.

Mental Attitude

- Take a firm decision in mind that your next 10 minutes or half hour or even much more (as you grow in experience) is dedicated to meditation and you will neither want nor do anything during that period.

- Forget your external identity like being a father, mother, official status, etc., for the time being and just be a simple being, pure and untainted.
- Do not be judgmental or critical and do not analyze in between the benefits you may get. Take a "let go" attitude and decide that whatever happens, let it happen. Accepting everything contained in the moment, both outside and inside your body, is important.
- Do not concentrate intensely. Take a light, effortless attitude.
- Be alert enough to prevent drifting off to sleep. Meditation is actually walking through a ridge, where on one side simple thoughts or turbulent thoughts may unknowingly carry you away and on the other side when thoughts calm down or become nil, you may fall to sleep. It is only if you maintain the awake state that you can experience meditation.
- It has to be understood that in the initial days of practice, just a temporary calming down of mind may be the only benefit, for many. There are persons with hyperactive mind, for whom even this calming down of mind can be attained only with difficulty. Results of meditation have great interpersonal variations, and there may be persons for whom it may not be apt or easy.

MEDITATION STEPS

Each step to be done slowly with ample time for contemplation and for experiencing:
- Gently close your eyes (closed eyed meditation may be beneficial for most people in early stages, except in specific situations or in specific types of meditations).
- Notice the sounds around you. Just notice them and leave them. Just be pleasant on them. Do 'not think much or analyze about the source of sound, whether it is good or bad, etc. Just know it as pleasant waves of the nature, in the infinite background of silence. New sounds may come to your attention. Just attend them…wish them with a smile and leave them… Accept everything around you…it is just right…that is how it has to be… Be pleasant and peaceful…
- Feel relaxed and relax all your muscles one by one from toes to head or vice versa. Think about each muscle, relax it, keep the attention there for a few seconds, and be pleasant…. Relax the muscles of your right foot and toes…right calf…right thigh…. Relax

the muscles of left foot and toes...left calf...left thigh...abdomen... chest.... Relax the right hand and fingers...right forearm...right upper arm...right shoulder.... Relax the left hand and fingers...left forearm...left upper arm...left shoulder.... Relax the neck muscles.... Relax the small muscles of face, except for leaving a gentle smile on your face...and enjoy the feel.... Do not fall into sleep while you relax like this.... Just enjoy it and be aware.... For an advanced meditator, this relaxation of muscles automatically happens, once he falls into meditation.

- Feel the sensations from head to foot or vice versa. Keep the attention in your body parts one by one. No need to think...just feel it, witness it, accept it, and leave it...imagine that all the sensations are pleasant.
- Feel your respiratory movements without altering them. Leave them to their natural rhythm and just feel them. Experience the gentle touch of incoming air, with full of life, to your delicate nostrils. Feel the air leaving you only to come back as long as universe decides you to be alive...as long as nature wants you to be in this form...enjoy the loving touch by the nature and its fondling through the fresh air coming in and going out....
- Imagine that your mind is like an infinite sky and your thoughts are small clouds in it. Understand that you are not the small thought clouds but you are the infinite sky in which it arises and vanishes. Shift the attention from the thoughts to the infinite background from which thoughts arise...know that it is the real you, from which the thoughts arise.... Know the real you.... Be pleasant and peaceful....
- Think about the infinite dimensions of your mind. Your mind can reach anywhere at any time...you experience the whole universe in your mind. Your mind is vast and has thoughts and blankness. Search for the blank areas of your mind, like the cloudless areas of infinite sky, and go deep into it. Go into the peaceful calm areas deep inside you...feel the peace and joy of knowing yourself deeply....
- Watch for any thoughts and if there is any, do not go after them, but understand that you are not the thought, but you are the one who experienced the thought...shift the attention to the experiencer or witness inside you...which is the real you...which is the deeper consciousness which experience everything...which is your true self.

CHAPTER 20: Meditation: An Experience beyond Words

- Know that even your body, your official status, family, and anything else is just add-ons to the real you.
- Imagine blankness...and go deeper and deeper into that peaceful blankness.
- Feel the peace deep inside and realize that without anything else, you yourself are peaceful and happy.
- Go deep into the blank areas of your mind...feel that it is infinite, beyond time and space...you can travel millions of years backward or forward in this peaceful blankness deep inside you...and you can travel millions of miles peacefully and blissfully....
- From birth until now, your body, mind, thoughts, and attitude have changed. It will change again. Think about the unchanging witness inside you, which saw all these changes...it is the real you....
- Deep inside, be peaceful with you....
- Once you are peaceful, you may consider autosuggestions to correct the behavioral or attitude defects in you, which leads to stress. This has to be done only with the help of an experienced clinical psychologist or psychiatrist. If it is a guided meditation, the guide can give individualized suggestions. Philosophical messages can also be used.
- As the experience of meditator increases, he can reach the peaceful and pleasant thoughtless areas deep inside the mind more and more easily and can stay there blissfully without any disturbing thoughts for more and more time.
- In the initial stages, thoughts on one side and sleep on other extreme can hinder the true experience of meditation and it may be difficult to find a balance.
- When thoughts arise, do not get worried, but just accept the fact that you had a thought, and then go beyond. Also understand that this is a normal happening in early days of meditation.
- Many a time, we will know that we were driven by a thought wave, only sometime after being in that thought. Whenever we realize that we were taken off by a thought, think about the infinite background from which the thought aroused...the background which is also the real experiencer or witness inside you, which watched the thought...the background which is the real you also... fix the mind again in the stillness deep inside...in the peaceful blankness...in the bliss (if you have started experiencing it).
- When you feel that you had enough meditation for today, or after a fixed time (as set with a gentle and pleasant nondisturbing alarm

or a person entrusted to gently alert you), you can slowly open the eyes. In a guided meditation, the guide gives the instruction to open the eyes. Wait for some time before you slowly stand up. Avoid brisk and violent movements for a few minutes.
- It is always better to start with short sessions, i.e., meditation for 5-10 minutes, once or twice a day, before expanding the duration and increasing the frequency, which can be done as one gains more experience and develops more interest.

The so-called blissful states may be experienced only after years of practice, and sometimes never for many, so never make it a target for meditation. In early stages, get satisfied with the peaceful pleasant feel or at least the calming down of mind. Initially, the peaceful feel may be achieved only during the actual meditation session and is likely to be lost while you involve in other activities. It is only after practicing it for a long time that you may be able to maintain that peace, emotional stability, and bliss during routine activities also and thus actually "live in meditation".

CONCLUSION

The techniques of meditation may be diverse, and the most useful one for each person may differ, but all of them is intended to have only one conclusion, i.e., a more peaceful and meaningful life. But to conclude like that, one should not forget to invest a lot in the form of whole hearted and persistent practice.

FURTHER READINGS

1. Tolle E. Stillness Speaks, 1st edition. Mumbai: Yogi Impressions Books Pvt Ltd; 2003.
2. Tolle E. The Power of Now, 1st edition. Mumbai: Yogi Impressions Books Pvt Ltd; 2001.
3. Tejomayananda S. Meditation: A Vision, 1st edition. Mumbai: Central Chinmaya Mission Trust; 2003.
4. Tejomayananda S. Dhyanaswarupam, 1st edition. Mumbai: Central Chinmaya Mission Trust; 1997.
5. Pinto NV, Sarmento VDSM, Sousa R, Girão ÁC, Frota MA. School-Based meditation in adolescents: an integrative literature review. Int J Adolesc Med Health. 2023;35(2):159-65.
6. Feruglio S, Matiz A, Pagnoni G, Fabbro F, Crescentini C. The Impact of Mindfulness Meditation on the Wandering Mind: A Systematic Review. Neurosci Biobehav Rev. 2021;131:313-30.

7. Schutte NS, Malouff JM, Keng SL. Meditation and telomere length: a meta-analysis. Psychol Health. 2020;35(8):901-15.
8. Basso JC, McHale A, Ende V, Oberlin DJ, Suzuki WA. Brief, daily meditation enhances attention, memory, mood, and emotional regulation in non-experienced meditators. Behav Brain Res. 2019;356:208-20.
9. Nakamura Y, Lipschitz DL, Kuhn R, Kinney AY, Donaldson GW. Investigating efficacy of two brief mind-body intervention programs for managing sleep disturbance in cancer survivors: a pilot randomized controlled trial. J Cancer Surviv. 2013;7(2):165-82.
10. Serpa JG, Taylor SL, Tillisch K. Mindfulness-based stress reduction (MBSR) reduces anxiety, depression, and suicidal ideation in veterans. Med Care. 2014;52(12 Suppl 5):S19-24.
11. Rutledge T, Nidich S, Schneider RH, Mills PJ, Salerno J, Heppner P, et al. Design and rationale of a comparative effectiveness trial evaluating transcendental meditation against established therapies for PTSD. Contemp Clin Trials. 2014;39(1):50-6.
12. Davis K, Goodman SH, Leiferman J, Taylor M, Dimidjian S. A randomized controlled trial of yoga for pregnant women with symptoms of depression and anxiety. Complement Ther Clin Pract. 2015;21(3):166-72.
13. Fjorback LO . Mindfulness and bodily distress. Dan Med J. 2012;59(11):B4547.
14. Froeliger B, Garland EL, McClernon FJ. Yoga meditation practitioners exhibit greater grey matter volume and fewer reported cognitive failures: results of a preliminary voxel-based morphometric analysis. Evid Based Complement Alternat Med. 2012;2012:821307.
15. Kabat-Zinn J, Wheeler E, Light T, Skillings A, Scharl M, Cropley TG, et al. Influence of mindfulness-based stress reduction intervention on rates of skin clearing in patients with moderate to severe psoriasis undergoing phototherapy and photochemotherapy. Psychosom Med. 1998;60:625-32.
16. Kabat-Zinn J. Full Catastrophe Living, 2nd edition. London: Piatkus Books; 2013.
17. Kabat-Zinn J. Wherever You Go, There You Are: Mindfulness Meditation. In: Everyday Life, 2nd edition. New York: Hachette Books; 2005.
18. Zegal ZV, Williams JMG, Teasdale JD. Mindfulness-based Cognitive Therapy for Depression, 2nd edition. New York: Guilford Press; 2012.
19. Epel E, Daubenmier J, Moskowitz JT, Folkman S, Blackburn E. Can meditation slow rate of cellular aging? Cognitive stress, mindfulness, and telomeres. Ann N Y Acad Sci. 2009;1172:34-53.
20. Khalsa DS. Stress, Meditation, and Alzheimer's Disease Prevention: Where The Evidence Stands. J Alzheimers Dis. 2015;48(1):1-12.

CHAPTER 21

Mindfulness-based Therapies for Dermatological Disorders

Mahesh MM

> **Key Messages**
> - Dermatological disorders can significantly affect an individual's mental health.
> - Mindfulness-based therapy is a holistic approach for addressing both the psychological and physical elements of dermatological disorders.
> - Mindfulness, attempts to minimize the impact of the patient's thoughts by changing their relationship to thoughts rather than modifying the content.
> - This chapter illustrates the use of mindfulness-based therapies as an adjunct for the management of psychological elements of dermatological issues.

INTRODUCTION

Dermatological disorders encompass a wide range of conditions that affect the skin, hair, and nails, impacting millions of individuals. Significant morbidity occurs worldwide as a result of skin and subcutaneous illness. Skin disorders cause a large amount of disability even if they have a low fatality rate. In the Global burden of disease study 2017, skin disease ranked 10th. These disorders can have significant physical and psychological effects on those who suffer from them. Dermatological disorders can significantly impact an individual's mental health. Patients may experience anxiety, depression, social isolation, and decreased self-esteem due to their skin condition. These psychological effects can exacerbate the physical symptoms and hinder effective treatment.

While traditional medical treatments are often effective in managing the physical symptoms, the psychological impact of dermatological disorders is sometimes overlooked. A holistic approach to addressing both the psychological and physical elements of dermatological disorders is provided by mindfulness-based therapies. It is a complementary approach that takes psychological and emotional elements of these disorders, while the conventional medical therapies emphasize on managing the physical symptoms. This chapter examines the use of mindfulness-based therapies as an adjunct therapy for the management of psychological elements of dermatological issues, with a focus on their potential advantages and significance in improving general patient care.

Psychodermatology studies the relationship between the mind and skin. Psychological states that are linked to skin conditions can be classified into three main groups (proposed by Koo and Lebwohl, 2001)—(1) Psychophysiological disorders, (2) Primary psychiatric disorders, and (3) Secondary psychiatric disorders. For example, stress can worsen psoriasis, a psychophysiological condition. Psychological issues such as depression and anxiety were more prevalent in psoriasis patients. If we look into the psychoneuroimmunology explanation, the stress leads to psoriasis exacerbation due to the alteration in the function of hypothalamic-pituitary-adrenal (HPA) axis and in the cortisol level. This will lead to a change in the production of proinflammatory cytokines that are involved in the pathogenesis of psoriasis.

MINDFULNESS-BASED THERAPIES: AN OVERVIEW

Mindfulness-based therapies, rooted in ancient Buddhist practices, have gained widespread recognition in recent years for their potential to promote overall well-being and alleviate a range of physical and psychological health conditions. Kabat-Zinn (1990) defined mindfulness as "paying attention in a particular way; on purpose, in the present moment, and non-judgmentally." Mindfulness-based therapies focus on cultivating mindfulness, which involves paying non-judgmental attention to the present moment. Mindfulness-based Stress Reduction (MBSR) and Mindfulness-based Cognitive Therapy (MBCT) are two well-established mindfulness-based interventions. MBSR, developed by Jon Kabat-Zinn in the late 1970s, helps individuals manage stress and chronic pain. MBCT, a more recent adaptation, integrates mindfulness practices with cognitive behavioral therapy (CBT) techniques to prevent relapse in individuals with recurrent depressive disorders. Later specific protocols were developed for anxiety, obsessive-compulsive disorder (OCD), substance abuse disorders, etc. However, MBCT is imparted within a cognitive framework that involves exercises and techniques aimed at recognizing patterns linked to a particular condition. This includes understanding how emotions, thoughts, and behaviors interplay in sustaining anxiety or depression.

THE PROCESS OF MINDFULNESS IN SKIN DISORDERS

The underlying mental mechanisms of mindfulness suggest that reality can be apprehended through present-moment physical and bodily perception, as emphasized in mindfulness-based interventions. In contrast, cognitive behavioral therapy operates on the premise that reality is perceived through cognitive processes. The objective of CBT is to cultivate a metacognitive perspective, empowering patients to identify and challenge unhelpful or negative thought patterns, as highlighted by Westbrook, Kennerley, and Kirk in 2011. Reaching a metacognitive state, according to mindfulness-based interventions, enables people to recognize the connections between their thoughts, feelings, and behaviors. Then, by improving attention control and engaging in mindfulness training, the person have the option to stay in the present moment and experience the physical sensations rather than automatically reverting to negative thought patterns. Contrary to mindfulness-based therapies, CBT promotes cognitive challenge.

It has been shown that mindfulness practice increases our ability to focus and sustain our attention. This has relevance to dermatological patients, whose distress may be exacerbated by having their focus repeatedly pulled to the itchy sensation. Itching and scratching cycles can be painful and irritating; therefore, the goal of practicing mindfulness is not just to escape this sensation but rather to treat it with the same level of attention as other elements of experience. We can more clearly examine our own thought processes and ideas as thoughts by practicing mindful awareness. This may enable us to respond to them less automatically and more deliberately. It may also make it possible for us to ponder less distressingly, ineffectively, endlessly, or ruminatively. For instance, a person with dermatological issues might become more conscious of their fear that others are staring at their skin and better able to discern whether this is indeed the case in any given circumstances. In order to accomplish what is most important, they may also be better equipped to decide whether to avoid or enter a scenario where this might occur. We can more clearly examine our own thought processes and identify our ideas as thoughts by practicing mindfulness awareness. This may allow us to respond to them less automatically and more deliberately. There are a number of reasons to believe that MBCT may be especially useful for treating anxiety-related issues.

- Unlike conventional CBT, mindfulness attempts to minimize the impact of the patient's thoughts by changing their relationship to their thoughts rather than modifying the content of the patient's thoughts by confirming undesirable predictions.
- Second, mindfulness can minimize unhelpful rumination which has been found to maintain both anxiety and depression. Mindfulness assist the patients to develop general attentional control skills, so they may overcome the habit of paying excessive attention to body sensations, which causes escalation of anxiety through ruminating possible implications of these sensations.

RATIONALE FOR MINDFULNESS-BASED THERAPIES IN SKIN DISORDERS

- The main objective of mindfulness-based therapies is to create a new, more accepting relationship with experience (i.e., the patient able to accept the thoughts/sensations as it is).
- Mindfulness-based therapies will be expected to have an impact on many of the mechanisms associated in the persistence of negative emotions within the cognitive behavioral frameworks proposed by Salkovskis and Warwick in 2001, which include hypervigilance to bodily sensations and misunderstanding of signals such as intolerance of worry, rumination, uncertainty, and avoidance. In the following text, we will go through various ways in which MBCT might influence these systems:
  1. *Reacting versus responding*: In CBT model conceptualizations, responses to anxiety triggers, such as noticing a bodily sensation and giving it a negative interpretation, include oscillating between avoidance and suppression as well as

ruminating on the sensation's potential meaning. Such reactions have the consequence of escalating concern and upholding worry. This is typical of the doing mode of thinking, which tries to find unhelpful solutions to the "problem" of suffering in order to reduce unpleasant emotional experiences. As a result, for instance, noting shortness of breath can bring up thoughts of the person's burial. This increases the anxiety and the feeling of uncertainty about the future, which worsens the shortness of breath and causes other bodily symptoms that increase the anxiety and magnifying the body sensations. The use of coping mechanisms such as trying to cover up or avoid the sensations, images and accompanying emotions, or obsessing about possible causes for the symptom, are then engaged in an effort to alleviate the distress. This negative thought (worrying/rumination) increases/maintains the emotional issues, but the evidence shows that the mindfulness-based therapies are effective in reducing it. Thoughts and images are not intended to be changed; mindfulness-based therapies rather aim to lessen their impact by promoting a decentered approach to both of them and the response that results from them. The goal is to stop the spiral of escalation that may otherwise result in rumination, chronic avoidance, or anxious preoccupation. This ability to digest events in a distinct mental mode ("being" rather than doing) opens the door to the potential of choosing how to react in a flexible manner as opposed to reacting in a habitual manner. The ability to approach and engage with the event rather than run away from it is of utmost importance in the MBCT approach in building flexibility of reactions to stressful experiences.

2. *Engagement with present moment:* In anxiety or in depression, the patient is living with thoughts connected to their future- or past-oriented incidents. These patients experience unhappiness or is disconnected with their present and it leads to negative emotions. Way et al. (2010) demonstrated that a long-term disconnection with the present moments develop a chronic over reactivity of limbic system and to stress and emotional reactivity. One of the goals of mindfulness-based therapies are to reclaim the enjoyment of everyday life experiences, which is incompatible with the self-and future-focused elaborations that are typical of anxiety issues.

Normally, a mindfulness-based therapy protocol begins with the evaluation of patient's suitability for the program, also develops an individual problem formulation, considers how mindfulness-based therapy can be useful, and goes over what to expect throughout the course. According to Segal et al. (2002), the remaining sessions are given in a group setting across 8/12 weekly sessions lasting 2 hours each. Participants are expected to commit to the course by engaging in daily practices and other homework assignments. The interaction with the participants is similar to that of a teacher with a class, and the topics of conversation are frequently related to what the participants have noticed during the mindfulness and other activities. Other than the educational aspects, all the protocols are incorporated with different mindfulness activities such as mindfulness of the breath, raisin exercise, body scan meditation, mindfulness of the movement, mindfulness of the sound, touch, etc. The script of the basic practice is given below.

Mindful Breath

Mindful breathing is a simple yet powerful mindfulness meditation technique that can help you become more present and reduce stress and anxiety.

Procedure

- *Find a comfortable position*: It is essential to be in a comfortable position, so that you can fully focus on your breath. Sitting or lying down is preferable because it reduces distractions and allows for relaxation.
- *Choose your eye position:* While you can practice mindful breathing with your eyes open, many people find it easier to maintain their focus with their eyes closed. Closing eyes can help you redirect your attention inward.
- *Focus on your breath*: Direct your attention to your breath. Observe the natural rhythm of your inhales and exhales. Pay close attention to the physical sensations associated with breathing, such as the rise and fall of your chest or the feeling of air passing through your nostrils.
- *Stay present*: As you focus on your breath, it is common for your mind wander. When you notice thoughts drifting, gently bring

your attention back to your breath without judgment. This process of redirecting your focus is a fundamental aspect of mindfulness practice.
- *Focus on sensations*: Dive deeper into your observation by noticing the specific sensations associated with each breath. These sensations might include the expansion and contraction of the abdomen or chest, the feeling of the air moving in and out, or the temperature of the breath. Pay attention to these sensations one breath at a time.
- *Continuous awareness*: Keep your awareness focused on the breath, maintain a continuous awareness as one breath ends and the next one begins. This flow of attention helps you stay fully present in the moment.

Raisin Exercise: Procedure

- *Holding*: First, take a raisin and hold it in the palm of your hand or between your finger and thumb. Imagine that you have just dropped in from Mars and have never seen an object like this before in your life.
- *Seeing*: Take time to really focus on it; gaze at the raisin with care and full attention. Let your eyes explore every part of it. Examine the highlights where the light shines, the darker hollows, the folds and ridges, and any uneven parts or unique features.
- *Touching*: Turn the raisin over between your fingers, exploring its texture. Try doing this with your eyes closed if that enhances your sense of touch.
- *Smelling*: Hold the raisin beneath your nose. With each breath in, take in any smell, aroma, or fragrance that may arise. As you do this, notice anything interesting that may be happening in your mouth or stomach.
- *Placing*: Now slowly bring the raisin up to your lips, noticing how your hand and arm know exactly how and where to position it. Gently place the raisin in your mouth; without chewing, noticing how it gets into your mouth in the first place. Spend a few moments focusing on the sensations of having it in your mouth, exploring it with your tongue.
- *Tasting*: When you are ready, prepare to chew the raisin, noticing how and where it needs to be for chewing. Then, very consciously, take one or two bites into it and notice what happens in the aftermath. Place close attention to any waves of taste that come

from it as you continue chewing. Without swallowing yet, notice the bare sensations of taste and texture in your mouth and how these may change over time, moment by moment. Also pay attention to any changes in the raisin itself.
- *Swallowing*: When you feel ready to swallow the raisin, see if you can first notice the urge to swallow as it comes up, so that even this is experienced consciously before you actually swallow the raisin.
- *Following*: Finally, see if you can feel what is left of the raisin moving down into your stomach, and sense how your body as a whole is feeling after you have completed this exercise.

Body Scan Meditation

Body scan meditation involves paying focused and nonjudgmental attention to each part of your body, starting from your toes and moving up to the top of your head. It is a great way to relax, reduce stress, and increase body awareness.

Procedure

Begin by finding a comfortable and quiet place to sit or lie down. Close your eyes if you feel comfortable doing so. Take a few deep breaths in through your nose and out through your mouth to help you relax. Allow yourself to be fully present in this moment.
- *Toes*: Bring your attention to your toes. Notice any sensations in your toes—warmth, tingling, or tension. Breathe into your toes, allowing them to relax. Imagine any tension melting away with each breath.
- *Feet*: Now, shift your focus to your feet. Feel the soles of your feet against the floor or bed. Pay attention to any sensations, and with each breath, let go of any tension or discomfort you might be holding in your feet.
- *Ankles and calves*: Continue to move your attention up to your ankles and calves. Notice any sensations, any tightness, or relaxation. Breathe into this area and release any tension as you exhale.
- *Knees and thighs*: Shift your awareness to your knees and thighs. Feel the weight of your legs against the surface you are on. Notice any sensations in your knees and thighs. Breathe into this area, letting go of any tension.

- *Hips and pelvis*: Now, move your attention to your hips and pelvis. Notice how they make contact with the surface beneath you. Feel any sensations in this area, and as you breathe, allow any tension to dissolve.
- *Lower back and abdomen*: Bring your awareness to your lower back and abdomen. Notice the rise and fall of your abdomen with each breath. If you notice any tightness or discomfort, let it go with your exhale.
- *Chest and upper back*: Shift your focus to your chest and upper back. Become aware of your breath as it moves in and out of your chest. Feel the expansion and relaxation with each breath.
- *Shoulders and arms*: Move your attention to your shoulders and arms. Notice any sensations, any areas of tension. Breathe into this space, allowing your shoulders and arms to feel heavy and relaxed.
- *Hands*: Bring your awareness to your hands. Notice any sensations in your fingers and palms. If there's any tension, let it melt away with your breath.
- *Neck and throat*: Shift your focus to your neck and throat. Feel any sensations in this area, any tightness or relaxation. Breathe into your neck and throat, allowing them to soften.
- *Face*: Now, bring your attention to your face. Notice any sensations in your forehead, cheeks, and jaw. Allow your face to relax completely, letting go of any tension.
- *Head*: Finally, bring your attention to the top of your head. Feel the sensations at the crown of your head. Breathe into this area, allowing any remaining tension to dissolve.

Take out a few moments to simply rest in this state of relaxation and awareness. Notice how your body feels as a whole. When you are ready, slowly begin to reawaken your body, wiggling your fingers and toes, and gently opening your eyes. The body scan meditation can be as short or as long as you like, depending on your available time and preferences. It's a practice that can help you become more attuned to your body, reduce stress, and cultivate mindfulness in your everyday life.

Normally a mindfulness-based CBT protocol for skin disorder can be outlined as:

- *Session 1:* Introduction to MBCT for skin disorder (introduction, overview of the course, introduction to mindfulness, discussion on the relationship between stress, emotions, and skin disorders such as psoriasis)

- *Session 2:* Recognizing automatic pilot (understanding the autopilot mode, mindfulness of breath and sensations)
- *Session 3:* Becoming an observer of thoughts—recognizing thought patterns related to psoriasis
- *Session 4:* Mindfulness of body and breath—body scan meditation, mindful yoga
- *Session 5:* Acceptance and self-compassion—exploring self-compassion and self-criticism, and self-compassion meditation
- *Session 6:* Working with difficult emotions—identifying and working with difficult emotions related to psoriasis and emotion-regulation strategies
- *Session 7:* Relapse prevention and follow-up—strategies to prevent relapse and manage stress, creating a personal plan for managing psoriasis and stress
- *Session 8:* Integration and moving forward—sharing experiences and progress, maintaining a mindfulness practice and resources for ongoing support

Throughout the program, participants are encouraged to maintain a daily mindfulness practice, complete weekly homework assignments, and keep a journal to track their progress and experiences.

By enhancing awareness of internal mental and physical states, mindfulness can empower individuals to attain a heightened sense of command over their thoughts, emotions, and actions in the present moment. Being more attentive to the sensations of eating has the potential to heighten our enjoyment of food and enrich our gratitude for the chance to satisfy our hunger. Mindfulness can additionally assist individuals in tuning into hunger and fullness signals, thereby helping to prevent overeating or engaging in "emotional eating." As expressed by mindfulness expert, Jon Kabat-Zinn, "When we taste with attention, even the simplest foods provide a universe of sensory experience."

Developing a consistent mindfulness meditation practice, including mindful breathing, can lead to better results over time. It helps train your mind to be more present and resilient, making it easier to use this technique during challenging situations. Remember that mindfulness is a skill that improves with practice.

CONCLUSION

The intended effects of mindfulness-based therapies are to decrease negative automatic threat appraisals and promote approach-coping mechanisms and increase the patient's adaptability responses to the symptoms. Mindfulness-based therapies do not try to question the basis of cognitions. Theoretically, mindfulness could lessen stress levels, which in turn, could reduce the severity of the condition through the hypothalamic-pituitary-adrenal axis cortisol immune system route. Mindfulness also helps the people to reduce the quality of life impairment and promote acceptance-based coping mechanisms. The mindfulness-based practices help the patient to enhance the physical and psychological well-being.

FURTHER READINGS

1. Teasdale WM, Segal JZ, Kabat-Zinn J. Eating One Raisin: A First Taste of Mindfulness. The Mindful Way through Depression: Freeing Yourself from Chronic Unhappiness. New York: Guilford Press; 2007.
2. Heeren A, Philippot P. Changes in ruminative thinking mediate the clinical benefits of mindfulness: Preliminary findings. Mindfulness. 2011;2:8-13.
3. Hutton J. How can mindfulness help patients with skin conditions. Dermatol Nurs. 2016;15(3):32-5.
4. McManus F, Surawy C, Muse K, Vazquez-Montez M, Williams JMG. A randomized clinical trial of mindfulness-based cognitive therapy versus unrestricted services for health anxiety (hypochondriasis). J Consult Clin Psychol. 2012;80(5):817-28.
5. Michalak J, Hölz A, Teismann T. Rumination as a predictor of relapse in mindfulness-based cognitive therapy for depression. Psychol Psychother: Theory Res Pract. 2011;84(2):230-6.
6. Muse K, McManus F, Hackmann A, Williams M, Williams M. Intrusive imagery in severe health anxiety: Prevalence, nature and links with memories and maintenance cycles. Behaviour research and therapy. 2010;48(8):792-8.
7. Salkovskis PM, Warwick HM. Meaning, Misinterpretations, and Medicine: A Cognitive. In: Starcevic V, Lipsitt DR. Hypochondriasis: Modern Perspectives on an Ancient Malady. UK: Oxford University Press; 2001. pp. 202-222.
8. Segal ZV, Teasdale JD, Williams JM, GemarMC. The mindfulness-based cognitive therapy adherence scale: Inter-rater reliability, adherence to protocol and treatment distinctiveness. Clin Psychol Psychother. 2002;9(2):131-8.
9. Segal ZV, Williams JMG, Teasdale JD. Mindfulness based cognitive therapy for depression: A new approach to preventing relapse. New York: Guilford Press; 2002.
10. Surawy C, McManus F, Muse K, Williams JMG. Mindfulness-based cognitive therapy (MBCT) for health anxiety (hypochondriasis): Rationale, implementation and case illustration. Mindfulness. 2015;6:382-92.

11. Teasdale JD, Segal ZV, Williams JMG. How does cognitive therapy prevent depressive relapse and why should attentional control (mindfulness) training help? Behav Res Ther.1995;33:25-39.
12. Way BM, Creswell JD, Eisenberger NI, Lieberman MD. Dispositional mindfulness and depressive symptomatology: correlations with limbic and self-referential neural activity during rest. Emotion. 2010;10(1):12-24.
13. Wells A (Ed). Hypochondriasis and health anxiety. Cognitive therapy of anxiety disorders. Chichester: Wiley; 1997.
14. Wells A, White J, Carter K. Attention training: Effects on anxiety and beliefs in panic and social phobia. Clin Psychol Psychother. 1997;4(4):226-32.
15. Westbrook D, Kennerley H, Kirk J. An Introduction to Cognitive Behaviour Therapy: Skills and Applications. USA: Sage; 2011.

CHAPTER 22

Drug Treatment of Psychodermatological Conditions

Harish M Tharayil

> **Key Messages**
> - Psychiatric comorbidity is common in many dermatological conditions. Antipsychotics, antidepressants, mood stabilizers, and anxiolytics may be needed for their management.
> - Watch for emergence of Parkinsonian side effects/dystonia in the first few weeks of starting antipsychotic drugs.
> - Antipsychotics are indicated in delusions (e.g., infestations, body odor) and hallucinations (tactile, visual or auditory).
> - Mild sedation may occur during the initial days after starting most psychotropic drugs. Patients have to be warned about this.
> - Antidepressants are used in the management of depression and anxiety.
> - Benzodiazepines can be used for short-term relief of anxiety (3–4 weeks) and better to avoid for long-term use due to high risk of dependence and abuse.
> - Mood stabilizers are used for acute treatment and prophylaxis in bipolar disorders.
> - Z drugs are used for insomnia if it is not fully responding to primary drugs such as antipsychotics or antidepressants.

Note: The following descriptions are only brief notes on few psychotropic drugs and do not claim to be authoritative textbook or reference material on psychopharmacology. It is a handbook for providing basic information. Though written based on information available in different standard textbooks and other sources, this information has to be cross-checked and corroborated with other more authentic sources before being used on individual patients.

Individual doctor has to exercise extreme caution while using psychotropic drugs on patients under his care and has to familiarize themselves by reading such sources or undergoing further practical/clinical training.

INTRODUCTION

Psychiatric symptoms in dermatological disorders can be treated using different modalities. These include medications and psychosocial therapies. Both approaches are helpful individually and in some situations can be combined with more benefit to the patient. The major psychiatric problems seen in these patients are anxiety, depression, and psychotic symptoms (delusions and erroneous beliefs, tactile or other hallucinations). Medications are highly effective in all these conditions.

Newer drugs are being added to the list of psychotropic drug making it a bit difficult for an average practitioner to be up-to-date in this area. Hence, it is better to familiarize with a few drugs from each class and use them repeatedly to gain confidence.

A basic dictum in psychopharmacology:
- *Start low*: Start with a low dose. This will ensure that side effects such as sedation are minimized. Many patients are afraid to take drugs that affect their mental functions for various reasons. The uneducated accept these drugs more readily than the educated class. Usual reasons are fear of excessive sedation, fear of being dependent on the drug, and in some persons, a refusal to accept that they have a mental illness.
- Some clinicians may start these drugs without revealing the true nature of the drug because of many reasons. These include fear that the patient may refuse to accept the idea of psychological causation for their symptoms or fear of nonadherence. Lack of time limits, the busy clinician's desire to address all the concerns of the patient. An open discussion addressing these fears is the best way to deal with all these issues. It is always better to be honest with patients. In this era of information explosion, they may definitely find out more about the drug they are taking as it is only a matter of a few clicks on the keyboard of a computer. This can lead to loss of trust and break in the therapeutic alliance.

- *Go slow*: Titrate upward slowly. Rapid uptitration again increases the risk of side effects. The brain's neurotransmitter system adjusts to the presence of the drug in a few days, and hence, most side effects, especially sedation is not felt after the initial 3-5 days. Increasing the dose every 3-5 days is the best option for most psychotropic drugs.
- *Continue to go*: Do not stop at the first report of symptom reduction. This is only response (or remission) and not recovery. Response is defined as the reduction in intensity of the symptoms after the drug use started. Remission is defined as around 50% reduction of the symptoms on a standard rating scale used to measure that particular symptom. For example, a reduction of score by 50% on the Hamilton depression rating scale from the baseline in a given patient.
- *Taper off slowly*: When stopping these drugs, taper off gradually. This is because many drugs give rise to discontinuation symptoms on abrupt cessation. This could be serious [like neuroleptic malignant syndrome (NMS) on sudden withdrawal of antipsychotics to vomiting when antidepressants are stopped]. Hence, place the patient under follow-up till the drug is fully stopped and for few more weeks to detect any signs of relapse or recurrence.
- *Always think beyond drugs*: Recovery is a slower process and many other factors other than drugs and compliance have to be looked. Providing opportunities to discuss problems they face, allowing ventilation of pent up emotions, offering support, etc., help to improve therapeutic alliance and hasten recovery.

WORKING CLASSIFICATION

A simple classification of psychotropic drugs based on the major actions:
- Antipsychotics—earlier called major tranquilizers. These are drugs used in major psychotic disorders such as schizophrenia, bipolar disorder
- Antidepressants—drugs used for treatment of condition with depressive and anxiety symptoms
- Anxiolytics—for relief of anxiety symptoms
- Mood stabilizers—drugs used for control of manic phase of bipolar disorders. These are also used for preventing recurrence of mood episodes in such patients

- Anti-Parkinsonian agents—usually used to prevent occurrence of extrapyramidal symptoms in patients who are receiving antipsychotic drugs
- Stimulants—used for treatment of attention deficit hyperactivity disorder (ADHD) in children
- Drugs useful in addictions—used as anticraving agents/deterrents for maintaining abstinence preventing relapse in addiction medicine
- Drugs used in dementia
- Adjuvants.

Only few drugs from the following groups shall be included in this brief overview:
- Antipsychotics
- Antidepressants
- Anxiolytics—Benzodiazepines (BDZ)
- Non-BDZ hypnotics
- Mood stabilizers
- Anti-Parkinsonian agents
- Adjuvants

CHOOSING A DRUG: SOME TIPS

Choice of drugs in psychopharmacology is usually based on:
- *Diagnosis*: Diagnosis is made based on the prominent symptoms reported by the patient and confirmed by the clinician after thorough assessment of the mental state of the patient. Underlying organic disorders, which may have a role in causation, have to be ruled out before concluding that the condition is a primary psychiatric disorder.
- *Target symptoms*: These are the symptoms present in a patient leading to the consultation for disease/distress/disability. In psychiatry, these could be anxious mood, worries, depressed mood, feelings of worthlessness and fatigue, insomnia, reduced appetite, weight loss, and suicidal ideations. Findings on the mental status examination such as delusions, hallucinations, and thought disorders, and can also be target symptoms. Obsessions and compulsions are the target symptoms in obsessive compulsive disorders (OCDs). Thus, target symptoms vary depending on the diagnosis. However, no patient will have all the typical symptoms of the condition he is suffering from and many patients have atypical

or unusual symptoms not fully explainable by their diagnosis. Hence, all the symptoms to be addressed during treatment of an individual patient have to be accurately identified and listed at the start of the treatment. This also helps to monitor progress besides helping with the choice of the drugs. Appropriate rating scales can be used to determine severity and assess progress on follow-up.
- *Side effect profile*: The prescribing doctor should have a clear idea of the important side effects of the molecule he has chosen. In some situations, the side effects can be used beneficially in a patient. For example, the anticholinergic action of a tricyclic antidepressant (TCA) can reduce psychogenic vomiting in a depressed or anxious patient. Similarly, antihistaminic effects may help to improve appetite in some patients. Sedation is beneficial in some agitated patients, especially in the early phase of treatment.
- *Patient preferences*: Many of these conditions are chronic or recurring. It is better to deal with the patient using the chronic illness mode. In such conditions, the clinician has to discuss with the patient and sometimes consider or accept the suggestion put forward by him or her. This also increases adherence to treatment.
- Basic medical/surgical conditions if any have to be considered before choosing drug. For example, atypical antipsychotics like olanzapine and clozapine are better avoided in obese patients and those with diabetes mellitus or with high risk of developing this.
- *Drug interactions, especially cytochrome P450 (CYP450) system*: Most drugs including many psychotropic drugs are metabolized by enzymes from this system. This has to be borne in mind while prescribing to persons who are already on other medications.
  - Treatment is planned based also on the severity of symptoms, availability of drugs, and cost. In general, it can be said that older drugs (typical antipsychotics, TCAs, diazepam, etc.) are cheaper than the newer drugs of the same group [atypical antipsychotics, serotonin selective reuptake inhibitors (SSRIs), clonazepam, etc.].
  - Education of the patient and family is vital to ensure compliance and follow-up of care.
  - Concerns regarding adverse effects to be discussed and other options considered.
  - It may be good to seek their ideas about the cause of illness in some situations.

- Dose is titrated on the basis of response and side effects.
- Psychosocial interventions and behavioral modifications can be used with good benefit, especially before the onset of the action of the drug.

ANTIPSYCHOTICS

These drugs act by blocking the dopamine receptors in various regions of the brain. Based on their affinity for the D2 receptor, they are classified as typical and atypical. Typicals include phenothiazines, thioxanthenes, and few others. Phenothiazines are the most widely used ones and are divided in to three based on their side chain—chlorpromazine (aliphatic), fluphenazine (piperazine), and thioridazine (piperidone). The most commonly used parenteral antipsychotic to control aggression/violence in an acute setting is haloperidol. This is a typical drug belonging butyrophenone family. It is usual dose for this indication is 5–10 mg given IM or IV. The atypicals act on other subtypes of dopamine receptors as well as on some of the serotonin receptors.

Typical Antipsychotics

- *First-generation drugs*: Mainly act by blocking D2 receptors.
- *Chlorpromazine*: Usual dosage is 50–900 mg. Sedation, increased appetite, acute dystonia, parkinsonism, etc., are the common side effects.
- *Trifluoperazine*: Usual dose range is 5–30 mg. Though effective, it is not used less commonly nowadays. Hence, availability may be an issue.
- *Thioridazine*: Usual dose range is 50–400 mg. It is not widely used now due to reports of cardiac toxicity and risk of developing retinitis pigmentosa.
- *Haloperidol*: Usual dosage is between 2.5 and 20 mg. Acute dystonia and Parkinsonism are the usual side effects. Sedation is not as severe as with chlorpromazine. It is available in injectable form, and hence, can be used in acute excitement.
- *Fluphenazine*: Usual dose range is 2–15 mg. Tablets are not freely available. It is the most common antipsychotic used as a depot injection.

Atypical Antipsychotics

These are also called second-generation antipsychotics (SGA).

It is also called serotonin-dopamine antagonists (SDAs) as they act on the dopamine and serotonin systems.

It is easy to divide them into two groups based on the similarity of their names.

- *Dons include*:
  - Risperidone: Usual dose range is 0.5–8 mg/day in two divided doses
  - Ziprasidone
  - Iloperidone
  - Lurasidone

  This group has increased propensity for extrapyramidal symptoms such as acute dystonia, Parkinsonism. Increased prolactin secretion may lead to amenorrhea and galactorrhea in females. This may lead to gynecomastia and sexual dysfunctions in males.

- *Pines include*:
  - *Olanzapine*: Usual dose range is 2.5–20 mg/day in two divided doses. An injectable form is also available.
  - *Quetiapine*: Usual dose range is 12.5–30 mg in single or two divided doses.
  - *Clozapine*: Used in resistant cases. Side effects include agranulocytosis, sedation, weight gain, and metabolic syndrome. It is an atypical drug. Monitoring of total and differential leukocyte counts needed to be done periodically to detect low WBC count especially, neutropenia. It can also cause myocarditis.

  This group has higher propensity to produce weight gain, leading to higher risk of developing diabetes mellitus and coronary heart disease.

- *Newer drugs*:
  - *Aripiprazole*: Usual dose range is 2.5–15 mg/day in single or two divided doses. It has a much more favorable side effect profile as it has very little risk of developing extrapyramidal and metabolic side effects compared to other atypical drugs.
  - *Brexpiprazole*: Partial agonist of D2. Structurally similar to Aripiprazole.
  - *Cariprazine*: D3/D2 receptor partial agonist Acts on 5 HT 1A, @B, @A, 2C too. Available in 1.5–6 mg doses.

- *Depot preparations:*
  - Depot fluphenazine 12.5-50 mg IM once in every 2 or 3 weeks
  - Depot haloperidol 50/100 mg monthly once deep IM
  - Aripiprazole extended-release injections

Indications

Delusional disorders such as monosymptomatic hypochondriac psychosis (including dysmorphophobic delusions), delusional parasitosis, other conditions with delusions (delusions of body odor, halitosis, etc.) and/or hallucinations, and severe agitation.

In Psychiatry

Schizophrenia, manic phase of bipolar disorder, severe depression with psychotic features in both bipolar and unipolar depression, organic psychoses, and delirium.

Mechanism of Action of Antipsychotics

- First-generation drugs are predominantly dopamine D2 type receptor blockers. This gives the therapeutic effect and extrapyramidal symptoms.
- SGAs are serotonin and dopamine blockers. Added benefit claimed is the efficacy against negative symptoms in schizophrenia.
- Choice of drug is based on side effect profile, age, and present clinical situation.
- In addition to this, both these drugs also act on other neurotransmitters. This causes following side effects:
  - Sedation, weight gain—histamine blockade
  - Constipation, urinary retention—anticholinergic action
  - Sexual dysfunction—raised prolactin
  - Cardiac/hypotension—sympatholytic

Side-effects

- Acute neurological—sedation, increased risk for seizures, Parkinsonism, dystonia, akathisia, and neuroleptic malignant syndrome.

- Acute dystonia and other extrapyramidal syndromes:
  - Dystonia is a painful contraction of a small group of muscles, develops with oral drugs within 24–72 hours. With IM or IV administration it happens within minutes
  - Can be treated with anticholinergic IV (usually injection promethazine IM/IV)
  - Response within 5–15 minutes. Oral trihexyphenidyl has to be started in such patients
  - Other extrapyramidal symptoms include—Oculogyric crisis, torticollis
  - Retrocollis, tongue protruding, grimacing
  - Treatment is with anticholinergics for dystonia
  - Differential diagnosis (D/D): Conversion disorder, other movement disorders
- *Drug-induced Parkinsonism*:
  - Develops within 5–90 days of starting antipsychotics
  - Features: Tremor, rigidity (lead pipe/cogwheel), akinesia/hypokinesia, postural instability. Other features—shuffling gait, stooped posture, drooling of saliva, mask-like face
- *Treatment*:
  - Treated with anticholinergics such as benzhexol, trihexyphenidyl, and procyclidine
  - Continued treatment is needed
- *Akathisia*:
  - Most distressing and under recognized side effect. Subjective and objective feeling of restlessness, more in lower limbs with urge to move the legs
  - Movements are swinging of legs, rocking off of foot, pacing
  - Inability to sit or stand still
  - Develops within four weeks
  - D/D: Anxiety disorder, aggravation of psychosis
- *Treatment*:
  - Reduce dose of drug (or slower increase of dose)
  - Propranolol, benzodiazepines such as diazepam, lorazepam
  - Switch to atypical or to clozapine if there is no improvement

Neuroleptic Malignant Syndrome

- Hyperpyrexia, muscle rigidity, altered mental status, autonomic dysfunction symptoms like fluctuating blood pressure, myolysis leading to myoglobinuria, and renal shutdown

- Usually develops soon after initiation or dose hike of antipsychotic. Can happen immediately after sudden stoppage, especially if the patient was on higher doses
- Leukocytosis, elevated C-reactive protein (CRP), high erythrocyte sedimentation rate (ESR)
- Risk factors—high-potency antipsychotics, high dose, use of depot, past similar episode, age < 40 years, male
- *Treatment*:
    - Stop the offending drugs
    - General supportive measures, attention to feeding and hydration, cooling blanket
    - Watch urine output and color, cardiac monitoring, alkalization of urine
    - Intubation and ventilatory support, dialysis if needed
    - Specific treatment
    - Bromocriptine, amantadine, levodopa, dantrolene
    - Dantrolene sodium, dopamine agonists such as bromocriptine, and benzodiazepines

Chronic Neurological: Tardive Dyskinesia, Tardive Akathisia

- Tardive syndromes—Tardive dyskinesia—late appearing, involuntary, choreoathetoid movements, orofacial region
- Risk factors—long-term exposure to antipsychotics, older age, female sex, diagnosis of mood disorder, cognitive disorders, and typical drugs
- *Treatment*:
    - Usually unsuccessful, use SDAs, especially clozapine, no anticholinergics
    - Use low-potency drugs in smaller dose, if TD persist use cholinergic drugs
    - Benzodiazepines, propranolol, vitamin E, etc., have also been tried
- *Nonneurological side effects*: Blood count changes, skin rash, hepatic dysfunction, cardiac problems, postural hypotension, weight gain, and prolactin release.
- *With atypical like*: Clozapine/Olanzapine—metabolic syndrome, and diabetics mellitus.

DEPRESSION

Diagnosis

Five out of the following symptoms for 2 weeks:
1. Either depressed mood or markedly diminished interest or pleasure to be present (plus 2 or 3 from below)
2. Weight loss/gain
3. Insomnia/hypersomnia
4. Psychomotor retardation/agitation
5. Fatigue/loss of energy
6. Feelings of helplessness, hopelessness and worthlessness, or excessive or inappropriate guilt
7. Poor concentration/indecisiveness
8. Recurrent thoughts about suicide/death

Antidepressants

Mechanism of action: Most of the antidepressants act by modifying the monoamine neurotransmitter systems such as serotonin, norepinephrine, and dopamine.

Monoamine Oxidase Inhibitors

There is another class of drugs called monoamine oxidase (MAO) inhibitors. These are also now available in Indian market. Tranylcypromine is a nonselective MAO inhibitor used as an antidepressant. Selegiline is a MAO B inhibitor used mostly in Parkinsonism.

Indications

Depressive disorder, generalized anxiety disorder, panic disorder, phobias, OCD, premature ejaculation, ADHD, chronic pain syndrome, anticraving in alcohol use (SSRIs):
- *Older ones—tricyclics*: Imipramine, amitriptyline, dothiepin (dosulepin)
- *Main disadvantages*: Response takes longer time, usually 3-6 weeks
- *Side effects*: Sedation, anticholinergic side effects such as dry mouth, urinary retention, orthostatic hypotension, sexual dysfunction, cardiac conduction abnormalities, especially in

overdose, manic switch, tremors, gastrointestinal (GI) upsets, and constipation

Newer drugs: SSRIs
- Escitalopram, fluoxetine, sertraline, and fluvoxamine
- Most commonly used drug is *escitalopram*—90% of clinical response occurs with starting dose, high-dose causes increased side effects, faster onset of action, side effects are less, chance of manic switch is less compared to TCA, side effects are less with low starting dose:
  - Most selective SSRI
  - About 10% of patients will not be able to tolerate even a low dosage.
- *Fluoxetine* is available as capsules of 10, 20 and 40 mg, Liquid preparations contains 20 mg/5 mL:
  - Given in OD dose, usually in the morning (it can cause insomnia)
  - Usual dose is 20-40 mg/day for all conditions except OCD, which may require higher doses up to 60-80 mg/day
  - Starting dose is 20 mg/day
  - Effect may be seen after the 1st week and full therapeutic response occurs around 4 weeks.
- *Sertraline* available as tablet 25 mg, 50 mg, and 100 mg:
  - Given OD, starting dose is 25-50 mg OD, if patient do not respond after 1-3 weeks, increase dose 50 mg/weekly to a maximum of 200 mg.
- *Fluvoxamine* is available as tablets 50 mg, and 100 mg:
  - More effective for OCD
  - Starting dose is 50 mg HS, increase the dose after 1 week
  - Therapeutic dose is 50-300 mg. When the dose is >100 mg, give in divided dose.

Side effects of SSRIs:
- Agitation, restlessness
- Insomnia
- Low appetite, gastrointestinal upset—so better given after food
- Headache—usually felt frontally, more with fluoxetine
- Erectile dysfunction—all SSRIs equally cause this, usually continue as long as the drug is taken
- Weight gain in some patients
- Seizures (in 0.1 to 0.2%)—more with higher dose

- Insomnia and sedation—fluoxetine—insomnia, escitalopram—sedation, sertraline—both
- Electrolyte imbalance—hyponatremia, allergic reaction—rash, serotonin syndrome.

Newer drugs—serotonin and norepinephrine reuptake inhibitors (SNRIs):
- *Venlafaxine* (37.5-150 mg):
  - Faster onset of action, available as capsules and tablets 37.5 mg, 75 mg, 150 mg. Extended release forms also available.
  - Usually given in BD or OD dose, usual response occurs below the dose of 225 mg, mild dose act as anxiolytic
  - Common side effect is nausea, vomiting and hypertension in higher dose ranges.
- *Duloxetine* (20-80 mg):
  - Claimed to be more useful in patients with pain and other somatic symptoms
  - Side effects of SNRIs
  - Sedation, constipation, increased appetite, weight gain, and dyslipidemia
  - Serotonin syndrome

Newer drugs— noradrenergic and specific serotonergic antidepressants (NaSSAs):
- *Mirtazapine:*
  - Available as 7.5 mg, 15 mg, and 30 mg tablets
  - More anxiolytic and sedative than SSRIs
  - Causes weight gain

Newer drugs—dopamine-norepinephrine uptake inhibitors (DNRI):
- *Bupropion*—available as extended release tablets of 150 mg and 30 mg:
  - Also used in smoking cessation 15-450 mg
  - May cause seizures in higher doses
  - Less risk of manic switch reported

Antidepressant Discontinuation Syndromes

Withdrawal symptoms can occur following stoppage of most classes of antidepressants. It could be severe anxiety and agitation, vomiting, insomnia, etc., with TCA. With SSRI, it could be reemergence of anxiety, restlessness, and GI upsets.

A new antidepressant called *Vilazodone* belonging to the class SPARI (serotonin partial agonist and reuptake inhibitor) has entered Indian market recently. It is said to have a faster onset of action and lack of sexual dysfunction. Recommended dose ranges from 10 to 40 mg/day in two doses.

New addition: Vortioxetine is a newly available drug. It is a serotonin receptor modulator. It is available in 10 mg and 20 mg oral preparations. Starting dose is 10 mg. Lack of sexual side effects is one advantage of this molecule.

Anxiolytics/Hypnotics— Benzodiazepines (BDZ):
- Diazepam/chlordiazepoxide/alprazolam/clonazepam/nitrazepam/flurazepam/oxazepam
- Since BDZ drugs have tolerance and a chance of leading on to dependence, it is wiser to choose antidepressants for long-term treatment of anxiety disorders
- Usual dose range—diazepam 5-40 mg, clonazepam 0.25-1 mg, lorazepam 1-8 mg
- Nitrazepam, oxazepam, and flurazepam are more sedating than others
- Alprazolam is the most dependence-prone drug, though all have this risk
- Tolerance develops faster necessitating dose hike and this leads to difficulty in reducing dose leading to dependence
- Avoid prescribing these drugs for >4-6 weeks at a stretch as the risk of dependence is high. Patients may also have a tendency to self-medicate by purchasing it like an over-the-counter drug. It is better to warn patients of the severe difficulty they may experience in future by doing this.

Hypnotics/Non-BDZ hypnotics— Z drugs:
- Zopiclone/Eszopiclone
- Zolpidem—plain and CR
- Zaleplon

Mood stabilizers—bipolar disorders:
- *Lithium*: Oldest mood stabilizer. Blood level testing needed
  - Blood level 0.6-0.8 for therapy in acute mania and 0.8-1.5 mEq/mL for prophylaxis of further mood episodes
  - Side effects—tremors, increased thirst, polyuria
  - Long-term—hypothyroidism, renal

- In pregnancy—Ebstein's anomaly in the fetus
- Lithium can precipitate or worsen dermatological conditions such as acne, psoriasis, etc.
- Can cause hair loss
- Anticonvulsant
- Sodium valproate—dose 200 mg to 2 g. No titration needed:
  - Side effects—blood count, hepatic involvement, skin rash, hair loss
  - If there is/or more than three previous episodes
  - In episodes of mixed polarity/dysphoric mania
  - More effective in preventing manic episodes than depressions
- Newer anticonvulsants:
  - Lamotrigine—more effective in preventing bipolar depressive episodes
  - Carbamazepine/Oxcarbazepine—dose titration needed
  - Side effects include ataxia, hepatic, agranulocytosis, rash, and Stevens-Johnson syndrome.

Anti-Parkinsonian agents:
- Trihexyphenidyl/Benzhexol
- Usual dose 2-12 mg
- May cause dependence/urinary retention
- Procyclidine usual dose 2.5-15 mg
- *Drugs useful in addictions*:
  - Anticraving agents: Naltrexone – 50 mg (partial opioid antagonist), Baclofen sustained release form 20 mg to 40 mg [gamma-aminobutyric acid type B ($GABA_B$) agonist], Acamprosate (333 mg and 666 mg tablets) [acting through N-methyl-D-aspartate (NMDA) system]. Acamprosate is used only in alcohol use disorders. Others can be used in alcohol and other substance also.
  - Deterrent: Disulfiram (250-500 mg) for alcohol dependence. It may lead to serious and even fatal reaction if alcohol is consumed with 24-48 hours of taking this drug. Hence, special consent is needed along with intimation to the family or care giver.
  - Deterrents for maintaining abstinence preventing relapse in addiction medicine.

Drugs used in disorders of sexual functions:
- Sildenafil
- Tadalafil

Catatonia

This is a syndrome characterized by excitement or stupor. Stupor is a state in which the patient is mute, immobile, and unresponsive. Excitement is characterized by purposeless and often unprovoked aggression. Other signs include rigidity, waxy flexibility, negativism, posturing, and abnormal involuntary movement. It could commonly occur in mood disorders and psychotic conditions. Organic conditions have to be ruled out by physical examination and appropriate investigations before deciding they are due to psychiatric conditions. Lorazepam is used as a first-line drug, irrespective of the etiology. Antipsychotics may be sued to control aggression. Antidepressants or antipsychotics can be chosen based on the primary diagnosis. Electroconvulsive therapy (ECT) is a good option in this condition.

Adjuvants:
- L Thyroxine—as an augmenting agent along with antidepressants
- Propranolol—used along with anxiolytics for relief from physical symptoms of anxiety
- Selegiline—as an augmenting agent in various *psychotherapies*

CONCLUSION

Comorbid psychiatric disorders are common in patients with dermatological conditions. Subthreshold symptoms are also seen in many if proper screening is done. Anxiety, worries, sadness, erroneous beliefs, etc., are usually present. Effective pharmacologic and psychosocial treatment methods are available. Combination of these approaches offer synergistic effect. These measures can be combined with dermatological treatments. Equipping doctors in screening for mental health problems can improve detection of these problems and their timely management.

FURTHER READINGS

1. Sadock BJ, Sadock VA, Ruiz P. Kaplan & Sadock's Synopsis of Psychiatry, 11th edition. India: Wolters Kluwer; 2014.
2. Sadock BJ, Sadock VA (Eds). Kaplan & Sadock's Comprehensive Textbook of Psychiatry, 9th edition. New York: Lippincott Williams & Wilkins; 2009.

CHAPTER 23

Dermatological Adverse Effects of Psychotropic Medications

Savitha Soman

> **Key Messages**
> - Adverse cutaneous drug reactions (ACDRs) can occur to any drug, especially to all classes of psychotropics.
> - Most of them are fortunately mild; however, a few can be life-threatening.
> - Early recognition and timely management are very important.

INTRODUCTION

Psychodermatological disorders can be divided into "psychophysiological disorders, primary psychiatric disorders, secondary psychiatric disorders, and cutaneous sensory disorders". Psychotropic agents of different classes are used in the treatment of several of these conditions and often implicated as causative agents in the others. The commonly prescribed psychotropic drugs and their uses are summarized in **Table 1**.

Adverse cutaneous drug reactions (ACDRs) are the most frequent adverse events in patients on medications. Psychotropics are frequently implicated, with a prevalence of 5%. The incidence is about 0.1%, of which 3.3% are life-threatening events. As psychotropic agents are very commonly prescribed in both psychiatric and other medical settings, this association poses a significant problem.

An adverse cutaneous reaction to a drug is defined broadly as "any undesirable change in the structure or the function of the skin, its appendages, or mucus membranes". Most of these are type B reactions which are unpredictable, idiosyncratic, and often not dependent on drug dosage. While most ACDRs are self-limiting or easily treatable, the severe reactions can be life-threatening.

CHAPTER 23: Dermatological Adverse Effects of Psychotropic Medications

Table 1: Classification and indications of psychotropic agents.

Class of drugs	Examples	Indications
Antipsychotics (neuroleptics)	• *Typical*: Haloperidol, Pimozide, Chlorpromazine • *Atypical*: Risperidone, Olanzapine, Quetiapine, Aripiprazole	Psychotic illnesses (delusional parasitosis, olfactory reference disorder)
Mood stabilizers	Lithium, antiepileptics (sodium valproate, carbamazepine, lamotrigine)	• Bipolar disorder • Aggression
Antidepressants	• *TCA*: Amitriptyline, Imipramine, Dothiepin, Doxepin • *SSRI*: Fluoxetine, Sertraline, Paroxetine, Escitalopram • *SNRI*: Duloxetine, Venlafaxine • *NaSSA*: Mirtazapine • *NDRI*: Bupropion	Depression, anxiety disorders, OCD, trichotillomania, body dysmorphic disorder, chronic pruritus
Anxiolytics	• *BZDs*: Clonazepam, Lorazepam, Chlordiazepoxide, Alprazolam • *Serotonin 1A partial agonist*: Buspirone	Anxiety disorder

(BZD: benzodiazepine; NaSSA: noradrenergic selective serotonin antidepressant; NDRI: norepinephrine dopamine reuptake inhibitor; SNRI: selective norepinephrine reuptake inhibitor; SSRI: selective serotonin reuptake inhibitor; TCA: tricyclic antidepressant)

All classes of psychotropics can cause skin reactions. As the psychotropic armamentarium is growing, it becomes important for both the dermatologists and the psychiatrists to know the cutaneous adverse effects associated with these drugs and learn ways to manage and prevent them.

CUTANEOUS ADVERSE EFFECTS WITH SPECIFIC DRUG CLASSES

Antipsychotics

About 0.029% is the incidence of skin rash associated with these agents, the most common being photosensitivity and pigmentation. Chlorpromazine and other phenothiazine derivatives are chiefly implicated. Rates of rash with risperidone and olanzapine are 2% and 1%, respectively. Allergic rash with newer antipsychotics like aripiprazole has also been reported. Oral suspensions or solutions of haloperidol, fluphenazine, and thioridazine have been known to cause contact dermatitis.

Antidepressants

A study with a big sample size of 109,000 found the incidence of ACDR with antidepressants to be 0.054. Exanthematous eruptions and urticaria were the most common reported types. Large drug surveillance programs have reported a low prevalence of rashes with tricyclic antidepressants (TCA). With selective serotonin reuptake inhibitors (SSRIs), 0.051% incidence of ACDRs have been reported. Petechiae, ecchymosis, hyperpigmentation, alopecia, and hyperhidrosis are commonly seen. Selective norepinephrine reuptake inhibitors (SNRIs) are relatively safer, though hyperhidrosis has been a frequently reported complaint. 1% of patients on mirtazapine have reported itching and rash. Severe skin complications like erythema multiforme (EM), Stevens-Johnson syndrome (SJS), Lyell's syndrome [toxic epidermal necrolysis (TEN)], acute generalized exanthematous pustulosis (AGEP), and drug-induced hypersensitivity syndrome (DIHS) are also known with different antidepressant classes. There have also been reports of antidepressant combinations leading to skin rash.

Mood Stabilizers

While a low incidence of skin rash (0.23% only) was found in a pooled sample of 208,401 patients, most of the serious reactions can be laid at the door of the mood stabilizers, carbamazepine and lamotrigine being the chief culprits. Oxcarbazepine, while being popularized as a safer drug, had demonstrated similar ACDR in a small case series. 0.01% incidence of rash is seen with lithium therapy. Since management of severe bipolar disorders may require use of more than one mood stabilizer concurrently, the risk of ACDRs in severely ill patients is higher.

Anxiolytics

Exanthematous eruptions are the most common ACDRs. Skin eruptions have been found at a rate of 4.2 and 3.8 per 1,000 for chlordiazepoxide and diazepam, respectively, while 4% of patients on alprazolam report the same.

Table 2: Commonly used psychotropics and common cutaneous adverse effects.

Drug	Cutaneous adverse effect
Chlorpromazine	• Pigmentation • Photosensitivity reactions
Haloperidol	• Pigmentation • Contact dermatitis • Injection site reactions
Lithium	Exacerbation of psoriasis, acne, follicular hyperkeratosis, alopecia, verrucous growths
Sodium valproate	Alopecia
Carbamazepine	• Erythema multiforme • SJS
Lamotrigine	• EM • SJS, TEN
Antidepressants	• Urticaria • Exanthematous rash • Bullous reactions • Hyperhidrosis
Anxiolytics	Exanthematous rash

(EM: erythema multiforme; SJS: Stevens–Johnson syndrome; TEN: toxic epidermal necrolysis)

Drug Additives

Rash due to allergic reactions may sometimes be due to the additives in the generic psychotropics. Tartrazine has been chiefly implicated, with urticaria, bronchospasm, and purpura being the presenting symptoms.

Table 2 lists the commonly used psychotropics and their cutaneous adverse effects.

CROSS REACTIONS

Potential cross-reactions may cause more harm than good when switching psychotropics due to an ACDR; hence, a clinician needs to be aware of this pitfall. Since SSRIs, especially paroxetine, fluoxetine, and sertraline, seem to display some cross-reactivity, it is suggested that another class of antidepressant be used if switching from an SSRI. Chlorpromazine has shown no cross-reactivity with other phenothiazines. Carbamazepine and valproate are known to demonstrate cross-reactivity. Isolated skin rashes due to carbamazepine have been successfully managed with desensitization.

RISK FACTORS

Since most of the ACDRs are idiosyncratic, it is difficult to predict the occurrence of the same. However, research has identified people who are at a higher risk of developing these cutaneous adverse effects. The winter season seems to confer an extra risk, where though the exposure to sunlight is at its lowest, it also probably means low vitamin D levels. Both admitted and outpatient data have revealed that women have a 50% higher risk, presumably due to hormonal influences affecting the immune system and/or altered drug metabolism. There is a racial difference; the African-American patients are the most affected, varying rates of drug metabolism being a possible reason. Elderly individuals are at a higher risk, which may be partly due to polypharmacy as well as declining renal and liver function. Immunocompromising conditions like HIV increase the risk for more serious reactions, as also viral infections, multiple medical comorbidities, and concurrent substance use. High initial loading doses and rapid uptitration increase the risk of ACDRs, suggesting a dose-dependent association in these cases. Among the antiepileptic drugs, immunologic mechanisms seem to have an important role. Human leukocyte antigen (HLA)-B 1502 and HLA-B 1508 in those of Indian origin, HLA-A 3101 in Japanese and Northern European natives, and HLA-B 1511 in Thai, Japanese, and Han Chinese individuals are notable examples of this association, with these groups showing an increased sensitivity to the use of carbamazepine. Patients with manic illness also seem to have more ACDRs, presumably due to use of antiepileptics as mood stabilizers.

In a case–control study using data from a 1993–2014 pharmacovigilance program in psychiatry that compared 594 cases of ACDR (cases) to 8,085 (controls), it was found that ACDRs were more common in women, especially those below the age of 50 years. Other risk factors found were a diagnosis of substance use and use of drugs like maprotiline, carbamazepine, lamotrigine, and clomethiazole.

MORPHOLOGY OF CUTANEOUS LESIONS

Adverse cutaneous drug reactions can be conceptualized as common and benign, severe and life-threatening, as well as other cutaneous reactions to psychotropics.

Common Adverse Reactions

Pruritis

Pruritus or itch is generally seen as a secondary symptom; however, it can also be a primary side effect of all classes of psychotropics.

Exanthematous Lesions

Exanthematous lesions are the most common ACDRs with psychotropic agents. They can occur with any class of psychotropics but are seen more commonly with mood stabilizers. The initial eruption occurs within a fortnight of drug initiation and generally disappears within 2 weeks of stopping the drug. Occasionally, there is spontaneous resolution.

Urticaria and Angioedema

Urticaria is the second most common ACDR that can occur following any psychotropic use, usually within minutes to days after starting a drug. The lesions fade quickly but new ones arise. There may be accompanying angioedema and anaphylaxis.

Fixed-drug Eruption

Fixed-drug eruptions can occur with any class of psychotropic. They appear within hours of initiating the drug and typically resolve within several weeks after stopping the drug. Recurrent drug eruptions can cause hyperpigmentation.

Photosensitivity

Psychotropics can cause photosensitivity in response to UV light exposure, leading to grayish purple discolorations and hyper-pigmentation. Phototoxic or photoallergic reactions may occur.

Alopecia

Alopecia has been associated with all psychotropic classes and can begin either at once or even a few months after drug initiation. Lithium and valproate are chiefly implicated.

Pigmentation

Several TCAs may cause a brown, gray, or blue discoloration in areas exposed to the sun; hair and nail changes may also occur. Pigmentation starts after long exposure to the drug and fades away just as slowly. SSRIs rarely cause generalized pigmentation. Among antipsychotics, chlorpromazine is mainly held responsible.

Severe and Life-threatening

Erythema Multiforme

Erythema multiforme (EM) is associated mainly with mood stabilizers, begins within a few days of drug initiation, and may be the forerunner of more serious adverse reactions.

Stevens–Johnson Syndrome (SJS) and TEN

Mood stabilizers are chiefly implicated, though there are reports with SSRIs, amoxapine, and antipsychotics as well.

Drug Hypersensitivity Vasculitis

Drug hypersensitivity vasculitis is a rare adverse effect reported with some antidepressants and antipsychotics, causing necrosis of the walls of blood vessels, and begins within a few weeks of starting the drug.

Erythroderma (Exfoliative Dermatitis)

Symptoms start in the first few weeks after drug initiation, either as a dermatitis or as progression from an earlier benign skin eruption.

Erythema Nodosum

Erythema nodosum is a rare acute inflammatory reaction to some antidepressants, presenting as painful nodules.

Drug Rash with Eosinophilia and Systemic Symptoms (DRESS) Syndrome

DRESS syndrome is an idiosyncratic reaction that presents with fever, hepatitis, eosinophilia, exanthema, atypical circulating lymphocytes, and lymphadenopathy, at least three of which are essential to make a diagnosis. It is commonly associated with aromatic antiepileptic agents.

General Conditions Associated with Psychotropic Medications

Acneiform eruptions, psoriasiform reactions, and hyperhidrosis have been reported with all classes of psychotropic agents. Seborrheic dermatitis is reported mainly in the context of antidepressant and mood stabilizer use. Lichenoid reactions can be seen due to phenothiazines, propranolol, and carbamazepine. Hidradenitis suppurativa and acne conglobata secondary to lithium have been reported. Rarely, mycosis fungoides secondary to antidepressant use has been evident. Valproate has been known to cause morphea, both localized and generalized variants. Benzodiazepine use has been implicated in systemic lupus erythematosus, Sweet's syndrome, and hirsutism.

These adverse effects are summarized in **Table 3**.

DIAGNOSIS

An algorithm has been proposed to assess the drug-adverse effects relationship: (1) Previous experience with the drug in a general population, (2) alternative etiologic candidates, (3) timing of events, (4) drug levels or evidence of overdose, (5) patient reaction to discontinuation, and (6) patient reaction to rechallenge.

A clear history focusing on exposure to drug, timeline encompassing the first and last use of the drug and when the eruptions occurred, past and family history of drug hypersensitivity reactions, improvement after cessation of the drug, and a detailed physical examination can aid in diagnosis. The cutaneous findings must be clearly documented. The most likely offenders are drugs started in

Table 3: Benign and serious ACDRs to psychotropic agents.

Reaction	Clinical presentation	Drugs implicated
Pruritis	Generally secondary to other drug reactions	All classes of psychotropics
Exanthematous rashes	Macules and maculopapular lesions, sore throat, associated with pain, 3–14 days after starting drug	All classes
Urticaria	Migratory wheals with/without angioedema and anaphylaxis, begins minutes to hours after drug initiation. May be the harbinger of an SJS	All classes
Fixed-drug eruption	Edematous oval or round plaques with itching, bullae may be present, begins few to 24 hours after starting drug. Residual dusky brown macules	All classes
Photosensitivity	Exaggerated sunburn (phototoxic) or generalized skin eruptions (photoallergic reactions)	Mostly antipsychotics, chiefly chlorpromazine. Benzodiazepines
Alopecia	Occurs at varying times after starting the drug, nonscarring, recovers with drug discontinuation	Valproate, lithium, most antipsychotics, and antidepressants
Pigmentation	Skin, eyes, nails, and teeth; occurs with long-term use	Antipsychotics like chlorpromazine, TCAs, venlafaxine (hypopigmentation), SSRIs, anticonvulsant mood stabilizers

Continued

Continued

Reaction	Clinical presentation	Drugs implicated
Erythema multiforme	Polymorphous rashes, less than 20% body involvement, typically on extremities, classical target lesions. Begins within days of drug initiation	• Antiepileptic mood stabilizers • Rarely antipsychotics and antidepressants
SJS	Flu-like symptoms with mucocutaneous involvement, 20% body area involvement in the first 48 hours	• Antiepileptic mood stabilizers • Rarely antipsychotics and antidepressants
Toxic epidermal necrolysis	Bullae with more than 20% body involvement, mucous membrane affected. First 2 months of treatment	Mostly anticonvulsants
Drug hypersensitivity vasculitis	Palpable purpura on legs and ankles, necrosis of blood vessel walls, begins few weeks after drug initiation	Clozapine, lithium, carbamazepine, diazepam, chlordiazepoxide, trazodone
Erythroderma	Generalized itching, redness, flaking of skin; in the first few weeks of treatment	All classes
Erythema nodosum	Painful red deep-seated nodules, acute reaction	Paroxetine and venlafaxine
DRESS syndrome	Drug eruption, eosinophilia, lymphadenopathy, multiple organ involvement, 1–8 weeks after starting drug	Almost exclusively anticonvulsant related

(ACDRs: adverse cutaneous drug reactions; DRESS: drug rash with eosinophilia and systemic symptoms; SJS: Stevens–Johnson syndrome) the 6 weeks prior to the reaction and drugs taken intermittently. Red flags that must alert the clinician to serious ACDR include high fever, facial and tongue swelling, pain, difficulty breathing, erosions of mucous membrane, blisters with skin detachment, palpable purpura, and lymph node enlargement. It is also vital to differentiate these ACDRs from self-inflicted skin lesions. Laboratory tests may be indicated only if there is suspicion of other organ system involvement.

TREATMENT

Once an ACDR is diagnosed, the offending drug is generally withdrawn. If removal of the drug is not possible due to the severity of the underlying psychiatric condition, dose reduction may be tried. This has been found to work in the case of drugs like lithium and carbamazepine. Often, the doctor and the patient can discuss the risk and benefits of continuing versus stopping the drug and take an informed decision. Low initial doses and slow hike in doses can prevent ACDRs to a certain extent, especially in the case of carbamazepine. Supportive measures are instituted to combat the ACDR. Topical or systemic antihistamines are prescribed for pruritis, topical steroids for mild-moderate rash, and systemic steroids for more severe reactions. In case of hyperhidrosis, dose reduction, switching to a different agent, and/or use of topical aluminum chloride hexahydrate are the available options. Drugs like glycopyrrolate, benztropine, and clonidine may be used if symptoms are severe. If mild alopecia is seen, the drug need not be stopped. If severe, one can change to another drug to improve adherence. If there are any red flags, the drug should be stopped immediately, a dermatology consultation taken, and patient hospitalized if symptoms are severe. Oral or IV steroids and IV immunoglobulin are administered in cases of SJS and TEN. Educating the patient about avoiding skin irritants may prevent ACDRs to a certain extent and informing them of early warning signs of ACDRs aids in early detection.

CONCLUSION

While ACDRs are not specific to psychotropic agents, it is well known that all classes of psychotropics can lead to ACDRs. Most of them fortunately are mild; however, a few can be life-threatening.

Clinicians must be aware of the cutaneous adverse effects of the various psychotropic agents, educate their patients about them, start medications at low doses and hike them slowly, avoid polypharmacy, and be mindful of cross-reactions. Supportive measures must be initiated once an ACDR sets in; hospitalization may be mandated for severe adverse effects. Discontinuation of the offending drug is the first step; if this is impossible due to the nature of the underlying psychiatric illness, dose reduction is tried. Rechallenge with the offending drug is the exception rather than the rule. With our knowledge of the various risk factors like ethnicity and HLA type predisposing individuals to cutaneous hypersensitivity reactions, preventive measures may become the order of the day. There have been recommendations to do a genetic testing before starting particularly notorious drugs like carbamazepine as well as a warning label on the product against using it in individuals with a specific HLA type; however, these strategies are yet to be made universal or cost effective. At present, close monitoring for possible side effects in vulnerable individuals during the initial months of psychotropic treatment is the best recommended strategy.

FURTHER READINGS

1. Koo JYM, Lee CS (Eds). General approach to evaluating psychodermatological disorders. In: Psychocutaneous Medicine: Basic and Clinical Dermatology. New York: Marcel Dekker; 2003. pp. 1-12.
2. Ghosh S, Behere RV, Sharma PSVN, S Savitha. Relevant issues in pharmacotherapy of psycho-cutaneous disorders. Indian J Dermatol. 2013;58(1):61- 4.
3. Svensson CK, Cowen EW, Gaspari AA. Cutaneous drug reactions. Pharmacol Rev. 2001;53:357-79.
4. Srebrnik A, Hes JP, Brenner S. Adverse cutaneous reactions to psychotropic drugs. Acta Dermato Venereol Suppl. 1991;158:9-12.
5. Lange-Asschenfeldt C, Grohmann R, Lange-Asschenfeldt B, Engel RR, Ruther E, Cordes J. Cutaneous adverse reactions to psychotropic drugs: Data from a multicentre surveillance programme. J Clin Psychiatry. 2009;70(9):1258-65.
6. Drake LA, Dinehart SM, Farmer ER, Goltz RW, Graham GF, Hordinsky MK, et al. Guidelines of care for cutaneous adverse drug reactions. American Academy of Dermatology. J Am Acad Dermatol. 1996;35(3):458-61.
7. Bliss SA, Warnock JK. Psychiatric medications: Adverse cutaneous drug reactions. Clin Dermatol. 2013;31:101-9.
8. Satanove A. Pigmentation due to phenothiazines in high and prolonged dosage. JAMA. 1965;191(4): 263-8.
9. McMorran WS, Krahn LE. Adverse cutaneous reactions to psychotropic drugs. Psychosomatics. 1997;38:413-22.

10. Nath S, Rehman S, Kalita KN, Baruah A. Aripiprazole induced skin rash. Industrial Psychiatry J. 2016;25(2):225-7.
11. Warnock JK, Knesevich JW: Adverse cutaneous reactions to antidepressants. Am J Psychiatry. 1988;145:425-30.
12. Warnock JK, Morris DW. Adverse cutaneous reactions to antidepressants. Am J Clin Dermatol. 2002;3(5):329-39.
13. Schwartz TL. Diaphoresis and pruritis with extended-release Venlafaxine. Ann Pharmacother. 1999;33(9):1009.
14. Mitkov MV, Towbridge RM, Lockshin BN, Caplan JP. Dermatologic side effects of psychotropic medications. Psychosomatics. 2014;55:1-20.
15. Herstowska M, Komorowska O, Cubata WJ, Jakuszkowiak-Wojten, Gałuszko-Węgielnik M, Landowski J. Severe skin complications in patients treated with antidepressants: a literature review. Postepy Dermatol Alergol. 2014;31(2):92-7.
16. Tuman TC, Tuman BA, Sereflican B, Yidlirim O. J Mood Disord. 2016;6(2):91-2.
17. Beran RG. Cross-reactive skin eruption with both carbamazepine and oxcarbazepine. Epilepsia. 1993;34(1):163-5.
18. Li LM, Russo M, O'Donoghue MF, Duncan JS, Sander JWAS. Allergic skin rash with Lamotrigine and concomitant Valproate therapy: Evidence for an increased risk. Arquivos de Neuro-Psiquiatria. 1996;54:47-9.
19. Edwards GJ. Adverse effects of anti-anxiety drugs. Drugs. 1981;22(6):495-514.
20. Arndt KA, Jick H. Rates of cutaneous reactions to drugs: A report from the Boston Collaborative Drug Surveillance Programme. JAMA. 1976;235(9):918-23.
21. Desmond RE, Trautlein JJ. Tartrazine (FD and C yellow 5) anaphylaxis: a case report. Ann Allergy. 1981;46:81-2.
22. Krasowska D, Szymanek M, Schwartz RA, Myslinski W. Cutaneous effects of the most commonly used antidepressant medication, the selective serotonin reuptake inhibitors. J Am Acad Dermatol. 2007;56(5):848-53.
23. Cogrel O, Beylot-Barry M, Vergier B, Dubus P, Doutre MS, Merlio JP, et al. Sodium Valproate induced cutaneous pseudolymphoma followed by recurrence with Carbamazepine. British J Dermatol. 2001;144(6):1235-8.
24. Eames P. Adverse reactions to Carbamazepine managed by desensitisation. Lancet. 1989;1(8636):509-10.
25. Bigby M, Jick S, Jick H, Arndt K. Drug-induced cutaneous reactions: a report from the Boston Collaborative Drug Surveillance Program on 15.438 consecutive inpatients. 1975-1986. JAMA. 1986;256:3358-63.
26. Ives TJ, Bentz EJ, Gwyther RE. Dermatologic adverse drug reactions in a family medicine setting. Arch Fam Med. 1992;1:241-5.
27. Hajjar ER, Hanlon JT, Artz MB, Lindbald CI, Pieper CF, Sloane RJ, et al. Adverse drug reaction risk factors in older outpatients. Am J Geriatr Pharmacother. 2003;1(2):82-9.
28. Thong BY, Tan TC. Epidemiology and risk factors for drug allergy. Br J Clin Pharmacol. 2011;71(5):684-700.
29. Schnyder B, Pichler WJ. Mechanisms of drug induced allergy. Mayo Clinic Proc. 2009;84(3):268-72.

30. Greil W, Zhang X, Stassen H, Grohmann R, Bridler R, Hasler G, et al. Cutaneous adverse drug reactions to psychotropic drugs and their risk factors: a case-control study. Eur Neuropsychopharmacol. 2019;29:111-21.
31. Nigen S, Knowles SR, Shear NH. Drug eruptions: approaching the diagnosis of drug-induced skin diseases. J Drugs Dermatol. 2003;2:279-99.
32. Kimyai-Asadi A, Harris JC, Nousari HC. Critical overview: adverse cutaneous reactions to psychotropic medications. J Clin Psychiatry. 1999;60:714-25.
33. Tan E, Grattan C. Drug-induced urticaria. Exp Opin Drug Saf. 2004;3:471-84.
34. Harth Y, Rapoport M. Photosensitivity associated with antipsychotics, antidepressants and anxiolytics. Drug Saf. 1996;14(4):252-9.
35. Uehlinger C, Barrelet L, Touabi M, Baumann P. Alopecia and mood stabilisers: Two case reports. Eur Arch Psychiatr Clin Neurosci. 1992;242(2-3):85-8.
36. Weber MB, Recuero JK, Almeida CS. Use of psychiatric drugs in dermatology. Anais Brasileiros de Dermatologia. 2020;95(2):133-43.
37. Warnock JK, Morris DW. Adverse cutaneous reactions to mood stabilizers. Am J Clin Dermatol. 2003;4(1):21-30.
38. Mufaddel A, Osman OT, Almugaddam F. Adverse cutaneous effects of psychotropic medications. Exp Rev Dermatol. 2013;8(6):681-92.
39. Fleming P, Marik PE. The DRESS syndrome: The great clinical mimicker. Pharmacotherapy. 2011;31(3):332
40. Lamer V, Lipozenčić J, Turcić P. Adverse cutaneous reactions to psycho-pharmaceuticals. Acta Dermatovenerol Croatica. 2010;18:56-67.
41. Garnis-Jones S. Dermatologic side effects of psychopharmacologic agents. Dermatol Clin. 1996;14(3):503-8.
42. Aithal V, Appaih P. Lithium induced hidradenitis suppurativa and acne conglobata. Indian J Dermatol Venereol Leprol. 2004;70:307-9.
43. Cerroni L, Fink-Puches R, El-Shabrawi-Caelen L, Soyer HP, LeBoit PE, Kerl H. Solitary skin lesions with histopathologic features of early mycosis fungoides. Am J Dermatopathol. 1999;21(6):518-24.
44. Karimpour H, Karimpour S, Zamani MJ, Nikfar S, Rezaie A, Hajarolasvadi N, et al. Toxic reactions to chronic use of benzodiazepines: An overview. Int J Pharmacol. 2005;1(4):376-82.
45. Kramer MS, Leventhal JM, Hutchinson TA, Feinstein AR. An algorithm for the operational assessment of adverse drug reactions. I. Background, description, and instructions for use. JAMA. 1979;242(7):623-32.
46. Deandrea D, Walker N, Mehlmauer M, White K. Dermatological reactions to lithium: a critical review of the literature. J Clin Psychopharmacol. 1982;2(3):199-204.
47. Chadwick D, Shaw MD, Foy P, Rawlins MD, Turnbull DM. Serum anticonvulsant concentrations and risk of drug induced skin eruptions. J Neurol Neurosurg Psychiatry. 1984;47(6):642-4.
48. Cheshire WP, Fealy RD. Drug induced hyperhidrosis and hypohidrosis: Incidence, prevention and management. Drug Saf. 2008;31(2):109-26.
49. Gautam M. Alopecia due to psychotropic medications. Ann Pharmacother. 1999;33(5):631-7.

CHAPTER 24

Psychodermatology Liaison Clinic

Shrutakirthi D Shenoi, Varsha Gowda VM

> **Key Messages**
> - Psychodermatological disease requires liaison approach.
> - Dermatologist, psychiatrist, and clinical psychologist are involved in management.
> - Patient receives standard dermatological treatment along with psychiatric drugs/nonpharmacological or psychological supportive care.

INTRODUCTION

The role of skin–mind connection is becoming important in the management of dermatological conditions. Stress is known to precipitate certain disorders such as alopecia areata and vitiligo. Stress can also aggravate conditions such as psoriasis, atopic dermatitis, idiopathic pruritus, and urticaria. It is well-known that nearly 30% of chronic dermatoses have associated psychiatric comorbidities such as dysthymia, anxiety, and compulsive disorders. For holistic management, patient has to be treated for his apparent skin problem as well as the apparent mental state. A dermatologist either because of his busy schedule or due to inexperience may be unable to recognize and handle the emotional problems of the patients. It is in this instance that liaising becomes essential.

Psychodermatology is a branch of dermatology that bridges the skin and mind. Here, the dermatologist liaises with a psychiatrist and a clinical psychologist. Liaison clinics generally function in a hospital setting. The dermatologist initially sees the patients. Patients suspected to be having psychodermatological condition are referred to the clinic. The clinical psychologist and psychiatrist independently interview the patients and discuss their findings and management plan with the dermatologist.

The concept of liaison clinic is popular in Europe. There are reports of the functioning of such clinics in India, Israel, and Singapore. The advantages of a liaison clinic are three-fold. Firstly, patients get the benefit of consulting three specialists at a single session. Secondly, the hesitation and bias of visiting the psychiatry department are overcome. Thirdly, patients get both dermatological and psychological treatment.

SCOPE

The basis of the psychocutaneous disorders is that the brain and skin have a common ectodermal origin. The bidirectional brain and skin influences are mediated by neurotransmitters, hormones, and neuropeptides. In the liaison clinic, both inpatients and outpatients are seen. Typical issues include:
- *Psychodermatological cases*:
  - Primary psychiatric disorders with skin manifestations, e.g., delusions of parasitosis, trichotillomania, dermatitis artefacta, and body dysmorphia
  - Secondary psychiatric conditions, i.e., skin diseases with secondary psychiatric manifestations such as dysthymia in psoriasis and vitiligo
  - Psychophysiologic, e.g., skin diseases precipitated or aggravated by stress such as urticarial and alopecia areata
- Patients with iatrogenic psychiatric problems, e.g., steroid psychosis secondary to high-dose therapy, especially in pemphigus
- Patients with unexplained skin symptoms, e.g., generalized itching, burning sensation, or skin pain
- Patients who have attempted suicide or self-harm
- Patients who wish to undergo alcohol or tobacco deaddiction
- Patients with specific phobias without skin disease, e.g., patients with history of sexual exposure with or without sexually transmitted disease with venereophobia and HIV phobia.

LIAISON CLINICS

- Psychodermatology liaison clinic at Kasturba Medical College, Manipal, Karnataka, India
- Psychodermatology liaison clinic at Kozhikode Medical College, Kozhikode, Kerala, India
- Psychodermatology liaison clinic at GGS Medical College, Faridkot, Punjab, India
- Psychodermatology clinic, Kaplan Medical Center, Rehovot, Israel
- The Psychodermatology service at The Royal London Hospital, United Kingdom
- Psychodermatology clinic in Detroit, Michigan, USA
- Psychodermatology clinic, Changi General Hospital, Singapore

SAMPLE OF A CASE RECORD IN A LIAISON CLINIC

Case 1: Primary Psychiatric Disorder with Skin Manifestations

Dermatology Notes

An 83-year-old male patient visited the clinic with history of feeling of insects crawling across his skin and itching, especially over scalp, groin, and legs. He used to scratch the skin and also repeatedly brushed away imaginary insects. On detailed examination, no evidence of parasitic infestation was found. Diagnosis of delusion of parasitosis was made.

Psychiatry Notes

An 83-year-old male presented with sensation of insects crawling over scalp, groin, and legs. On psychiatric examination, he had mild anxiety. No signs of depression were detected. He had the delusion that his body was invaded by insects.

Impression: Delusion of parasitosis.

Treatment: Risperidone (2 mg) + Trihexyphenidyl (2 mg) was prescribed to be administered once at night and was asked for a follow-up visit after 2 weeks.

Case 2: Secondary Psychiatric Disorder

Dermatology Notes

A 43-year-old male presented with 15-year history of itchy skin lesions, with lesions initially appearing over the scalp, later over the rest of the body. He received ultraviolet light therapy and methotrexate in the past. Multiple erythematous scaly plaques appeared all over trunk and limbs affecting 30% BSA with nail pitting. This condition was diagnosed as psoriasis vulgaris.

Psychiatry Notes

A 43-year-old male working as agriculturist stayed in a joint family, and was diagnosed with psoriasis for last 15 years.

For last 10 years, his wife had stayed away from him. She did not allow him to touch her, kept his utensils and clothes separately and considered him untouchable. She humiliated him and complained that her life was spoilt because of him. She kept nagging him and slept separately. She did not cooperate with his treatment. He felt humiliated due to her attitude. At functions/gatherings, he tried to hide his lesions by wearing full-sleeves shirt and buttoned his collar. He says he was alive because of his children, otherwise he would have committed suicide. He had nonpervasive sad mood and low self-esteem.

- *Impression*: Dysthymia
- No psychotropics at time of presentation to the clinic
- Required "Couple therapy"

Clinical Psychology Notes

Patient was diagnosed to have psoriasis for the past 15 years. Marital discord was present along with interpersonal conflict secondary to skin condition. Wife was worried about the disease getting transmitted to other family members. Interaction between patient and his children was cordial and children were supportive.

Wife was made understood about the nature of the illness. Supportive counseling was provided to patient and his wife.

ADVANTAGES OF PSYCHODERMATOLOGY APPROACH

- Treatment response is good.
- Patient's sufferings are minimized.
- Patient satisfaction is excellent.
- Addressing psychosocial impact of dermatoses improves patient's quality of life.

DIFFICULTIES ENCOUNTERED AT LIAISON CLINIC

- Shortage of resources and difficulties in the pricing.
- High rate of missed appointments due to long travelling hours and limited liaison clinics.

CONCLUSION

Establishing a psychodermatology liaison clinic is a practical approach of dealing with dermatology patients who have significant psychological issues.

FURTHER READINGS

1. Shenoi SD, Prabhu S, Nirmal B, Petrolwala S. Our experience in a psychodermatology liaison clinic at Manipal. Indian J Dermatol. 2013;58:53-5.
2. Gould WM, Gragg TM. A dermatology-psychiatry liaison clinic. J Am Acad Dermatol. 1983;9:73-7.
3. Orion E, Feldman B, Ronni W, Orit BA. A Psychodermatology clinic. The concept, the format and our observations from Israel. Am J Clin Dermatol. 2012;13:97-101.
4. Chung WL, Ng SS, Koh MJ, Peh LH, Liu TT. A review of patients managed at a combined psychodermatology clinic: A Singapore experience. Sing Med J. 2012;53:789-9.
5. Brar BK, Brar SK, Puri N, Arora H. Psychodermatology liaison clinic at a tertiary care centre in north India. Sch J App Med Sci. 2016;4:2795-8.
6. Seale L, Gaulding JV, Porto D, Prabhakar D, Kerr H. Implementation of a psychodermatology clinic at a major health system in Detroit. Int J Womens Dermatol. 2018;7:227-9.

CHAPTER 25

Research in Psychodermatology: Unveiling the Mind–Skin Connection

Isabella Tan, Mohammad Jafferany

> **Key Messages**
> - This chapter explores multifaceted dimensions inherent to the domain of psychodermatology research.
> - Discusses the assistance and collaboration from international agencies.
> - Pioneer associations activities like European Society for Dermatology and Psychiatry and the Association for Psychoneurocutaneous Medicine of North America are explained.

INTRODUCTION

Psychodermatology stands as an emerging and interdisciplinary field at the forefront of scientific inquiry, dedicated to unraveling the intricate interplay between mental health and dermatological conditions. In recent years, this growing area of study has garnered increasing attention and momentum, driven by the growing recognition among researchers and healthcare professionals of the influence exerted by psychological factors upon the realm of skin health. This chapter is dedicated to the exploration of the multifaceted dimensions inherent to the domain of psychodermatology research. By shedding light on this intricate relationship, the intention is to underscore the importance of psychodermatology in the context of improving the lives of individuals grappling with the challenges posed by psychologically influenced skin disorders.

SCOPE OF PSYCHODERMATOLOGY RESEARCH

Psychodermatology, an interdisciplinary domain that investigates the relationship between the human psyche and skin, has witnessed a remarkable surge in attention and scholarly interest over recent years. Unlike traditional dermatology, which primarily focuses on the superficial aspects of skin health, psychodermatology delves into the profound connections that exist between emotional well-being and the overall health of the skin.

This advancing field has not only broadened our understanding of dermatological conditions but also uncovered new avenues for their treatment, particularly those influenced by psychological factors. The realization that mental states and emotional well-being significantly impact skin health has become increasingly evident. As a consequence, researchers have been spurred to explore innovative and holistic interventions that transcend the conventional treatment paradigms, with the primary goal of alleviating the burden of dermatological conditions shaped by the intricate interplay between mind and skin.

Psychodermatology has evolved from a niche area of study to a pivotal discipline, bridging the gap between psychology and dermatology. It offers promise in terms not only of enhancing our comprehension of the underlying mechanisms but also in providing more effective and comprehensive care for individuals grappling with the complex and often challenging interface of mental and dermatological health. Through this synergy between psychology and dermatology, psychodermatology will pave the way toward a brighter and more promising future for those in need of integrated healthcare.

Areas of Research

In the realm of psychodermatology research, several key areas of investigation have emerged. One prominent focus involves the exploration of how psychological factors exert their influence on the development and aggravation of various skin conditions. Stress, in particular, has undergone extensive scrutiny due to its role in conditions such as psoriasis. It is well documented that chronic stress can trigger the release of proinflammatory cytokines, thereby exacerbating skin inflammation and potentially serving as a catalyst for the onset or worsening of dermatological disorders. Furthermore, anxiety and depression have also been closely associated with the exacerbation of skin conditions, underscoring the imperative need for comprehensive mental healthcare within the field of dermatology.

Additionally, psychodermatology research extends its reach into the realm of psychotherapeutic interventions, with cognitive-behavioral therapy (CBT) emerging as a prominent approach. CBT in psychodermatology aims to address the emotional and cognitive factors that contribute to skin conditions. It empowers individuals with a repertoire of coping strategies and stress management techniques, ultimately leading to a reduction in the severity of skin-related symptoms. A growing body of evidence underscores the efficacy of CBT in enhancing the overall quality of life for individuals grappling with psychodermatological issues.

Furthermore, a critical facet of psychodermatology research involves an in-depth exploration of the neurobiological mechanisms that underlie the mind–skin connection. Among these mechanisms, cortisol, the body's primary stress hormone, potentially plays a crucial role. Elevated levels of cortisol, often associated with chronic stress, have been shown to exert a detrimental impact on skin health. Research in this area seeks to elucidate the pathways through which cortisol and other neurobiological factors influence the development and progression of skin conditions. By shedding light on these precise mechanisms, researchers aspire to identify potential therapeutic targets that could revolutionize the management and treatment of psychodermatological disorders.

Assistance and Collaboration from International Agencies

Collaboration with international agencies has undeniably played an instrumental role in elevating the stature of psychodermatology research to a global platform. Among these organizations, the World Health Organization (WHO) and the National Institutes of Health (NIH) have emerged as key catalysts in advancing the frontiers of knowledge within this field.

The involvement of these international agencies has yielded a multitude of benefits, not the least of which is the facilitation of knowledge exchange and data sharing across geographical borders. Psychodermatology, being a field with profound implications for human well-being, stands to gain immensely from the diverse insights and experiences brought forth by researchers, clinicians, and healthcare professionals from various corners of the globe.

Moreover, the presence of international agencies has contributed to the enrichment of the global perspective on psychodermatology. The cross-cultural collaboration of ideas has allowed the field to transcend geographical and cultural boundaries. Such a diverse viewpoint is invaluable, particularly in a discipline that deals with the interplay of psychological and dermatological factors, which can be influenced by myriad cultural, societal, and environmental variables.

Perhaps one of the most significant contributions of international agencies to psychodermatology is their role in promoting the development of standardized approaches to both research and treatment. Through the establishment of guidelines, best practices, and common research protocols, WHO and NIH can enable researchers and clinicians worldwide to adopt a unified framework when addressing psychodermatological issues. This standardization will not only enhance the quality and rigor of research but may also facilitate the comparability of findings across different regions, ultimately leading to more robust evidence-based practices.

As these agencies continue to foster this synergy, the future of psychodermatology holds the promise of greater inclusivity, enhanced efficacy, and a more comprehensive approach to addressing the challenges posed by the intersection of mind and skin.

Funding

Securing funding for psychodermatology research is a crucial step in advancing our understanding of the mind–skin connection. There are various avenues available for researchers to obtain the financial support necessary to advance their investigations.

- *Government grants*: Governmental bodies often allocate funds for scientific research, including psychodermatology. Researchers can apply for grants from agencies dedicated to healthcare and dermatology, which typically undergo a peer-review process. Government support also brings a level of credibility to the project.
- *Private foundations*: Private foundations with a focus on health and medical research are valuable sources of funding. These organizations are often motivated by a strong philanthropic

mission to improve human health. Psychodermatology researchers can explore partnerships with such foundations to secure financial backing for their work.
- *Pharmaceutical companies*: Pharmaceutical enterprises invested in dermatological therapies are keen on supporting research that can lead to innovative treatments and therapies. Collaborating with these companies can provide access to significant resources, including funding, laboratory facilities, and opportunities for clinical trials. Such partnerships can accelerate the translation of research findings into practical applications.
- *International agencies*: International agencies, such as the WHO and the NIH, have recognized the importance of psychodermatology research. They offer research grants that facilitate the continuation and progress of impactful projects. In addition to financial support, the endorsement of these agencies lends global recognition and validation to psychodermatology research endeavors.

While securing funding for psychodermatology research may present challenges, it is an achievable endeavor with the right strategies and partnerships in place. Researchers in this field have a range of options to explore, from government grants and private foundations to collaborations with pharmaceutical companies and support from international agencies. These resources not only provide financial backing but also contribute to the credibility and global impact of psychodermatology research efforts.

Psychodermatology Fellowships

Psychodermatology fellowships can serve as valuable resources for aspiring researchers and clinicians in this field. These fellowships can provide a structured platform for individuals to bridge the gap between dermatology and psychology, equipping fellows with the knowledge and skills required to conduct high-quality research and deliver effective patient care.

Psychodermatology fellowships, particularly those offered by the ESDaP (European Society for Dermatology and Psychiatry), serve as invaluable resources for aspiring researchers and clinicians in this specialized field. ESDaP's fellowship program provides a structured and immersive platform for individuals seeking specialized training and mentorship in psychodermatology, making it a pivotal development in medical training.

ESDaP's fellowship program equips fellows with a profound understanding of the intricate relationship between the human mind and the skin, offering knowledge that forms the foundation for their careers as researchers or clinicians. In the medical world, these two disciplines often operate in parallel, but ESDaP's fellowships create a synergy, enabling fellows to integrate psychological insights into their dermatological practice. This integration recognizes the inseparable link between emotional well-being and skin health, leading to a more comprehensive understanding of patient's conditions.

Psychodermatology fellowships are a vital resource for those aspiring to make a difference in the lives of individuals grappling with psychodermatological issues. These fellowships offer a means to bridge the gap between dermatology and psychology and provide a platform for specialized training and mentorship, ultimately advancing the field of psychodermatology.

APMNA

The Association for Psychoneurocutaneous Medicine of North America (APMNA) is a central organization dedicated to promoting psychoneurocutaneous medicine, a field that explores the interplay between the mind and the skin, as well as the role of psychoneuro-immunology in skin diseases. APMNA consists of dermatologists, psychiatrists, psychologists, and allied health professionals, all committed to advancing the understanding of this intricate connection. APMNA's core mission includes the following:

- *Advocating high-quality care*: APMNA champions the delivery of top-notch care for dermatology patients, emphasizing a holistic and patient-centered approach by acknowledging the psychological aspects of skin health.
- *Fostering a holistic approach*: The organization promotes a holistic approach to addressing chronic skin diseases, recognizing the importance of considering both physical and psychological dimensions in effective treatment.
- *Providing a forum for ideas*: APMNA serves as a vibrant platform for professionals from diverse backgrounds to exchange ideas in psychoneurocutaneous medicine. It encourages dialogue and collaboration, fostering a multidisciplinary approach to research and patient care.

- *Supporting education and research*: APMNA actively supports the advancement of psychocutaneous education and research by providing resources and opportunities for learning and investigation, contributing to the growth of knowledge in this evolving field.

Furthermore, APMNA is in collaboration with global dermatology to celebrate World Psychodermatology Day. This annual event, held on the third Saturday of November every year, is a virtual gathering, which underscores the importance of psychoneurocutaneous medicine and its global impact.

Psychodermatology Activities and Research Advancements

The field of psychodermatology is dynamic and continually evolving. Activities within this field encompass a wide range of endeavors, including the following:

- *Research advancements*: Ongoing research endeavors in psychodermatology aim to unravel the mechanisms connecting the mind and skin. This includes the exploration of genetic predispositions, immune system responses, and the impact of lifestyle factors on skin health.
- *Clinical practice*: Psychodermatology has found its way into clinical practice, where healthcare providers are increasingly recognizing the importance of addressing mental health concerns in dermatology consultations. Integrated care models are being developed to provide holistic treatment for patients.
- *Patient support*: Support groups and online communities have emerged to provide a platform for individuals dealing with psychodermatological issues to share experiences, coping strategies, and emotional support.
- *Patient education*: Educational initiatives target both patients and healthcare providers, raising awareness about the mind-skin connection and the available resources for managing psychodermatological conditions.

CONCLUSION

In conclusion, psychodermatology research is expanding our understanding of the intricate relationship between the mind and the skin. It delves into the impact of psychological factors on skin conditions, explores innovative therapeutic interventions, and investigates the neurobiological mechanisms at play. Collaboration with international agencies, the availability of diverse funding sources, and the support of organizations like APMNA have propelled the field forward.

For aspiring researchers and clinicians, psychodermatology fellowships have the potential to offer a structured path to specialization, while regular meetings and activities within the field facilitate knowledge exchange and research advancements. With a growing body of evidence and a commitment to improving the lives of individuals with psychodermatological issues, psychodermatology holds immense promise for the future of dermatological care. It is a field where science and compassion intersect to provide holistic solutions for individuals grappling with the mind–skin connection.

FURTHER READINGS

1. Jafferany M, Franca K. Psychodermatology: Basics concepts. Acta Derm Venereol. 2016;96(217):35-7.
2. Brown GE, Malakouti M, Sorenson E, Gupta R, Koo JY. Psychodermatology. Adv Psychosom Med. 2015;34:123-34.

Index

Page numbers followed by *b* refer to box and *t* refer to table.

A

Abacavir 51
Acamprosate 270
Acanthosis nigricans 144
Acne 63, 67, 99, 165, 193
 disability index 184
 excoriée 28, 102, 225
 quality of life 184
Acquired immunodeficiency
  syndrome 106
Acquired melanocytic nevi 121
Acrochordons 138
Actigraphy 154, 157
Activity 207
Acyclovir 52, 140
Adjustment disorder 1, 48, 55, 147, 148
Adrenal-medullary, sympathetic 64
Adrenocorticotropic hormone 3, 144
Aesthetic 101
 clinic 90
 dermatological 89*t*
 practice, procedures and
  indications in 87*t*
 psychology of 86
Aggression 51
Aging, chronological 138
Agitation 51, 52
 control 111
Agoraphobia 146
Akathisia 263, 264
Alazopram 134
Alcohol use disorders 270
Allergic reaction 268
Alopecia 278

Alopecia areata 12*b*, 63, 100, 225
Alprazolam 273
Alzheimer's disease 234
Ambience 91
Amitriptyline 134, 273
Amnesia 109
Amphotericin B 52
Anaerobic gram-positive cocci 115*t*
Anal eczema 44
Androgenetic alopecia 138, 145
Angioedema 144, 277
Angiokeratoma 121
Angioma 121, 138
Ankles and calves 251
Anogenital itch 115
 causes for 115*t*
Anogenital pruritus
 acute 115
 chronic 115
Anticraving agents 270
Antidepressant discontinuation
  syndromes 268
Antidepressants 134, 256, 258, 266, 273-275
 use of 118
Antiepileptics 273
Antihistamines 157
Antileprosy treatment 133
Anti-Parkinsonian agents 259, 270
Antipsychotics 256, 258, 273
 atypical 33, 262
 high-potency 265
 mechanism of action of 263
 second-generation 33
 types of 261
Antiretroviral medications 51, 108
 highly active 107

Anxiety 1, 43, 74, 108, 114, 120, 121, 124, 136, 145, 181, 189, 195, 234
  development of 141, 246
  screening questionnaires for 104
Anxiety disorder 55, 110, 128, 130, 269
Anxiolytics 134, 258, 273-275
Aripiprazole 262, 263, 273
Artefactual skin disorder 20
Arterial leg ulcers 143
Arterial ulcers 143
Association for Psychoneurocutaneous Medicine of North America 296
Atopic dermatitis 8, 64, 100, 153, 154, 165, 205, 225, 286
Atopic eczema 63
Attention deficit hyperactivity disorder 259
Autoerythrocyte sensitization 36
Autogenic training 213
Automatic pilot 253
Automatic thought 214
Awareness and education, lack of 77
Azidothymidine 108

B

Baclofen sustained release 270
Bacterial
  infections 140
  vaginosis 115
Bacteroides species 115
Baldness 87
Beauty
  and aging 84
  and hair 84
  fairness and perception of 83
  standards and body image 77
Behavioral
  activation 199
  competence 33
  generalization of 33
  modification of 221
  problems 179
  techniques for habit reversal 196
  therapy 219, 227
Benzhexol 270
Benzodiazepines 28, 134, 158, 256, 259, 269
  receptor agonists 158
  short-acting 135
Bergen Insomnia Scale 157
Bier's spots 121
Bipolar affective disorder 110
Bipolar disorder 121, 258, 269
  manic phase of 263
Bizarre 24
Blood pressure
  diastolic 234
  systolic 234
Body dysmorphic delusions 21, 40
Body dysmorphic disorder 12*b*, 44, 83, 92, 101, 113, 114, 118
Body image 199
  and self-esteem 188, 199
  and self-esteem, addressing 197, 199
Body mass index 144
Body odor delusion 21, 263
Body scan meditation 251
Botulinum toxin type-A 84
Brain
  -derived neurotrophic factor 49
  imaging, functional 7
Breath
  exercises 158
  focus on 249
Brexpiprazole 262
Bromhidrosis 38
Building resilience 198
Bupropion 268, 273
Burning mouth syndrome 12

C

Calcitonin gene-related peptide 4, 6
Candida 115
Candida phobia 111
Cannabinoids 3
Carbamazepine 118, 270, 275
Cardiff Acne Disability Index 99, 183, 184
Cardiovascular diseases 234
Cariprazine 262
Catatonia 271
Catharsis 217
Central nervous system 2
   symptoms 181
Cephalosporins 51
Cheilitis factitia 30
Cherry angioma 138
Child behavior checklist 184
   detects emotional 179
Children's Dermatology Life Quality Index 103, 184, 195
Chlordiazepoxide 273
Chlorpromazine 261, 273, 275
Circadian rhythm 151
Citalopram 134
Citrine skin 138
Clinical
   observation 91
   practice 297
   psychology 289
Clomipramine 134
Clonazepam 135, 273
Clozapine 262, 265
Coccygodynia 117
Cognitive behavioural
   and information-based strategies 132
   interventions 196
   therapy 69, 119, 134, 191, 205, 206, 213, 293
      techniques 246
Cognitive-motor disorder, minor 109
Cognitive restructuring 33
   for negative thought patterns 196
Colloid milium 138
Combivir 51
Comfort, emphasis on 88
Concentration techniques 235
Concept, self-perception, 83
Confusion 51, 52
Constipation 263
Contact dermatitis 115
Conventional dermatological 89*t*
Coping 72
   mechanisms: double-edged sword 73
   skills 198
Corticosteroids 50, 51
Corticotropin-releasing hormone 2
Cortisol 144
   elevated levels of 293
Corynebacterium minutissimum 115
Cosmetic gynecology, growth of 119
Cosmetic surgery 81
Counseling
   importance of 191
   in psychodermatology, role of 191
   in redefining beauty standards, role of 202
Counselors 190
   exploring role of 191
Couple therapy 289
Crisis intervention and referral procedures 173
Culture-bound syndrome 124
Cupid's disease 111
Cutaneous
   bacterial infections 140
   dysesthesias 21

hypochondrias 44
lesions, morphology of 277
sensation, disturbances of 20
sensory disorders 19
Cutis rhomboidalis nuchae 138
Cytochrome P450 system 260
Cytokine interferon-gamma 5

D

Dapsone 52
Deep breathing 222
Deep necrosis 24
Deep trance 223
Deep wrinkles 138
Deeper psychopathology, dealing with 192
Deformity 129
Deliberate self-harm 107
Delirium 51, 52, 56, 109, 110
Delusion of parasitosis 37, 114, 205, 288
Delusional disorder 16, 263
Delusional infestation 12
Delusional parasitosis 21, 263
Delusions 51, 52, 111
Dementia, reversible 52
Dementia syndrome 109
Depersonalization 51t, 52t
Depot fluphenazine 263
Depot haloperidol 263
Depot preparations 263
Depressed mood 130
Depression 1, 48, 51, 52, 54, 74, 92, 104, 108, 110, 114, 120, 121, 136, 145, 180, 189, 195, 234, 266
  anxiety stress scale 181
  development of 141
  persistent 76
  severe 263
    levels of 121
  suicidality 52
  unipolar 263
Depressive disorder 128, 130
Dermatillomania 26, 102
Dermatitis 193
Dermatitis artefacta 24t, 102
Dermatitis artefacta syndrome 21, 22
Dermatitis Family Impact questionnaire 195
Dermatitis paraartefacta syndrome 21t, 22, 25
  patterns of 26t
Dermatological and aesthetic issues 98
Dermatological conditions 48t, 225
  understanding psychological impact of 165
Dermatological disease 10, 71, 88
  impact of 71
  like vitiligo 74
  treatment of underlying 104
  with psychiatric morbidity in elderly 138
Dermatological disorder 48, 49, 152, 192, 244
Dermatological illnesses 163, 166t
Dermatology Life Quality Index 182, 195
Dermatophytoses 115
Dermatoses 41, 115
  related with changes in physical appearance 99
  related with pathophysiological changes 99
  related with psychosexual changes 99
  result of compulsive disorders 43
  result of delusional illnesses and hallucinations 37
  self-induced 21, 102
Dhat syndrome 124
Diazepam 135, 269
Disability 129, 183
Discrimination 77

Disease coping skill training 69
Disease-specific scales 184
Disfigurement 52
Disorders
  category of 47
  symptomatology 27
Distraction techniques 199
Distress, patterns of 183
Disulfiram 270
Domain 103
Donor scar 96
Dopamine 3, 268
Dothiepin 273
Doxepin 134, 273
Drugs
  additives 275
  hypersensitivity vasculitis 278
  in psychopharmacology 259
  induced parkinsonism 264
  interactions 110
  rash with eosinophilia 279
  treatment of
    psychodermatological conditions 256
  used in
    addictions 259
    dementia 259
    disorders of sexual functions 270
Duloxetine 118, 268, 273
Dynias 117
Dyschromias 138
Dysesthesias 12
Dyshidrotic dermatitis 225
Dysmorphophobia 11, 16, 205
Dysmorphophobic delusions 263
Dyspareunia 117
Dyspigmentation 100
Dysthymia 76, 289
Dystonia 263, 264
  acute 264

E

Ecosyndrome 40
Eczema 139, 153, 193
  area and severity index 64
  disability index 183
  hand 48, 49
  lead to 44
  recurrent 63
  stress-related worsening of 64
  symptoms of 64
  washing 21, 43, 44
Education and eating 104
Efavirenz 51*t*
Ekbom's syndrome 37
Elasticity, loss of 138
Electroconvulsive therapy 172, 271
Electrolyte imbalance 268
Emotional 214
  connection 76
  fallout 76
  regulation 198
  space, safe 197
Enacted stigma 129
Energy, loss of 130
Engulf 76
Epidermal barrier
  defects 139
  function 64
Epidermatillomania 26
Erectile dysfunction 267
Erythema
  multiforme 278
  nodosum 278
Erythroderma 278
Erythromelalgia 225
Escitalopram 134, 273
Estazolam 158
Estrogens 51*t*
Eszopiclone 158, 269
Euphoria 51*t*

European Society for Dermatology and Psychiatry 295
Exacerbation 18
Exanthematous lesions 277
Excoriation disorder 20, 27
Exfoliative dermatitis 278
Expectations, types of 90
Eye
  fixation method 222
  position 249

F

Facial skin disease rosacea 155
Factitious disorders 21, 114
Family
  counseling 104
  members 75
  therapy 69, 219, 229
Fat deposits 87
Fatigue 130
Favre–Ricochet syndrome 138
Fear 129
Fearfulness 52
Feel sensations 240
Feeling restless 146
Feet 251
Female genital mutilation 121
Fine wrinkles 138
Fluoroquinolone antibiotics 51
Fluoxetine 134, 172, 267, 268, 273
Fluphenazine 261
Flurazepam 158, 269
Fluvoxamine 134, 172, 267
Fostering holistic approach 296
Fox–Fordyce
  disease 99
  spots 120
Funding 294
Fungal infections 141

G

Gabapentin 117
Gamma-aminobutyric acid type B agonist 270
Gardner–Diamond syndrome 22, 36
Gardnerella vaginalis 115
General health questionnaire 180
Generalized anxiety disorder 108
Genital
  arousal disorder, persistent 117
  dermatillomania 121
  self-mutilation in males 122
Geriatric depression scale 180
Glutamate 3
Glutamate gamma amino butyric acid 3
Gratitude and mindfulness 200
Grimacing 264
Group therapy 219
Guilt, excessive 130

H

H1 antihistamines 51
H2 antihistamines 51
Habit
  control motivation 206
  reversal 69, 205, 206
    techniques 32
  therapy 32
Hair
  excess 87
  loss 100
    causes of 100
  pulling, episodes of 31
  transplantation 95
Halitosis 263
Hallucinations 51t, 52t, 111, 263

Hallucinatory state 223
Haloperidol 261, 273, 275
Hamilton anxiety scale 181
Hamilton depression rating scale 180
Hansen's disease 128
Health survey, short form 182
Healthcare set-up, adolescent 104
Healthy body exists 226
Help seeking behavior 173
Herpes zoster 68, 140, 141
Hidradenitis suppurativa 49, 99
Hips and pelvis 252
Histamine 4
   levels 155
Holistic healthcare 136
Homeostatic sleep drive 151
Hopelessness 164
Hormonal mechanisms 150
Hospital anxiety depression scale 181
Human development, crucial stage in 98
Human immunodeficiency virus 106
   associated cognitive disorders 108, 109
Human leukocyte antigen 276
Human sleep 151
Hyperacusis 52t
Hyperpigmentation 101
Hyperpyrexia 264
Hypersomnia 130
Hypertension 234
Hypertensive ischemic leg ulcers 143
Hypnos, Greek God of Sleep 221
Hypnosis 69, 225
   induction of 222
   myths and realities 225t
   stages of 222

Hypnotherapy 134, 219, 221, 226
   benefits of 224
Hypnotics
   off label 159
   trance 223, 223t
Hypochondriacal 124
   delusions 21, 39
Hypochondriacal disorder 21, 41
Hyponatremia 268
Hypothalamic-pituitary-adrenal axis 2, 62, 142

I

Idiopathic guttate hypomelanosis 138
Idiopathic pruritus 286
Ikoma's group 116
Illnesses, chronic 164
Iloperidone 262
Imipramine 134, 273
Imminent death, fear of 52
Immune function, impaired 188
Immune system, activated 139
Immunosenescence 140
Impression 289
Impulsive type 42
Infections 8, 115, 140
   asymptomatic 107
Infective conditions like scabies 153
Inhibit cytochrome P450 enzymes 172
Insane, paresis of 111
Insight, lack of 16
Insomnia 52, 130, 256, 267
   agitation, hallucinations, mania, depression 52
   and sedation 268
   prevalence in psoriasis ranges 154
   severity index 157

Institutional stigma 129
Insulin resistance, manifestations of 99
Integrates mindfulness practices 246
Integration and holistic care 197
Interdisciplinary domain 292
Interleukin 6
International Agencies 295
　assistance and collaboration 293
International Classification of Diseases 20
Interpersonal
　relationship 15, 93
　sensitivity 120
Intricate relationship 291
Irritant dermatoses 24
Isoniazid 52
Isotretinoin 52
Itch and scratching 188
Itch-scratch cycle 62, 64

J

Jacobsons progressive muscle relaxation 133, 208

K

Ketamine 222
Knees and thighs 251
Korean glass skin 88
Koro syndrome 123
Kriya Yogas 237

L

Lamotrigine 270, 273, 275
Lemborexant 159
Leprosy 129
　affected person 133
　causation of 129
　counseling and psychoeducation in 133
　diagnosis of 133
　homes 130
　psycho social aspects of 132
Lesions, morphology of 24, 27
Lethargic state 223
Leukocytosis 265
Liaison
　approach 34
　clinics 288
　　sample of case record in 288
Lichen
　planus 66, 142
　simplex chronicus, primary 44
Lifespan 137
Life-threatening
　organic picture, severe 107
　severe 278
Light trance 223
Limbs, stiffness of 223
Lip-licker's dermatitis 30
Lithium 269, 270, 273, 275
Lorazepam 134, 271, 273
Lurasidone 262
Luster of nails, loss of 138

M

Male genital mutilation, prevalence of 122
Malignancy, afraid of 221
Malingering 21, 22, 35
Mania 51t, 52t, 110
Manu's battle with acne 201
Marital harmony 76
Maternal stress 63
Medical
　hypnotherapy 223
　illnesses, chronic 163
Meditations 222, 232, 234, 235, 242
　advanced states of 233
　based on activities 235
　experience beyond words 232
　exploring medical benefits of 234
　self-practiced 236

steps 239
systems 232
techniques of 242
Melasma 138, 144
Melatonin 159
Mental
  attitude 238
  disorders, diagnostic and statistical manual of 152
  health 86
    issues 74
  stress 188
Metabolic syndrome 265
Methotrexate 50
Migraine 234
Mind
  body connection 189
  body problem 81
  calming of 233
  face mirror of 1
Mindful
  breath 249
  stress reduction 69
Mindfulness and relaxation techniques 196
Mindfulness-based
  cognitive therapy 245
  stress reduction 196, 245
  therapy 244, 245
    for dermatological disorders 244
    in skin disorders, rationale for 247
Mindfulness in skin disorders, process of 246
Mindfulness meditation practice 253
Mind-skin connection, understanding of 294
Mirtazapine 268, 273
Mixed venous 143
Mobiluncus species 115
Moisturizer 158
Monoamine oxidase inhibitors 266

Monosymptomatic hypochondriac psychosis 263
Montgomery–Åsberg Depression Rating Scale 180
Mood stabilizers 258, 269, 273, 274
Morsicatio buccarum 29
Motivation
  and social support 207
  understanding 81
Mucocutaneous pain syndromes 117
Mucocutaneous skin syndrome 113
Multifaceted dimensions 291
Münchausen syndrome 22, 36
Münchausen-by-proxy syndrome 22, 36
Music, soft 158
Mycobacterium leprae 128
Mycoplasma hominis 115
Mycoses fungoides 153
Myths and misconceptions 225

N

N-acetyl cysteine 33
Nail
  biting 30
  chewing 30
Nail Psoriasis Quality of Life Scale 185
Naltrexone 34, 270
Narcolepsy 156
National Institutes of Health 151, 293
Natural killer 6
Navigating storm 72
Negative body image 72
Neoplasms 115
Nerve growth factor 6
Neurocognitive disorders 110
Neurodegenerative disorders 139
Neurodermatitis 225

Neurogenic cutaneous inflammatory 4
Neurogenic inflammation 4
Neuro-immuno-cutaneous-endocrine 1, 2
Neuroleptic malignant syndrome 258, 263, 264
Neuroleptics 273
Neurolinguistic programming 230
Neurons 3
Neuropeptides 3
Neuropsychiatric conditions 132
Neuropsychological impairment 109
Neurotic excoriations 26
Nevirapine 51
Nightmares 51
Nitrazepam 269
Nocturnal
 emissions 124
 itching 158
 pruritis 153
 variations 116
Noncontagious nature 220
Nonneurological side effects 265
Nonrapid eye movement 151, 234
Nonsteroidal anti-inflammatory drug 51
Noradrenergic and specific serotonergic antidepressants 268
Norepinephrine uptake inhibitors 268
Nortriptyline 134
Nummular eczema 225

O

Obsessive-compulsive behaviors 74
Obsessive-compulsive disorder 74, 92, 108, 120, 121, 205, 246, 259
Obstructive sleep apnea 156
Oculogyric crisis 264

Olanzapine 25, 118, 262, 265, 273
Onychophagia 30, 102
Onychotemnomania 30
Onychotillomania 30, 102
Opioid agonist tramadol 118
Orchidynia 117
Orexin receptor antagonists 159
Organ of expression 72
Oxazepam 134, 269
Oxcarbazepine 270

P

Pain 234
Pain syndrome, chronic 266
Painful bruising syndrome 20, 36
Painful ecchymoses syndrome 36
Panic attacks, depression 51
Panic disorder 108
Paranoia 52*t*
Paranoid ideation 120
Parasitic 115
Parasomnias 157
Paroxetine 273
Paroxetine sertraline 134
Partially guided self-practiced meditation 236
Participation scale 183
Patient education and empowerment 172
Patient–doctor interaction 10
Peaceful living 233
Pediatric symptom checklist 184
Pelvic floor rehabilitation 117
Pemphigus 49
Penile size dissatisfaction 120
Penodynia 117
Perceived stigmatization questionnaire 183
Peripheral arterial disease 143
Peripheral nerves 62
Person-Centered Dermatology Self-Care Index 195
Phobias 74

Phobic anxiety 120
Photoaging 138
Photosensitivity 277
Pigmentary problems 87
Pigmentation 278
Pimozide 25, 273
Pittsburgh Sleep Quality Index Scores 155
Placing 250
Plaque, chronic 49
Polycystic ovarian syndrome 99
Polymorphic 24, 27
Polysomnography 157
Postorgasmic illness syndrome 122
Postpartum depression 63
Posttest stress 108
Posttraumatic stress disease 121
Post-traumatic stress disorder 108, 234
Posture 238
Pranayama 235-237
Pregabalin 118
Pregnancy 63
Prenatal distress 63
Procainamide procaine penicillin G 52
Procaine derivatives 52
Proctodynia 117
Proinflammatory cytokines 292
Promethazine 264
Prominent veins 121
Propranolol 271
Prostatodynia 117
Prurigo nodularis 68, 153
Pruritus 6, 153, 277
  in elderly 139
Pseudo-knuckle pads 29
Pseudo stellate scars 138
Psoriasis 8, 49, 64, 74, 141, 153, 165, 192, 205, 286
  adolescent 185
  arthritis quality of life scale 185
  disability index 183, 195
  early-onset 65
  etiology of 64
  index of quality of life 185
Psyche and genitals 113
Psychiatric
  comorbidity 119, 256
  condition 7, 282
  illness
    indicator of 163
    secondary 12
  morbidity 48, 128
  problems 107
    iatrogenic 287
  symptoms 44
Psychiatric disorder 11, 54, 271
  longer-term 108
  management of 109
  prevalence of 48*t*
  primary 11, 16, 18, 19, 21*t*
    cutaneous manifestations 18
    with dermatological symptoms 194
    with skin manifestations 288
  secondary 11, 19, 49, 50, 195, 289
    in dermatology patients 47
    treatment-emergent psychiatric conditions 50
Psychocutaneous disorders 287
  management of 219
Psychocutaneous medicine 18
Psychodermatological
  conditions 192
  disease 286
    primary 12
  disorders 272
    classification of 11*t*
    secondary 12, 19
  illness, primary 12
  issues in geriatric population 136
Psychodermatologists use rating scales 185
Psychodermatology 11, 18, 291, 292
  activities and research advancements 297

advantages of 290
assessment tools and questionnaires in 178
case-taking in 10
complexity and circularity in 94
counseling 16, 189, 190, 196, 201, 202
  assessment and evaluation in 194
  employs 196
  holistic approach to skin and mind 186
family and social support in 200
liaison clinic 286, 290
research 297
  endeavors 295
  extends 293
  scope of 292
  studies 245
  understanding skin-mind connection 186
Psychoeducation 69, 219, 221
Psychogenic
  excoriations 102
  pruritus 42
    subtypes of 42t
  purpura 36, 63, 66
Psychogenital disorders, primary 114
Psychological
  adverse effects 51, 52
    of dermatological medications 51t
  and neuropsychiatric complications of HIV and STD 106
  basis 23, 27
  behavior 91
  comorbidities secondary to genital dermatoses 114
  distress, presence of 195
  effects of genital mutilation 121
  expectations 89
  impact 194
    of skin disease on family: hidden scars 75
    on skin health 187
  interventions 133, 171
    in psychodermatological conditions 205, 219
  morbidity 145
  needs 90
  procedures, useful 112
  reactions, acute 108
  symptoms 47
  therapy on cognitive behavior therapy 110
Psychology, assessment of 90
Psychomotor retardation 130
Psychopharmacology
  medications 17
  role of 134
Psychophysiologic skin disorders 62, 63
Psychophysiological disorders 11, 19, 194
  involving genitals 114
  management of 68
Psychoses 109
Psychosexual dermatoses 99
Psychosis 51, 52, 55, 110
  hallucinations, mania 52
Psychosocial
  distress 189
  reactions 52
Psychosomatic
  causes 92
  disorders 47
  primary care 69
  skin diseases 77
Psychotherapy 104, 205
  like psychoeducation 219
  techniques 218
Psychotropics 18
  and common cutaneous adverse effects 275t

medications 279, 280*t*
  classification of 258, 273*t*
  dermatological adverse effects of 272
Public Health Initiatives and Policy 174
Pure itch 116

Q

Quack handling poison 220
Quality of life 73, 182
  assessment of 103
  conventional tools for 103
  domains affected in adolescent dermatoses 103*t*
  health-related 73
  impaired 53, 128, 131
  instrument 185
  scores 64
Quazepam 158
Questionnaire, self-reporting 179, 180
Quetiapine 262, 273

R

Raisin exercise, procedure 250
Rapid eye movement sleep 151
Rating scales 180
Rationale response, use of 215
Reacting versus responding 247
Reaction 280, 281
Reassurance 217
Record sheet 207
Relaxation
  methods 158
  procedures 205-207
  strategies for self-care 197
  techniques 222
  therapy 69
Reminiscence group therapy 134

Research
  advancements 297
  areas of 292
  in psychodermatology 291
Restless legs syndrome 157
Retrocollis 264
Risperidone 25, 118, 262, 273, 288
Rosacea 63, 67
Rumination 248

S

Sadness interfering, persistent 15
Schizophrenia 258, 263
  diagnosis of 96
Scratching 158
Screening
  scales 180
  tools 179
Sebaceous hyperplasia 120
Seborrheic
  dermatitis 68, 99
  eczema 44
Sedation 263
Seeing 250
Seizures 267
  increased risk for 263
Selective serotonin reuptake inhibitors 33, 121, 134
Selegiline 271
Self-appreciation 200
Self-compassion 200
Self-conscious 90
Self-image, ideal 92
Self-talk, positive 199, 200
Semen contact allergy 123
Senile comedones 138
Sensations, focus on 250
Sensorimotor disorder 157
Sensory and psychological disorders 18
Separation anxiety disorder 146

Serotonin and norepinephrine
 reuptake inhibitors 268
Serotonin selective reuptake
 inhibitors 260
Serotonin syndrome 268
Sertraline 267, 273
Sertraline 268
Sex development, disorders of 122
Sexual
 dysfunction 120, 263
 intimacy 76
 relationships 230
Sexually transmitted disease 106,
 111, 125
Shoulders and arms 252
Sildenafil 270
Simulated skin disease 20
Skin
 and mucosa 26
 and psyche
  mind 62
  to psychodermatology 1
 barrier function 188
 changes in aging 138
 conditions 72, 166, 167
 diseases 74, 287
  and psyche of society 76
  role of
   psychoneuroimmunology
   in 296
  visible 188
 disorder 47, 199
  cultural context of 77
  self-inflicted 20
 impact on psychological well-
  being 188
 infections 155
 irritants 282
 lesion, infected 25
 picking disorder 121, 102
 picking impact scale 181
 picking syndrome 26, 27*t*
 surface, changes in 73
 tag 121

Sleep 150
 assessment of 157
 disorders 156
 disturbance 131, 150
  in cancer survivors 234
  in dermatology 150
 major phases of 151
 normal 223*t*
 physiology of 151
 problems 152
 questions regarding 157
 time shorter 154
 wake cycle 151
Small penis syndrome 113, 119
Smegma 121
Smelling 250
Social
 anxiety disorder 146
 history 91
 life 129
 media
  double-edged sword 101
  influence 88
  playing big role 80
 phobia 120, 146
 pressures 82
 situations, influence of 82
 stigma 128
  and isolation 188
 support 198
 withdrawal 1
Sodium valproate 109, 270, 273,
 275
Somatization disorder 21, 40, 41
Somatization, scores of 120
Somatoform autonomic disorders
 21
Somatoform disorder 21, 40, 41
 in dermatology 41*t*
Somatoform pain disorder,
 persistent 41, 21
Somnambulistic state 223
Soothing assurances 220
Specific skin diseases 78

Staphylococcus aureus 115
Stevens-Johnson syndrome 270, 278
Stigma 77, 78, 128, 182
   and social support, impact of 169
   causes for 129
   effects of 129
   fear of 73, 129
   perceived 128
   self-imposed 129
   types of 128
Stigmatization 53
Stimulants 259
Stimulus control 33
Stress 128, 131, 136, 147, 205
   activates hypothalamo-hypophyseal-adrenal axis 62
   acute or mild 4
   and barrier function of skin 7
   and fatigue, chronic 74
   and immune response 4
   and inflammation 187
   and psychoneuroimmunology 2
   and wound healing 7
   chronic or severe 5
   disturbs 142
   in lichen planus 63
   management 132
   on skin, effect of 6
   preceding 43
   related dermatology 205
   related mood disorders 110
   responders 65
   role of 220
Stressful situations 69
Stressors activate, major neural pathways 2
Stretch marks 87
Substance
   abuse 56
   abuse disorders 246
   use 181
Sudarshan kriya 235, 237
Suicidal
   ideation 195
   risk 183
   thoughts 128, 131
Suicidality 164
Suicide 53, 107, 109
   affecting behavior cognition scale 184
   and suicidality in dermatoses 165
   behaviors questionnaire-revised 183
   intent scale 184
   prevention in dermatological conditions 163
   relation to 165
   risk, using screening instruments for 174
   warning signs of 170, 174
Sunken eyes 138
Supportive
   counseling 197
   therapy 69, 205, 206, 217
Suprachiasmatic nucleus 151
Suvorexant 159
Swallowing 251
Symptom-based scales 179
Syndrome of unprovoked sexual arousal 117
Systematic desensitization 228
Systemic symptoms syndrome 279

T

Tadalafil 270
Taper off slowly 258
Tardive akathisia, chronic neurological 265
Tardive dyskinesia 265
   chronic neurological 265
Tardive syndromes 265
Tasting 250
Teaching adaptive coping strategies 198

Temazepam 158
Temperature biofeedback 212
Terminal illnesses 163
Thalidomide 52, 261
Thoughts 207
  program 253
Toes 251
Tongue protruding 264
Torticollis 264
Touching 250
Tourette-like syndrome 51
Transcendental meditation 236
Transcriptase inhibitors 109
Triazolam 158
Trichoteiromania 31, 35, 35*t*
Trichotemnomania 31, 35, 35*t*
Trichotillomania 11, 16, 20, 31, 35*t*, 35, 44, 102, 225
Tricyclic antidepressant 117, 134, 260
Trifluoperazine 261
Trihexyphenidyl 264, 270, 288
Tryptamine 4
Tumor necrosis factor 6

U

Unrealistic expectations 102
Unworthiness, feeling of 15
Urticaria 65, 144, 153, 205, 225, 277, 286

V

Valid questionnaires, using 157
Valproic acid 118
Varenicline 118
Vascular ulcers 142
Vedanta-based philosophical meditation 237
Venereological hypochondriasis 111
Venereophobia 120
  secondary 114
Venlafaxine 134, 268, 273

Venous leg ulcers 143
Vilazodone 269
Viral infections 140
Visha vydya-malayalam language 220
Visual analog scale 92
Vitiligo 63, 66, 193, 225
  impact scale 184
  life quality index 184
Vortioxetine 269
Vulnerable subpopulations 169
Vulvar pruritus 117
Vulvodynia 12*b*, 117

W

Warning signs 95
Weight gain 267
White cell count 109
Wickham's striae 142
Worrying 248
Worthlessness, feelings of 130
Wound healing 155
Wound-up, or on-edge 146

X

Xerosis 138

Y

Yale–Brown Obsessive-Compulsive Scale 181
Yoga 236, 237
  practicing 69

Z

Zaleplon 158, 269
Zidovudine 51*t*
Ziprasidone 262
Zolpidem 158, 269
Zopiclone 269
Zung anxiety scale 181
Zung depression scale 180

EU GSPR Authorised Reprsentative
Logos Europe, 9 rue Nicolas Poussin
1700, La Rochelle, France
Phone: +33 (0) 6 67 93 73 78
E-mail: contact@logoseurope.eu

www.ingramcontent.com/pod-product-compliance
Ingram Content Group UK Ltd.
Pitfield, Milton Keynes, MK11 3LW, UK
UKHW041658270226
468476UK00007B/115